Dedication

To my husband, Randy, for the wonderful life we share and to my children, Nicholas, Diana, and Michael, who bring so much joy to my life.

M.P.

To my husband, Tony, and to my children, Joe, Anne, John, and Ellen for all of their patience and support.

C.S.

Contents

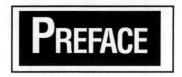

PREFACE

The *Pocket Companion for Luckmann's Core principles and Practice of Medical-Surgical Nursing* was developed as a quick reference guide for nurses and nursing students in the clinical setting based on content from Polaski and Tatro, *Luckmann's Core Principles and Practice of Medical-Surgical Nursing.* Information on over 300 adult medical-surgical diseases, disorders, and other topics is included and organized in a format closely following the main textbook. Each condition concludes with a reference to the page numbers in the textbook where more in-depth information can be found.

The *Pocket Companion* was developed to put concise, relevant information at your fingertips. Special features to help you quickly locate information include:

- consistently styled format with easily identified subject headers for each condition
- inclusion of only pertinent information for each condition with exclusion of routine nursing care
- separate listing of medical and nursing care
- alphabetical listing of conditions
- convenient pocket size
- comprehensive cross-referenced index with terms commonly used in clinical settings
- grouping of nursing interventions according to whether the patient is receiving medical or surgical treatment

All major prototypical disorders follow a format designed to assist the nurse to quickly locate information:

Overview—pertinent information such as a definition/brief description of the disorder, pathophysiology, incidence and risk factors.

Clinical Manifestations—signs and symptoms commonly seen in clients with the disorder.

Medical Management—prescribed medical interventions including pharmocological and dietary management.

Surgical Management—operative procedures performed for palliative or curative treatment.

Nursing Management—independent and collaborative nursing interventions specific for the condition. Interventions are grouped according to medical or surgical management where appropriate. For surgical interventions, routine pre- and postoperative care is not included, but found under "Perioperative Nursing Care", page 500.

Focused Discharge Care—discharge instructions for the client/significant other specific for the condition.

Several other concepts and therapies frequently encountered in the clinical setting were also included:

Mechanical Ventilation
Endotracheal Tubes
Tracheostomy
Blood Component Transfusion
Chemotherapy
Radiation Therapy
Perioperative Nursing Care
Enteral Nutrition
Closed Chest Drainage

To further assist you in your clinical practice, a list of NANDA nursing diagnoses are found on the inside covers.

Several appendices are found at the end of the book as additional sources of information:

A— Reference Laboratory Values
B— Analysis of Arterial Blood Gas Results
C— Blood Components

We realize the challenge of working in today's clinical setting with the complexity and multiplicity of patient care issues. We hope that the *Pocket Companion* will provide for you a source of information that will enhance your delivery of quality patient care.

Mary K. Palandri, RN, BSN
Catherine Rollman Sorrentino, RN, BSN

ACKNOWLEDGMENT

We would like to thank Thomas Eoyang, Vice President and Editor-in-Chief, Nursing Books, W.B. Saunders, for giving us this opportunity, and Francine Rosenthal, Assistant Developmental Editor, for her guidance, support, and unfailing good humor during this process.

Our thanks also to Alison Zaintz, The Production House, for her help in the preparation of this book.

Abdominal Aortic Aneurysm

OVERVIEW

- An aneurysm is a permanent localized dilation of an artery. A 50 per cent increase in the size of a vessel is the usual criterion. An aneurysm tends to enlarge gradually, and, if untreated, may rupture.
- The aorta is under greater stress than the rest of the arterial system because of its large diameter and exposure to high pressure during each systolic contraction. Abdominal aortic aneurysms (AAAs) occur about four times more often than thoracic aortic aneurysms.
- When an AAA reaches about 5 cm in diameter, it can usually be palpated. An AAA measuring 6 cm or greater in diameter has a 20 per cent chance of rupturing in one year.

CLINICAL MANIFESTATIONS

- most are asymptomatic; discovered on physical or x-ray examination
- awareness of a pulsating mass in the abdomen
- abdominal or back pain
- groin or flank pain

Ruptured AAA
- intense pain, typically in one or both flanks with radiation to the lower abdomen, groin or genitalia
- signs/symptoms of shock
- pulsating abdominal mass
- ecchymosis in the flank and perianal area
- decreased hemoglobin and elevated white blood cell count

MEDICAL MANAGEMENT

Surgery is usually not performed on clients with an asymptomatic AAA smaller than 4 to 5 cm.
- ultrasonographic examination every six months to determine any change in size
- antihypertensive therapy

SURGICAL MANAGEMENT

May be performed as an emergency (for ruptured AAA) or elective procedure.
- Excision is done through a midline incision that extends from the xiphoid process to the symphysis pubis. The aneurysm is exposed, clamps are applied above and below the area, the aneurysm is excised, and the segment is replaced with a Dacron graft.

NURSING MANAGEMENT

SURGICAL

In addition to routine preoperative care:
- Assess baseline peripheral pulses for comparison postoperatively.
- Administer fluids and vasoactive therapy (if ruptured AAA) and monitor for signs/symptoms of shock.

In addition to routine postoperative care:
- Assess pulses distal to graft at least hourly as ordered.
- Monitor for signs/symptoms of occlusion — change in pulses, severe pain, cool to cold extremity below graft, pallor or cyanosis.
- Monitor for signs/symptoms of complications, including:
  — myocardial infarction — clients often have underlying coronary artery disease
  — renal failure — secondary to ischemia sustained from decreased aortic blood flow
  — emboli in arteries of lower extremities or mesentery
  — bowel necrosis is exhibited as fever, leukocytosis, ileus, diarrhea and abdominal pain
  — spinal cord ischemia resulting in paraplegia, rectal and urinary incontinence, loss of pain and temperature sensation

FOCUSED DISCHARGE CARE

Instruct client regarding:

MEDICAL

- antihypertensive therapy
- signs/symptoms of enlarging aneurysm and need to notify physician of:
  — pulsating abdominal mass
  — abdominal or back pain
  — flank pain
- risk factor modification
- importance of follow-up ultrasound examinations

SURGICAL

- wound care
- activity restrictions
- signs/symptoms of ruptured bypass graft and need to notify physician of:
  — abdominal pain with intense back, flank and scrotal pain
  — pulsating abdominal mass
  — ecchymosis in the flank or perianal area
  — lightheadedness
  — nausea

(For more information, see pp. 806-808 of Polaski and Tatro, *Luckmann's Core Principles and Practice of Medical-Surgical Nursing.*)

Achalasia

OVERVIEW

- Achalasia is an idiopathic condition characterized by progressive increased dysphagia. It is due to impaired motility of the lower two-thirds of the esophagus.
- The lower esophageal sphincter (LES) fails to relax as it normally would with swallowing, causing food

and fluid to accumulate in the lower esophagus. When hydrostatic pressure exceeds the force of resistance of the LES, the contents pass into the stomach.

CLINICAL MANIFESTATIONS

Signs/symptoms increase in severity as achalasia progresses.
- dysphagia
- substernal pain, inability to belch (in early stages)
- regurgitation of undigested food

MEDICAL MANAGEMENT

Treatment is aimed at relieving the symptoms

- anticholinergic drugs, gastrointestinal hormones and calcium channel blockers to relax the LES or lower esophageal pressures
- analgesics for pain
- dietary changes (see Nursing Management)

SURGICAL MANAGEMENT

- esophageal dilation (also called bougienage) — dilating the lower esophagus and sphincter
- esophagomyotomy (Heller's procedure) — enlargement of the lower esophageal sphincter by incising the circular muscle fibers down to the mucosa. The incision is made via a thoracic approach, necessitating the use of chest tubes. Complications include reflux esophagitis and re-stenosis.
- gastrostomy tube placement — if the client will be unable to swallow for long periods

NURSING MANAGEMENT

MEDICAL

- Discuss dietary changes:
  — small frequent feedings
  — use of semisoft, warm foods rather than cold, hard foods
  — avoidance of hot, spicy or iced foods
  — avoidance of alcohol or tobacco
  — chewing all foods thoroughly

> — use of different positions to reduce pressure while
>   eating
- Instruct client to sleep with head of bed elevated.
- Daily weights.
- Administer prescribed analgesics.

SURGICAL

ESOPHAGEAL DILATION

- *Preoperative care*
  Instruct client regarding:
  - procedure is done while awake with a local anes-
    thetic and an analgesic or tranquilizer
  - taking slow, deep breaths during passage of the
    tube
  - there may be brief discomfort when bag is inflated
- *Postoperative care*—Monitor for signs of perforation
  (chest or shoulder pain, elevated temperature and
  subcutaneous emphysema). Report to physician immediately.

ESOPHAGOMYOTOMY (HELLER'S PROCEDURE)

- *Preoperative care*
  In addition to routine pre-operative care:
  - Discuss purpose and care of chest and nasogastric
    tubes.
- *Postoperative care*
  In addition to routine postoperative care:
  - Monitor thoracotomy incision for excessive bleed-
    ing. Maintain clean and dry dressings.
  - Maintain chest tube drainage system.
  - Monitor for respiratory distress.
  - Maintain nasogastric or gastric drainage system.
  - Administer prescribed analgesics.

FOCUSED DISCHARGE CARE

Instruct client regarding:

MEDICAL

- diet
- symptoms of respiratory complications related to
  esophageal reflux and aspiration

- sleeping with the head of bed elevated
- signs/symptoms of esophageal perforation
- signs/symptoms of infection
- signs/symptoms of respiratory complications
- care of gastrostomy tube
- wound care
- when to call physician

(For more information, see pp. 1017-1020 of Polaski and Tatro, *Luckmann's Core Principles and Practice of Medical-Surgical Nursing.*)

Acidosis, Metabolic

OVERVIEW

- Metabolic acidosis may be caused by two different mechanisms: accumulation of fixed acid or loss of base.
- When acidosis is the result of addition of fixed acid (as in lactic acidosis), bicarbonate is consumed in buffering. When acidosis is due to loss of bicarbonate, chloride levels increase to maintain electroneu-trality.
- Causes of metabolic acidosis include:
  - fixed acid excess:
    - renal failure — acid end products of protein metabolism cannot be excreted
    - diabetic ketoacidosis — ketoacids accumulate from lipid metabolism
    - lactic acidosis — lactic acid builds up as a consequence of anaerobic metabolism
    - ingested toxins (i.e., aspirin, antifreeze)
  - base deficit:
    - renal tubular acidosis — kidneys cannot reabsorb bicarbonate
    - carbonic anhydrase inhibitors:
      - Diamox — interferes with bicarbonate reabsorption in the kidney
    - enteric drainage tubes (e.g., ileostomy) — intestinal secretions high in bicarbonate are lost
    - diarrhea

CLINICAL MANIFESTATIONS

- hyperventilation (compensatory)

6

- drowsiness, confusion or coma
- headache
- pH below 7.35
- bicarbonate (HCO_3) less than 22 mm Hg
- $PaCO_2$ normal or slightly decreased
- hyperchloremia (base deficit)

MEDICAL MANAGEMENT

- determination/treatment of underlying cause
- sodium bicarbonate therapy
- electrolyte replacement therapy

NURSING MANAGEMENT

- Monitor respiratory status.
- Administer bicarbonate therapy as ordered (observe IV site, as bicarbonate is a tissue irritant).
- Position for optimal ventilation.
- Intervene to prevent pain, fever or anxiety (these will increase the respiratory rate).
- Assess neurological status and implement appropriate safety measures.
- Monitor laboratory results — arterial blood gases, electrolytes, BUN, creatinine.
- Monitor for signs/symptoms of electrolyte imbalance.
- Assess ability to perform activities of daily living.
- Plan scheduled rest periods.

FOCUSED DISCHARGE CARE

Discharge care is based on the etiologic factor(s) causing metabolic acidosis.

(For more information, see pp. 72-76 of Polaski and Tatro, *Luckmann's Core Principles and Practice of Medical-Surgical Nursing.*)

Acidosis, Respiratory

OVERVIEW

- Respiratory acidosis is nearly always due to hypoventilation.

- The rate of carbon dioxide excretion by the lungs depends upon the rate of alveolar ventilation. As ventilation increases (i.e., as tidal volume or respiratory rate increases), carbon dioxide excretion increases and pH rises. Conversely, when ventilation is decreased, less acid is excreted and pH falls.
- Etiologic factors of respiratory acidosis include:
  — COPD
  — neuromuscular disease:
    — Guillain-Barré Syndrome
  — myasthenia gravis
  — respiratory center depression:
    — drugs
      - barbiturates
      - sedatives
      - narcotics
      - anesthetics
  — central nervous system lesions:
    — tumor
    — stroke
  — iatrogenic disorders:
    — inadequate mechanical ventilation
    — carbon dioxide narcosis
  — excess carbon dioxide production:
    — hypermetabolism
      - sepsis
      - burns
  — excessive carbohydrate intake:
    — total parenteral nutrition (TPN)
    — enteral feeding

CLINICAL MANIFESTATIONS

- dyspnea
- disorientation or coma
- dysrhythmias
- pH below 7.35
- $PaCO_2$ above 45 mm Hg
- hyperkalemia — acidosis at the tissue level causes extracellular hydrogen ions to shift into the cell while potassium moves into the blood
- hypoxemia

MEDICAL MANAGEMENT

- determination/treatment of underlying cause

- ventilatory support
- electrolyte replacement therapy
- intravenous sodium bicarbonate

NURSING MANAGEMENT

- Monitor respiratory status.
- Position for optimal ventilation; reposition frequently.
- Encourage coughing and deep breathing. Suction PRN.
- Administer sodium bicarbonate therapy as ordered (observe IV site as bicarbonate is a tissue irritant).
- Monitor oxygen therapy.
- Monitor laboratory results — arterial blood gases, electrolytes, oxygen saturations.
- Assess cardiac status.
- Assess ECG for rhythm changes.
- Assess neurological status and institute appropriate safety measures.
- Monitor for signs/symptoms of hyperkalemia:
    — irregular, slow heart rate
    — ECG changes — tall T waves, widened QRS complexes, prolonged PR intervals
    — paresthesias
    — muscle twitches, cramps
    — weakness
- Assess ability to complete activities of daily living.
- Schedule activities to allow for rest periods.

FOCUSED DISCHARGE CARE

Discharge care is based on the etiologic factor(s) causing respiratory acidosis.

(For more information, see pp. 72-76 of Polaski and Tatro, *Luckmann's Core Principles and Practice of Medical-Surgical Nursing.*)

Acromegaly

OVERVIEW

- Acromegaly is a disease of adults that develops after closure of the epiphyses of the long bones. It is marked by increases in bone thickness and hypertrophy of the soft tissues.
- Acromegaly results from growth hormone secreting adenomas of the anterior pituitary glands.

CLINICAL MANIFESTATIONS

- coarsening of the facial features
- prognathism (protrusion of the jaw)
- broad hands with spade-like fingers
- headache, diplopia, blindness, and lethargy (due to compression of brain tissue by the tumor)
- in advanced cases, clients can suffer from associated hormonal disturbances, such as diabetes mellitus, goiter, Cushing's disease, etc.

MEDICAL MANAGEMENT

- irradiation of the pituitary gland to destroy tumor
- bromocriptine (Parlodel) to reduce the levels of growth hormone and decrease tumor size

SURGICAL MANAGEMENT

- The treatment of choice is a surgical hypophysectomy to remove the tumor (approach through inner aspect of upper lip). Partial or complete removal of the pituitary gland occurs during resection of pituitary tumors.

NURSING MANAGEMENT

SURGICAL

Postoperative Care
In addition to routine postoperative care:

- Assess for signs of cerebral edema and rising intra-cranial pressure:
  — elevated blood pressure
  — widened pulse pressure
  — decreased pulse rate
  — pupil changes
  — altered respiratory pattern
- Assess for signs of target gland deficiencies (the pituitary no longer produces tropic hormones):
  — adrenal insufficiency
  — hypothyroidism
  — diabetes insipidus (ADH deficiency)
- Assess for signs of meningitis (elevated temperature, headache, irritability, and nuchal rigidity).
- Provide frequent oral hygiene.
- Observe the client for rhinorrhea after nasal packing is removed (can indicate a cerebrospinal fluid leak).
- Encourage client to avoid coughing, sneezing, or blowing his nose.

FOCUSED DISCHARGE CARE

Instruct client regarding:
- importance of taking daily replacement hormones
- need for client/significant other to demonstrate medication injection technique if client not able to tolerate oral medications
- signs of under and over-dosage
- need to call for dosage adjustment if experiencing physical or emotional stress
- dietary modifications
- need to report persistent post-nasal drainage
- need to avoid sneezing, coughing, and bending from the waist for specified period of time
- need for Medic Alert bracelet and card.

(For more information, see pp. 1246-1249 of Polaski and Tatro, *Luckmann's Core Principles and Practice of Medical-Surgical Nursing.*)

Acute Myocardial Infarction

OVERVIEW

- Acute myocardial infarction (MI), also known as a heart attack, coronary occlusion, or "a coronary", is a life-threatening condition characterized by the formation of localized necrotic areas within the myocardium. MI usually follows the sudden occlusion of a coronary artery and the abrupt cessation of blood and oxygen flow to the heart muscle.
- The most common cause of MI is complete or nearly complete occlusion of a coronary artery due to ongoing atherosclerosis. The vessel lumen slowly occludes and is often blocked with a thrombus. When blood flow ceases abruptly, the myocardial tissue supplied by the artery becomes ischemic, and infarction follows. Other causes of acute occlusion are coronary artery spasm or hemorrhage into a plaque.
- MI can be considered the endpoint of coronary artery disease (CAD). Unlike the temporary ischemia that occurs with angina, prolonged unrelieved ischemia causes irreversible damage to the myocardium. Cardiac cells can withstand ischemia about 20 minutes before cellular death occurs. Because the myocardium is very metabolically active, signs of ischemia can be seen within 8 to 10 seconds of decreased blood flow. When the heart is not sustained with blood and oxygen, it converts to anaerobic metabolism with lactic acid as a byproduct. Myocardial cells are very sensitive to changes in pH and become less functional, leading to conduction system disorders, dysrhythmias and decreased contractility.
- Every year approximately 1,500,000 Americans fall victim to heart attacks. MI is the leading cause of death in America, resulting in an estimated 500,000 deaths each year.
- Approximately 45 per cent of all heart attack clients are under the age of 65 years and 5 per cent are under age 40 years.
- The risk factors that predispose a client to heart attack are the same as for all forms of coronary artery disease (see "Coronary Artery Disease", p. 189).

- The infarcted site is called the zone of infarction and necrosis. Around it is the zone of hypoxic injury. This zone is able to return to normal but may necrose if blood flow is not restored. The outermost zone is called the zone of ischemia; damage to this area is reversible.
- The most common sites of infarction are: (1) the anterior wall of the left ventricle near the apex, (2) the posterior wall of the left ventricle near the base, and (3) the inferior surface of the heart.

CLINICAL MANIFESTATIONS

- chest pain (cardinal symptom)
  — similar to angina but more severe in character and duration and unrelieved by nitroglycerin
  — may radiate to neck, jaw, shoulder, back or left arm
- hypotension
- gray facial color
- cold diaphoresis
- weak pulse
- peripheral cyanosis
- tachycardia or bradycardia
- lethargy
- increased temperature within 24 hours lasting 3-7 days
- great fear of death, apprehension
- nausea and vomiting
- dyspnea, orthopnea
- palpitations
- ECG changes — pathologic Q wave and serial ST-segment and T-wave changes

MEDICAL MANAGEMENT

The crucial time frame for salvage of the myocardium is the first six hours. Pain control is a priority. Continued pain is a sign of myocardial ischemia. Pain also stimulates the autonomic nervous system and increases preload, increasing myocardial demands.
- Acute attack:
  — analgesics and nitrates to alleviate pain
  — supplemental oxygen
  — invasive hemodynamic monitoring
  — bedrest and sedation to ease restlessness and fear

— anticoagulation therapy (reduce risk of embolism)
— continuous ECG monitoring
— anti-dysrhythmic therapy
— thrombolytic therapy (to lyse or dissolve the clot) — streptokinase, urokinase, tissue plasminogen activator (t-PA) and acylated plasminogen streptokinase activator complex (APSAC) — must be administered within 6 hours after the onset of chest pain, followed by five to seven days of heparin therapy
- Prevention of complications:
  (1) Dysrhythmias (major cause of death after an MI): ventricular premature beats, ventricular tachycardia and fibrillation, supraventricular tachycardia and heart block secondary to ectopic foci near the area of ischemia, conduction system interference or reperfusion of a previously ischemic area
     — continuous cardiac monitoring
     — oxygen therapy
     — prompt intervention for dysrhythmias (procainamide, lidocaine, etc.)
  (2) Cardiogenic shock — secondary to decreased myocardial contraction, dysrhythmias or sepsis
     — rapid pain relief
     — hemodynamic monitoring
     — intravenous fluid administration
     — vasopressors (levarterenol, dopamine, dobutamine, etc.)
     — oxygen therapy
     — antiarrhythmic therapy
  (3) Heart failure and pulmonary edema — secondary to decreased myocardial contraction
     — low-sodium diet
     — fluid restriction
     — digitalis therapy and diuretics
  (4) Pulmonary embolism — secondary to phlebitis of the legs or pelvic veins
     — anticoagulant therapy
     — range of motion exercises during bedrest
     — elastic stockings
  (5) Recurrent myocardial infarction — secondary to overexertion, embolization or further thrombotic occlusion
     — strict, progressive activity program
     — anticoagulation therapy

(6) Pericarditis — the inflamed area of infarction rubs against the pericardial surface, causing it to lose its lubricating fluid
— frequent assessment for early detection and intervention
— analgesics
— anti-inflammatory agents
- Cardiac rehabilitation program

NURSING MANAGEMENT

- Assess characteristics of chest pain and associated symptoms.
- Assess respirations and blood pressure.
- Obtain a 12-lead ECG.
- Administer analgesics and nitrates and monitor response to drug therapy.
- Administer thrombolytic therapy. See "Arterial Occlusion, Chronic", p. 61.
- Provide restful, quiet environment.
- Maintain continuous cardiac monitoring.
- Administer antidysrhythmics as ordered.
- Monitor serial serum enzyme levels.
- Assess apical pulse for murmurs, rub, S_3 and S_4.
- Monitor serum potassium levels.
- Monitor hemodynamic parameters - cardiac output, pulmonary artery pressures, etc.
- Assess for signs of decreased cardiac output (decreased urinary output, change in mental status, hypotension, etc.).
- Assess for signs of congestive heart failure (rales, rhonchi, S_3 and S_4, dependent edema, etc.).
- Administer supplemental oxygen.
- Monitor oxygen saturations and arterial blood gas results.
- Maintain progressive activity schedule per cardiac rehabilitation program.
- Monitor cardiopulmonary response to activity.
- Monitor effectiveness of stool softeners and laxatives to prevent straining.
- Facilitate dietary consult.
- Assist client in identifying own risk factors.

FOCUSED DISCHARGE CARE

Instruct the client regarding:
- disease process and treatment

- importance of risk factor modification -
  - — dietary restrictions — decreased cholesterol, decreased saturated fat, low-calorie
  - — smoking cessation
  - — blood pressure reduction
  - — stress management
- importance of cardiac rehabilitation program
- how to take pulse to monitor response to activity
- management of anginal episodes —
  - — lie or sit down
  - — take nitroglycerin tablets sublingually, 5 minutes apart
  - — if pain not relieved by 3 nitroglycerin, client is to be taken to emergency department
- activity limitations
- driving limitations
- importance of follow-up visits

(For more information, see pp. 684-691 of Polaski and Tatro, *Luckmann's Core Principles and Practice of Medical-Surgical Nursing.*)

Addison's Disease

OVERVIEW

- Addison's disease is a condition of hypofunctioning of the adrenal cortex as a result of a disorder within the adrenal gland.
- Addison's disease affects all age groups and both sexes.
- Seventy per cent of the cases are considered idiopathic. This condition may have an autoimmune basis. Sudden cessation of long-term use of exogenous steroids or bilateral adrenalectomy are two other possible causes of Addison's disease.
- Adrenal hypofunction causes decreased levels of mineralocorticoids (aldosterone), glucocorticoids (cortisol), and androgens.
  - — Aldosterone normally promotes conservation of sodium (and frequently water) and excretion of potassium. A deficiency of aldosterone causes

16

increased sodium excretion and the following: (1) water excretion increases, (2) extracellular volume is depleted (dehydration), (3) hypotension develops, (4) cardiac output decreases, and (5) potassium levels increase.

— Glucocorticoid deficiency causes decreased gluconeogenesis with resultant hypoglycemia and liver glycogen deficiency. Cortisol deficiency also results in failure to inhibit the anterior pituitary secretion of adrenocorticotropic hormone (ACTH), which increases levels of melanocyte-stimulating hormone (MSH), causing increased skin pigmentation.

— Androgen deficiency fails to produce symptoms in men because the testes supply adequate amounts of sex hormones. Women depend upon the adrenal cortex for an adequate secretion of androgens.

CLINICAL MANIFESTATIONS

The onset is usually insidious, and symptoms intensify as the disease progresses:
- fatigue
- weight loss, nausea, vomiting
- postural hypotension
- bronzed skin discoloration
- emotional disturbances range from mild neurotic symptoms to severe depression
- decreased resistance to emotional or physical stress.

MEDICAL MANAGEMENT

- Corticosteroid replacement
- For Addisonian crisis, medical management goals are to: (1) reverse shock, (2) restore blood circulation, and (3) replenish body with essential steroids.

NURSING MANAGEMENT

- Administer steroids as ordered.
- Monitor for signs of decreasing cardiac output.
- Monitor electrolyte levels and blood glucose results.
- Monitor intake and output.
- Assess for signs of infection as additional stress may necessitate an increase in steroid replacement dose.

- Monitor for signs and symptoms of Addisonian crisis:
  — sudden profound weakness
  — severe abdominal, back, and leg pain
  — hyperpyrexia followed by hypothermia
  — peripheral vascular collapse
  — coma
  — renal shutdown.
- Implement progressive activity schedule and monitor client's response.

FOCUSED DISCHARGE CARE

Instruct client regarding:
- actions of prescribed hormones
- importance of taking medications daily without fail (failure to take may precipitate an Addisonian crisis)
- signs of under and over-dosage of medication
- importance of hydrocortisone self-injection when unable to tolerate oral medication
- need for intramuscular self-injection kit to be available at all times
- intramuscular injection technique
- need for a Medic Alert bracelet and card
- need to call physician to have dosage increased when experiencing stressful situations, e.g., emotional upheavals, dental extractions, upper respiratory infections, etc.

(For more information, see pp. 1232-1236 of Polaski and Tatro, *Luckmann's Core Principles and Practice of Medical-Surgical Nursing.*)

Adult Respiratory Distress Syndrome (ARDS)

OVERVIEW

- Adult respiratory distress syndrome (ARDS) is a sudden, progressive pulmonary disorder characterized by severe dyspnea, hypoxemia and diffuse bilateral infiltrates.

- ARDS develops as a result of an insult, condition or noxious event that traumatizes the lung tissue. The insult may be directly to the lung or indirectly through other body systems.
- After the initial insult occurs, normal lung function is maintained for approximately 1 to 96 hours. Then hypoxemia rapidly develops and progresses with decreasing lung compliance and the development of diffuse lung infiltrates, atelectasis and pulmonary edema.
- There are approximately 150,000 cases of ARDS each year in the United States.
- Mortality rates are 30 to 60 per cent.
- Conditions at high risk of leading to ARDS are:
  — direct pulmonary trauma
    — pneumonia
    — lung contusion
    — fat embolus
    — aspiration
    — massive smoke inhalation
    — prolonged exposure to high concentrations of oxygen
  — indirect pulmonary trauma
    — sepsis
    — shock
    — multisystem trauma
    — disseminated intravascular coagulation
    — pancreatitis
    — drug overdose
    — massive blood transfusions
    — pregnancy-induced hypertension
    — increased intracranial pressure

CLINICAL MANIFESTATIONS

- increased respiratory rate, labored breathing
- air hunger, retractions, cyanosis
- adventitious breath sounds may or may not be present

MEDICAL MANAGEMENT

- endotracheal intubation with mechanical ventilation and use of positive end-expiratory pressure
- sedation to reduce anxiety and restlessness
- pharmacologic paralysis with pancuronium bromide

or curare if the client is "bucking the ventilator" and
sedation is ineffective
- inotropic agents to improve cardiac output and increase systemic blood pressure
- antibiotics if infection is present
- large doses of corticosteroids (controversial)

NURSING MANAGEMENT

- Follow principles of nursing management for clients
  with pneumonia, pulmonary edema and other pulmonary disorders affecting gas exchange (see specific disorders in *Pocket Companion*).
- Provide continuous mechanical ventilation (see "Mechanical Ventilation", p. 437).
- Provide emotional support and frequent updates to
  client and significant other.

FOCUSED DISCHARGE CARE

Discharge instructions will vary depending upon client
condition and post discharge needs.

(For more information, see pp. 597-599 of Polaski and Tatro,
Luckmann's Core Principles and Practice of Medical-Surgical Nursing.)

Agranulocytosis

OVERVIEW

- Agranulocytosis is an acute, potentially fatal blood
  dyscrasia characterized by profound neutropenia
  resulting in greater susceptibility to bacterial invasion.
- Agranulocytosis results either from the failure of
  granulocyte production to keep pace with destruction of cells or increased granulocyte destruction.
- Causes of agranulocytosis include:
  — agents that produce neutropenia when given in
    large doses over time (chemotherapy, radiation,
    benzene)

— agents that produce neutropenia only in clients sensitive to the drug (chlorpromazine, propylthiouracil, phenytoin, chloramphenicol, phenylbutazone)

CLINICAL MANIFESTATIONS

- severe fatigue, weakness
- sore throat, ulcerations of the pharyngeal and buccal mucosa
- dysphagia
- fever, severe chills
- weak, rapid pulse

MEDICAL MANAGEMENT

- identification/possible elimination of toxic agent or disease
    — agranulocytosis caused by toxic substances usually reverses within 2 to 3 weeks after withdrawal of the causative agent
- surveillance cultures (collected at predetermined intervals [i.e., weekly] for detection of infectious organisms)
- antibiotic therapy
- granulocyte transfusion therapy

NURSING MANAGEMENT

- Administer antibiotic and marrow stimulating therapy.
- Administer granulocyte replacement therapy. See "Blood Component Transfusion", p. 88.
- Maintain protective isolation.
- Monitor temperature and assess for signs/symptoms of infection.
- Monitor laboratory findings — CBC, WBC, culture reports, absolute granulocyte count.
- Encourage balanced diet with no fresh fruits or vegetables.
- Provide adequate rest.
- Provide meticulous oral and physical care.
- Avoid rectal suppositories and rectal temperatures.
- Obtain cultures as ordered.

FOCUSED DISCHARGE CARE

Instruct client regarding:
- disease process and treatment regime
- measures to prevent infection:
  — good personal hygiene
  — avoid crowds and people with known infectious disease
  — wear a mask in public
  — no fresh fruits, vegetables or raw meats
  — change air conditioner and furnace filters weekly
  — remove additional sources of bacteria found in standing water—fish tanks, flower vases, humidifier
  — well-balanced diet
  — adequate rest
- signs/symptoms to report to physician
- importance of follow-up laboratory and clinic visits

(For more information, see pp. 861-862 of Polaski and Tatro, *Luckmann's Core Principles and Practice of Medical-Surgical Nursing.*)

Airway Obstruction, Foreign Body

- Foreign bodies usually enter the right main bronchus because its orifice is slightly wider than that of the left main bronchus. It also lies in a more direct line with the trachea.
- Clinical manifestations of an aspirated foreign body include: severe dyspnea; hemoptysis; fever; atelectasis; pulmonary infection; excessive mucous production; harsh, brassy cough; wheezing; and inspiratory stridor. If the obstruction is complete or nearly complete and at the laryngeal level, clinical manifestations include: obvious respiratory distress, inability to speak, ineffective ventilation efforts and the international sign for distress (hands at the throat). Asphyxia follows rapidly.

- Complete airway obstruction is a life-threatening emergency requiring immediate intervention.
- The Heimlich maneuver and thrust techniques are used when clients are unable to speak, unable to elicit effective cough or are unconscious.
- For incomplete obstruction, the client may be placed in Trendelenburg's position so that the foreign body will not move any lower into the airway.
- Some foreign bodies lodged in the laryngeal area may be removed with grasping forceps inserted through a laryngoscope under local or general anesthesia.
- A bronchoscope and special grasping forceps are used for objects that are deeper into the airway.

(For more information, see p. 1573 of Polaski and Tatro, *Luckmann's Core Principles and Practice of Medical-Surgical Nursing*.)

Alkalosis, Metabolic

OVERVIEW

- Metabolic alkalosis may be caused by either abnormal loss of fixed acid or excess accumulation of bicarbonate.
- The above are interdependent because hydrogen excretion is accompanied by bicarbonate reclamation in the kidneys and in the gastric cells.
- Etiologic factors causing metabolic alkalosis include:
  — fixed acid loss:
    — hypokalemia secondary to diuretic or steroid therapy — when potassium is deficient, the kidneys excrete hydrogen in exchange for sodium and this in turn stimulates bicarbonate reabsorption
    — gastric fluid loss (vomiting, nasogastric suctioning) — hydrochloric acid is lost

— excessive bicarbonate intake:
    — overcorrection of acidosis with sodium bicarbonate
    — massive transfusion of whole blood — citrate anticoagulant used for storage is metabolized to bicarbonate
  — excessive bicarbonate reabsorption:
    — hyperaldosteronism—increased renal absorption of sodium and subsequent loss of potassium

CLINICAL MANIFESTATIONS

- hypoventilation (compensatory)
- dysrhythmias
- pH above 7.45
- hypokalemia
- hypocalcemia — in alkalosis, there are less hydrogen ions to occupy binding sites on blood proteins allowing calcium to bind to the sites, reducing the proportion of unbound calcium
- $PaCO_2$ normal or slightly increased

MEDICAL MANAGEMENT

- determination/treatment of underlying cause
- potassium replacement therapy
- calcium replacement therapy
- acidifying salts administration (in extreme cases) — ammonium chloride
- cardiac monitoring

NURSING MANAGEMENT

- Monitor respiratory status.
- Monitor cardiac status.
- Evaluate ECG for rhythm changes.
- Administer electrolyte replacement therapy.
- Monitor laboratory results — arterial blood gases, electrolytes.
- Monitor oxygen saturations.
- Monitor for signs/symptoms of hypokalemia:
  — thready, weak pulse
  — postural hypotension
  — ECG changes:

- — ST depression
        - — flattened or inverted T wave
        - — prominent U wave
        - — heart block
    - — anxiety, lethargy, confusion
    - — nausea, vomiting
- Monitor for signs/symptoms of hypocalcemia:
    - — anxiety, irritability
    - — paresthesias
    - — muscle twitching and cramps
    - — ECG changes:
        - — prolonged ST interval
        - — prolonged QT interval
    - — hypotension
    - — abdominal cramping
- Assess neurological status and implement appropriate safety measures.
- Assess ability to perform activities of daily living.
- Plan scheduled rest periods.

FOCUSED DISCHARGE CARE

Discharge care is based upon etiologic factor(s) causing metabolic alkalosis.

(For more information, see pp. 72-76 of Polaski and Tatro, *Luckmann's Core Principles and Practice of Medical-Surgical Nursing.*)

Alkalosis, Respiratory

OVERVIEW

- Respiratory alkalosis is caused by alveolar hyperventilation, in which excess carbon dioxide (CO_2) is eliminated. The most common cause of respiratory alkalosis is hypoxemia.
- Low levels of oxygen (PaO_2) in the blood are sensed by the peripheral chemoreceptors in the carotid bodies and aortic arch. These receptors then increase their rate of firing to the respiratory center in

the medulla, and rate and depth of ventilation increase.

- Etiologic factors that cause respiratory alkalosis include:
  — hypoxemia
    — emphysema
    — pneumonia
    — adult respiratory distress syndrome (ARDS)
  — impaired lung expansion:
    — pulmonary fibrosis
    — ascites
    — scoliosis
    — pregnancy
  — thickened alveolar-capillary membrane:
    — congestive heart failure
    — adult respiratory distress syndrome (ARDS)
    — pneumonia
    — pulmonary embolism
  — chemical stimulation of the respiratory center:
    — sepsis
    — high level of ammonia (hepatic failure)
    — high level of salicylates (aspirin overdose)
  — traumatic stimulation of the respiratory center:
    — central nervous system trauma
    — central nervous system tumor
    — increased intracranial pressure
    — stress
    — pain

CLINICAL MANIFESTATIONS

- tachypnea
- giddiness, dizziness, syncope, convulsions, or coma
- weakness, paresthesias, tetany
- pH above 7.45
- $PaCO_2$ below 35 mm Hg
- hypokalemia — in alkalosis, potassium shifts into the cell
- hypocalcemia — in alkalosis, there are less hydrogen ions to occupy binding sites on blood proteins allowing calcium to bind to the sites, reducing the proportion of unbound calcium

MEDICAL MANAGEMENT

- determination/treatment of underlying cause
- measures to increase carbon dioxide retention:
  — mechanical hypoventilation
  — carbon dioxide rebreathing
  — sedation
- ventilatory support
- electrolyte replacement therapy

NURSING MANAGEMENT

- Monitor respiratory status.
- Implement CO_2 retention measures as ordered.
- Assess for signs/symptoms of hypokalemia:
  — thready, weak pulse
  — postural hypotension
  — ECG changes:
    — ST depression
    — flattened or inverted T wave
    — prominent U wave
    — heart block
  — anxiety, lethargy, confusion
  — nausea, vomiting
- Assess for signs/symptoms of hypocalcemia:
  — anxiety, irritability
  — paresthesias
  — muscle twitches and cramps
  — ECG changes:
    — prolonged ST interval
    — prolonged QT interval
  — hypotension
  — abdominal cramping
- Monitor laboratory findings — arterial blood gases, electrolytes.
- Assess cardiac status.
- Assess ECG for rhythm changes.
- Assess neurological status and implement appropriate safety measures.
- Assess ability to perform activities of daily living.
- Schedule activities to allow for rest periods.
- Implement measures to prevent pain, fever or anxiety, if present (these increase respiratory rate).

FOCUSED DISCHARGE CARE

Discharge care is based on the etiologic factor(s) causing respiratory alkalosis.

(For more information, see pp. 72-76 of Polaski and Tatro,
*Luckmann's Core Principles and Practice of Medical-Surgi-
cal Nursing.*)

Alzheimer's Disease

OVERVIEW

- Dementia involves progressive change in personality and two or more areas of cognition, usually
  memory and one or more of the following: language,
  calculation, visual (spatial perception), judgment,
  abstraction. Dementia of the Alzheimer's type (DAT)
  comprises at least one-half of all the dementias.
- The actual cause of dementia of the Alzheimer's type
  has not been found.
- DAT occurs in 10 to 15 per cent of people over age 65,
  19 per cent of people over age 75, and 47 per cent of
  people over 85.
- Risk factors identified include: (1) increasing age, (2)
  familial tendency, and (3) environmental and metabolic factors.

CLINICAL MANIFESTATIONS

First Stage

- memory loss
- poor judgment and problem-solving skills
- personality changes — irritability, suspiciousness
  or indifference

Second Stage

- language disturbances — impaired word finding,
  circumlocution (talking around a subject), empty

spontaneous speech, paraphasia (words used in wrong context), echolalia (repetition of words)
- motor disturbances — apraxia (difficulty using everyday objects like a toothbrush)
- increased memory loss
- forgetfulness
- hyperorality (desire to take everything into the mouth to suck, chew, or taste)
- increased irritability and depression
- delusions, hallucinations
- psychotic behavior
- wandering
- occasional incontinence

THIRD STAGE

- virtual loss of all mental abilities
- minimal voluntary movement; limbs become rigid with flexor posturing
- frequent urinary and fecal incontinence
- lost ability for self-care

MEDICAL MANAGEMENT

- low-dose antipsychotic agents — haloperidol
- antidepressants — nortriptyline, desipramine

NURSING MANAGEMENT

- Adapt communication to the level of the client.
- Speak slowly and simply, with firm volume and low pitch.
- Assess nonverbal behavior.
- Intervene if client displays angry, hostile behavior by:
  — decreasing environmental stimuli
  — approaching in a calm, reassuring manner
  — taking care not to place any more demands on the client
  — distracting the client
  — making sure all verbal and non-verbal cues are congruent
  — using multiple sensory modalities (visual, auditory, and tactile) to communicate.
- Implement measures to enhance memory:

- — reorient as necessary
- — place a clock and calendar in client's room
- — allow client to reminisce
- — repeat instructions frequently.
- Institute appropriate safety measures:
    - — ensure that client cannot leave the premises without being noticed
    - — ensure that identification bracelet is worn at all times
    - — remove harmful objects.
- Encourage the client to do own activities of daily living as much as possible.
- Allow plenty of time to complete tasks.
- Anticipate elimination needs and schedule voiding and defecation times.
- Limit fluid intake after the dinner meal to decrease nocturnal incontinence.
- Provide emotional support to family members, particularly the caregivers.

FOCUSED DISCHARGE CARE

- Instruct the family regarding:
    - — disease process and prognosis
    - — providing a safe home environment
    - — communication techniques
    - — measures to enhance the client's memory and orientation
- Refer to available community resources—Alzheimer's Disease and Related Disorders Chapter, respite care, adult day care, and Home Health Care.

(For more information, see pp. 370-375 of Polaski and Tatro, *Luckmann's Core Principles and Practice of Medical-Surgical Nursing.*)

Amputation

OVERVIEW

- Extremity amputation is the surgical removal of all or part of an extremity. Clients with peripheral vascular

disease are the most frequent candidates for amputation of the lower extremities.
- Primary amputations are undertaken as definitive treatment for lower extremity ischemia. Secondary amputations follow a previous reconstructive vascular procedure. Amputations may also be required for acute limb-threatening conditions, mainly trauma, and for malignant tumors and congenital deformities.

SURGICAL MANAGEMENT

- Prior to amputation the physician determines:
  (1) client's physical condition
  (2) type of amputation to be performed
     — closed or "flap" — stump is covered with a flap of skin sutured over the end of it
       • performed when there is no evidence of infection
     — opened or "guillotine" — stump is not covered with a skin flap but left open to allow wound to drain
       • used when infection is present
       • requires a second surgery for stump closure once infection is eradicated
  (3) level of amputation — should be as distal as possible
  (4) peripheral vascular function test results
  (5) client's attitude toward amputation and rehabilitation potential
  (6) type of postoperative prosthetic-fitting and rehabilitation program

NURSING MANAGEMENT

In addition to routine preoperative care:
- Assist the client in dealing with anticipated loss and body image change.
- Prepare client for "phantom limb" sensation (sensation that missing limb is still present).
- Facilitate referral to social work or psychologist.

In addition to routine postoperative care:
- Assess for signs of bleeding or oozing.

- Elevate stump for the first 24 hours if ordered to control edema, then place flat on bed to prevent hip contracture.
- Assess incision for signs of healing.
- Encourage range of motion and muscle strengthening exercises.
- Follow weight-bearing guidelines prescribed by physician.
- Consult physical therapy for adaptive devices for ambulation, transfer techniques and exercise instructions.
- Assist the client in coping with the loss and integrating the prosthetic device into the total body image.

FOCUSED DISCHARGE CARE

Instruct client regarding:
- stump care:
  — inspect daily for redness, blistering or abrasions
    — use a mirror to examine all sides
  — perform daily stump hygiene
    — wash with mild soap, rinse and dry
    — do not use oils, creams or alcohol on the stump
    — wear woolen socks over the stump
    — put prosthesis on immediately when arising and keep on all day (once wound has healed completely) to reduce swelling
    — continue prescribed exercises to prevent weakness
- prosthesis care:
  — remove sweat and dirt daily from inside of socket with warm water and soap
  — never attempt to adjust prosthesis; consult a prosthetist
- available support groups and community resources

(For more information, see pp. 809-813 of Polaski and Tatro, *Luckmann's Core Principles and Practice of Medical-Surgical Nursing.*)

Amyotrophic Lateral Sclerosis

OVERVIEW

- Amyotrophic lateral sclerosis (ALS) is the most common of the motor neuron diseases.
- ALS involves degeneration of both anterior horn cells and the corticospinal tracts. Consequently, both upper and lower motor neuron signs and symptoms are seen. The sensory system is not involved.
- The onset of ALS usually occurs in middle age. Men are affected more often than women.
- Weakness typically begins in the upper extremities and progressively involves the upper arms and shoulders and then the muscles of the neck and throat. The trunk and lower extremities are usually not affected until late in the disease.
- Cognition, as well as bowel and bladder sphincters, remain intact, even when the client is totally debilitated.
- The course of the disease is relentlessly progressive. Death usually results from pneumonia due to respiratory compromise within 2 to 5 years.

CLINICAL MANIFESTATIONS

- weakness, fatigue
- muscle atrophy
- muscle twitching
- spasticity and hyperreflexia
- dysphagia (difficulty swallowing)
- dysarthria (slurred speech)
- shallow respirations
- ineffective cough

MEDICAL MANAGEMENT

- Supportive therapy is the only intervention for ALS.

NURSING MANAGEMENT

- Assess client's ability to perform self-care.

- Conserve client energy by spacing activities and allowing rest periods.
- Encourage fluid intake.
- Initiate aspiration precautions.
- Collaborate with physical and occupational therapy for exercises and adaptive devices for ambulation and self care.
- Allow plenty of time to complete activities.
- Assure that suction equipment is maintained at the bedside.
- Monitor respiratory status and laboratory arterial blood gas results.

FOCUSED DISCHARGE CARE

- Instruct the client/family regarding:
  — disease process and prognosis
  — need for respiratory support equipment in the home (oxygen, suction set-up) and training of household members in its use
  — methods to conserve energy
  — importance of avoiding exposure to anyone with respiratory infections
  — the need to use good posture and swallowing techniques while eating and drinking to avoid aspiration
  — use of abdominal muscles to enhance respiration when the intercostal muscles and diaphragm become weak
  — use of adaptive devices
  — the importance of follow-up pulmonary function tests and clinic visits
- Refer to available community resources (Home Health Care agency, ALS support groups).

(For more information, see pp. 382-383 of Polaski and Tatro, *Luckmann's Core Principles and Practice of Medical-Surgical Nursing.*)

Anemia, Acute Posthemorrhagic

OVERVIEW

- Acute posthemorrhagic anemia is a normocytic, normochromic anemia that develops after the rapid loss of red blood cells during a massive hemorrhage.
- The adverse effects of acute hemorrhage result from a rapid decrease in blood volume and red blood cells reducing the oxygen-carrying capacity of the blood and perfusion to vital organs. The severity of symptoms and the prognosis for acute hemorrhage depend upon (1) the rate of bleeding, (2) the site of the hemorrhage, and (3) the volume of blood lost.

CLINICAL MANIFESTATIONS

- restlessness
- dizziness, syncope
- thirst
- pallor
- diaphoresis
- rapid, thready pulse
- dramatic drop in blood pressure
- rapid, deep respirations, which later become shallow
- disorientation, coma

MEDICAL MANAGEMENT

- determination of and intervention to control hemorrhage
- fluid replacement therapy
- blood component replacement therapy
- oxygen therapy

NURSING MANAGEMENT

- Administer fluid and blood component therapies. See "Blood Component Transfusion", p. 88.
- Assess for signs/symptoms of decreased cardiac output.

- Monitor vital signs.
- Monitor laboratory findings — CBC.

FOCUSED DISCHARGE CARE

Acute anemia will be resolved prior to discharge.

(For more information, see p. 849 of Polaski and Tatro, *Luckmann's Core Principles and Practice of Medical-Surgical Nursing.*)

Anemia, Aplastic

OVERVIEW

- Aplastic anemia describes bone marrow that is severely hypoplastic ("empty"), that is, devoid of erythroid, myeloid and megakaryocytic cell lines. Hypoplastic bone marrow results in anemia, leukopenia and thrombocytopenia. When all three cellular elements are suppressed, the condition is known as pancytopenia.
- The etiologic agents that cause aplastic anemia inhibit mitosis (cell division) or block the synthesis of purines or nucleic acids and thus impede blood cell production.
- In about one-half the cases of aplastic anemia, the cause is unknown. Factors identified as causing aplastic anemia are an autoimmune reaction or direct injury by myelotoxins (such as medications that cause aplastic anemia as a side effect).

CLINICAL MANIFESTATIONS

NORMOCYTIC ANEMIA

- progressive fatigue, lassitude, dyspnea

GRANULOCYTOPENIA

- increased susceptibility to infection

- bleeding into the skin and mucous membranes
- hemorrhage

MEDICAL MANAGEMENT

- identification and withdrawal of the offending agent or drug
- blood product replacement therapy
- bone marrow transplantation if autoimmune phenomenon is suspected or bone marrow fails to regenerate with withdrawal of myelotoxic agents (See "Bone Marrow Transplantation", p. 92)
- steroid and androgen therapy to stimulate bone marrow activity
- oxygen therapy

NURSING MANAGEMENT

- Administer blood products as ordered. See "Blood Component Transfusion", p. 88.
- Monitor laboratory findings — CBC and platelet count.
- Monitor response to activity and provide rest periods.
- Maintain protective isolation.
- Monitor temperature and assess for other signs/ symptoms of infection.
- Assess for signs/symptoms of bleeding — hematest positive stools, petechiae, epistaxis, change in level of consciousness, abdominal pain, etc.
- Maintain bleeding precautions — electric razor, soft toothbrush, assisted ambulation, etc.

FOCUSED DISCHARGE CARE

Instruct client regarding:
- the importance of follow-up clinic appointments
- need to avoid exposure to others with infections
- signs/symptoms to report to physician
- importance of adequate rest
- precautions to prevent bleeding:
    — no contact sports

- soft toothbrush
- electric razor
- care when doing yardwork
- safety precautions

(For more information, see pp. 847-848 of Polaski and Tatro, *Luckmann's Core Principles and Practice of Medical-Surgical Nursing*.)

Anemia, Due to Chronic Blood Loss

OVERVIEW

- Anemia due to chronic blood loss is a chronic, microcytic, hypochromic anemia.
- The results of chronic bleeding are (1) continuous loss of small numbers of erythrocytes, usually replaced by the bone marrow, and (2) continuous loss of iron.
- The major causes of chronic blood loss include bleeding peptic ulcers, prolonged or excessive menses, bleeding hemorrhoids and cancerous lesions within the gastrointestinal tract.

CLINICAL MANIFESTATIONS

- asymptomatic — mild cases
- dizziness, headaches
- sensitivity to cold
- pallor
- palpitations
- weakness, fatigue

MEDICAL MANAGEMENT

Includes modalities generally recommended for anemia.

SURGICAL MANAGEMENT

Surgery may be needed to correct the chronic blood loss.

(For more information, see p. 849 of Polaski and Tatro, *Luckmann's Core Principles and Practice of Medical-Surgical Nursing.*)

Anemia, Folic Acid Deficiency

OVERVIEW

- Folic acid deficiency causes a megaloblastic anemia.
- Folic acid deficiency impedes the formation of DNA precursors, which causes abnormal maturation of red blood cells (megaloblasts), leukocytes and platelets.
- Factors causing folic acid deficiency include:
  — diet lacking in foods such as green leafy vegetables, liver, citrus fruits and yeast
  — alcoholism (due to (1) inadequate dietary intake of folic acid and (2) high levels of alcohol in the blood which partially block the response of the bone marrow to folic acid)
- Anemia due to folic acid deficiency has a slow, insidious onset.

CLINICAL MANIFESTATIONS

- thin and emaciated appearance
- fatigue, weakness
- palpitations
- pallor
- slight jaundice
- dyspepsia; smooth, beefy tongue
- angina

MEDICAL MANAGEMENT

- determination/treatment of underlying cause
- folic acid replacement
- vitamin C therapy (increases role of folic acid in promoting erythropoiesis)
- oxygen therapy
- dietary modification

NURSING MANAGEMENT

- Administer replacement therapy as ordered.
- Monitor laboratory findings — CBC, folate level.
- Monitor response to activity and provide rest periods.

FOCUSED DISCHARGE CARE

Instruct client regarding:
- importance of medication regime
- dietary modifications
- importance of follow-up clinic appointments
- available community alcohol cessation programs (if history of alcohol abuse)

(For more information, see pp. 846-847 of Polaski and Tatro, *Luckmann's Core Principles and Practice of Medical-Surgical Nursing.*)

Anemia, Glucose-6-Phosphate Dehydrogenase (G6PD) Deficiency

OVERVIEW

- Glucose-6-phosphate dehydrogenase (G6PD) is an important red blood cell enzyme. G6PD anemia is a genetic disorder that leaves red blood cells more susceptible to hemolysis after ingestion of medications and food classified as chemical oxidants (i.e., quinine, aspirin, sulfonamides, primaquine, phenacetin, Vitamin K derivatives, chloramphenicol, thiazide diuretics, fava bean). After exposure to any of these agents, the client with G6PD deficiency develops acute intravascular hemolysis lasting 7 to 12 days.
- Among Americans, G6PD deficiency affects about 20 per cent of the black population and 1 to 2 per cent of the white population. It is common among Sephardic Jews, Greeks, Italians and Arabs.

CLINICAL MANIFESTATIONS

Clients with G6PD deficiency may remain completely asymptomatic throughout their lives. Typically, symptoms develop after a stressor occurs.
- anemia
- jaundice (bilirubin accumulation)

MEDICAL MANAGEMENT

- identification and elimination of the food or medication precipitating the hemolytic reaction
- fluid replacement therapy

NURSING MANAGEMENT

- Administer fluid replacement therapy.
- Encourage adequate rest.
- Monitor laboratory findings — CBC, bilirubin levels.
- Encourage nutritious diet.

FOCUSED DISCHARGE CARE

Instruct client regarding:
- foods or medications that may precipitate an attack
- importance of adequate rest
- importance of screening family members

(For more information, see pp. 850-851 of Polaski and Tatro, *Luckmann's Core Principles and Practice of Medical-Surgical Nursing.*)

Anemia, Hemolytic

OVERVIEW

- Major hallmarks of hemolytic anemia are:
  - a shortening of the red blood cell life span
  - an abnormal increase in the number of red blood cells destroyed by macrophages
  - failure of the bone marrow to replace destroyed red blood cells

- Premature hemolysis of red blood cells results from:
  — trauma
    — external trauma or burns
  — prosthetic heart valve replacement (causes turbulence in blood flow)
  — chemical agents and medications — benzene, nitrates, potassium chlorate, lead, quinine, quinidine, methyldopa, penicillin
  — infectious agents
  — systemic diseases
  — hemolytic reactions
  — autoimmune disorders
- Hemolytic anemia may be acute or chronic.

CLINICAL MANIFESTATIONS

- dyspnea
- palpitations, tachycardia
- chronic fatigue
- pallor
- sore mouth and tongue
- angina
- anorexia
- headache, dizziness
- signs/symptoms of renal failure — due to excretion of increased load of blood cell degradation products

MEDICAL MANAGEMENT

- identification/elimination of causative factor
- oxygen therapy
- blood product replacement therapy
- corticosteroid therapy
- chelating agents such as calcium disodium edetate

NURSING MANAGEMENT

- Administer steroid therapy as prescribed.
- Administer blood products as prescribed. See "Blood Component Transfusion", p. 88.
- Monitor laboratory findings — CBC, renal panel, bilirubin levels.
- Monitor intake and output.
- Assess response to activity and provide rest periods.

FOCUSED DISCHARGE CARE

Instruct client regarding:
- importance of medication regime
- importance of rest
- need for follow-up clinic appointments

(For more information, see p. 848 of Polaski and Tatro, *Luckmann's Core Principles and Practice of Medical-Surgical Nursing*.)

Anemia, Iron Deficiency

OVERVIEW

- Iron deficiency anemia is associated with either inadequate absorption or excessive loss of iron; it is a chronic, microcytic, hypochromic anemia.
- An inadequate supply of iron needed to synthesize hemoglobin, decreases the oxygen-carrying capacity of heme. When this disorder becomes severe, the marrow produces red cells that are deficient in hemoglobin concentration and are hypochromic and microcytic.
- The poor of all nations suffer far more frequently from iron deficiency than do the middle and upper classes. Menstruating women and young children also are vulnerable to iron deficiency. These groups of clients must have a higher daily intake of iron for prevention of this deficiency. Iron deficiency anemia also occurs with chronic blood loss (peptic ulcers, ulcerative colitis).
- The major risk factor for iron deficiency anemia is inadequate nutrition.

CLINICAL MANIFESTATIONS

Mild cases may be asymptomatic.

- palpitations, tachycardia
- dizziness, headaches
- sensitivity to the cold

- brittle hair and nails
- weakness, fatigue
- pallor
- sore mouth and tongue
- dyspnea

MEDICAL MANAGEMENT

- determination/treatment of the underlying cause
- supplemental iron preparations —ferrous sulfate (Feosol), ferrous gluconate (Fergon), iron-dextran (Imferon)
- oxygen therapy
- dietary modification — increased iron

NURSING MANAGEMENT

- Administer ordered iron replacement therapy.
  - Oral iron salt replacement should be given with meals (to decrease gastric upset).
  - Liquid iron preparations should be taken through a straw (to prevent staining the teeth).
  - Intramuscular replacements should be given by Z-track technique (to prevent discoloration of the skin).
- Monitor response to activity and provide adequate rest periods.
- Encourage diet high in protein, iron and vitamins.
- Assess for signs of constipation (commonly seen during iron therapy).
- Monitor laboratory findings — CBC, iron levels.

FOCUSED DISCHARGE CARE

Instruct client regarding:
- importance of medication regime and specifics of administration
- dietary modifications—high in iron.
- measures to prevent constipation if on iron replacement (high fiber diet, stool softener, increased fluids)
- importance of follow-up clinic appointments

(For more information, see pp. 844-845 of Polaski and Tatro, *Luckmann's Core Principles and Practice of Medical-Surgical Nursing.*)

Anemia, Pernicious

OVERVIEW

- Pernicious anemia refers to anemia due to decreased absorption of vitamin B_{12}.
- The principal cause of impaired vitamin B_{12} absorption is intrinsic factor deficiency. Lack of intrinsic factor due to atrophy of the stomach's glandular mucosa is the basic defect in pernicious anemia.
- A major risk factor for the development of pernicious anemia is gastric resection. The parietal cells in the stomach secrete the intrinsic factor required for vitamin B_{12} absorption. The disease can also be congenital as a result of absence of the intrinsic factor.
- Major characteristics of pernicious anemia include:
  — abnormally large red blood cells (macrocytic anemia)
  — hypochlorhydria (deficiency of gastric hydrochloric acid)
  — neurologic and gastrointestinal symptoms
  — a fatal outcome unless the client receives life-long injections of vitamin B_{12}.
- Pernicious anemia mainly strikes men and women over the age of 50 years.

CLINICAL MANIFESTATIONS

- weakness, fatigue
- dyspepsia; smooth, beefy tongue
- palpitations
- shortness of breath
- pallor
- sensitivity to cold
- anorexia, nausea, weight loss
- disturbed nervous system function
- angina

MEDICAL MANAGEMENT

- determination/treatment of underlying cause
- vitamin B_{12} therapy (lifelong therapy)

- oxygen therapy
- dietary modifications

NURSING MANAGEMENT

- Administer replacement therapy as ordered.
- Monitor laboratory findings - CBC.
- Monitor response to activity and provide rest periods.

FOCUSED DISCHARGE CARE

Instruct client regarding:
- importance of lifelong therapy of monthly vitamin B_{12} injections
- importance of follow-up clinic appointments - clients with pernicious anemia are at risk for developing gastric carcinoma and should have a complete physical examination twice a year
- dietary modifications

(For more information, see pp. 845-846 of Polaski and Tatro, *Luckmann's Core Principles and Practice of Medical-Surgical Nursing.*)

Anemia, Sickle Cell

OVERVIEW

- Sickle cell anemia is a chronic, hereditary, hemolytic disorder. Sickle cell anemia primarily affects the world's black population.
- In sickle cell anemia, the red blood cells contain an abnormal hemoglobin, that is, hemoglobin S (HbS) instead of hemoglobin A (HbA). These abnormal cells assume a sickle, or crescent, shape when oxygen in the blood decreases. Once they "sickle," the red blood cells become rigid and may obstruct capillary blood flow, causing further hypoxia and, consequently, more sickling. The heavy concentration of misshapen cells during a sickling crisis makes the

blood abnormally viscous, which results in sluggish circulation. The organs most vulnerable to infarction and necrosis are the brain and kidneys, because of their constant demand for oxygen, and the bone marrow and spleen, because of their normally sluggish circulation.

- Sickle cell *trait*, generally a relatively mild condition, may produce few or no symptoms. It is present in clients who are heterogenous for sickle cell hemoglobin. When exposed to extreme stressors, the client with the trait may develop symptoms of sickle cell disease.
- Factors that result in hypoxia and may trigger a crisis include: climbing to high altitudes, flying in non-pressurized planes, exercising strenuously or undergoing anesthesia without proper oxygenation.
- Complications of sickle cell anemia include:
  — hemolytic anemia — secondary to destruction of sickle cells
  — cholelithiasis (gallstones) - due to elevated bilirubin from hemoglobin released during destruction of sickle cells
  — splenic infarction
  — renal medullary ischemia with diminished capacity to concentrate urine
  — pulmonary infarction
  — myocardial infarction
  — cerebrovascular accident
  — osteoporosis — secondary to proliferation of the bone marrow in an attempt to compensate for chronic anemia

CLINICAL MANIFESTATIONS

Sickle Cell Crisis

- dyspnea, cyanosis
- jaundice or pallor
- chest pain
- bone or joint pain
- systolic murmur
- signs/symptoms of increased intracranial pressure
- enlarged liver and spleen
- decreased urinary output
- edema

MEDICAL MANAGEMENT

- bedrest
- oxygen therapy
- fluid and electrolyte therapy
- sedation
- analgesics
- folic acid replacement — to prevent increased anemia

NURSING MANAGEMENT

- Administer oxygen therapy.
- Administer analgesics.
- Encourage rest.
- Administer fluid and electrolyte therapy.
- Monitor intake and output.
- Daily weights.
- Assess all body systems for evidence of complications.

FOCUSED DISCHARGE CARE

Instruct client regarding:
- preventing a crisis:
  — avoid high altitudes
  — avoid flying in non-pressurized planes
  — avoid becoming dehydrated
- signs/symptoms of complications and when to call the physician
- disease process
- need for genetic counseling
- need for follow-up laboratory and clinic visits

(For more information, see pp. 871-874 of Polaski and Tatro, *Luckmann's Core Principles and Practice of Medical-Surgical Nursing.*)

Aneurysm, Aortic - Ruptured or Dissecting

- An aneurysm is an outpouching of a vessel wall, usually due to arteriosclerotic changes or trauma

involving the tunica media (muscular layer of the artery).
- The aneurysm may be saccular ("balloons out") or fusiform (encircles the vessel).
- Aortic aneurysms may involve the thoracic aorta or abdominal aorta.
- In aortic dissection, blood separates the vessel layers and a larger portion of the vessel may be affected. In an expanding aneurysm, the aneurysm wall is still intact. Symptoms are caused by increased pressure on the surrounding structures.
- A rupture occurs when the vessel wall loses continuity.
- A ruptured or dissecting aneurysm is a surgical emergency.
- Assessment findings of a ruptured or dissecting aneurysm may include:
  — severe abdominal and back pain if the aneurysm is leaking
  — an enlarging abdominal girth with a palpable, pulsatile mass
  — leg numbness, tingling or loss of motor function
  — mottled cyanosis below the level of the aneurysm
  — profound hypotension
- Treatment is rapid surgical intervention.
- Nursing Management
  — Insert two to four large-bore intravenous lines.
  — Monitor vital signs continuously.
  — Monitor ECG.
  — Administer anti-hypertensives to minimize extension of the dissection.
  — Obtain blood for laboratory studies (including type and crossmatch for 10 to 20 units of whole blood).
  — Ensure that necessary instruments are available if needed for cross-clamping the aorta.
  — Transport the client to the operating room with resuscitative personnel in attendance and an emergency laparotomy tray on the stretcher.

(For more information, see pp. 1582-1583 of Polaski and Tatro, *Luckmann's Core Principles and Practice of Medical-Surgical Nursing.*)

Aneurysm (Intracranial) and Subarachnoid Hemorrhage

OVERVIEW

- Intracranial aneurysms are congenital, traumatic, arteriosclerotic, or septal weakenings or out-pouchings in vessel walls. Ninety per cent of aneurysms are congenital. Cerebral aneurysms most often occur on the circle of Willis.
- Aneurysms may weaken, leak or rupture and cause bleeding into the subarachnoid space. This is called subarachnoid hemorrhage (SAH).
- SAH also may be caused by head trauma, blood dyscrasias, intracranial tumors, vascular anomalies or central nervous system infection.
- Risk factors for SAH include: head trauma, hypertension and cocaine use.

CLINICAL MANIFESTATIONS

An aneurysm is usually asymptomatic until it ruptures.
- sudden, severe headache with vomiting
- loss of consciousness, confusion, lethargy
- seizures
- stiff neck; leg and back pain
- motor weakness
- coma (within hours)

MEDICAL MANAGEMENT

- use of albumin and vasopressors to induce hypertensive, hypervolemic hemodilution to minimize vasospasm and force blood through spastic vessels
- measures to decrease ICP:
  — dexamethasone (Decadron) and osmotic agents
  — elevating the head of the bed 20 to 30 degrees
  — maintaining a patent airway to prevent increased PCO_2.

SURGICAL MANAGEMENT

- clipping of the aneurysm through a craniotomy

NURSING MANAGEMENT

MEDICAL

- Provide calm, quiet environment.
- Assess client's response to family visits and adjust visiting schedule accordingly.
- Avoid sedation which interferes with accurate neurological assessment.
- Maintain aneurysm precautions:
  — elevate head of the bed 15 to 30 degrees, as prescribed
  — instruct client to avoid straining
  — place needed items within easy reach
  — assist with position changes
  — instruct client not to tighten muscles during moving or turning
  — instruct client not to rotate or flex the neck
  — instruct client that no isometric or active exercises are permitted
  — instruct client on avoidance of Valsalva's maneuver
  — avoid rectal stimulation or straining at stool
  — no enemas or rectal temperatures
  — administer stool softeners and mild laxatives as prescribed
- Monitor neurological status.
- Monitor hemodynamic status.

SURGICAL

See care of the client after craniotomy, "Intracranial Tumors", p. 403.

(For more information, see pp. 329-332 of Polaski and Tatro, *Luckmann's Core Principles and Practice of Medical-Surgical Nursing*.)

Angina Pectoris

OVERVIEW

- Angina pectoris is a term used to describe chest pain resulting from myocardial ischemia (lack of blood

supply). Myocardial ischemia develops if the blood supply through the coronary vessels or oxygen content of the blood is not adequate to meet metabolic demands.

- The cause of angina pectoris is coronary artery disease (CAD) or any other cardiac disease impeding blood flow. As vessels become lined and eventually occluded with atherosclerotic plaque, they lose their ability to dilate and supply the heart with blood.
- Conditions that cause angina fall into two categories: (1) conditions that decrease blood or oxygen supply to the heart -
  — atherosclerosis
  — arterial spasm
  — hypotension
  — aortic stenosis or insufficiency
  — anemia and hypoxemia
  — polycythemia (increased blood viscosity slows blood flow through coronary arteries)
  (2) conditions that increase demands on the myocardium
  — exertion
  — emotion
  — digestion of a large meal
  — anemia
  — hyperthyroidism
  — myocardial damage
  — hypertrophy of the myocardium
  — aortic stenosis/insufficiency
- Myocardial ischemia occurs when either supply or demand is altered. In some clients the coronary arteries can supply adequate blood when the client is at rest, but with increased demand, angina develops. Myocardial cells become ischemic within 10 seconds of coronary artery occlusion. After several minutes of ischemia, the heart's pumping function is reduced. The reduction of pumping deprives the ischemic cells of much needed oxygen and glucose. The cells convert to an anaerobic metabolism which leaves lactic acid as a waste product. As lactic acid accumulates, pain develops. Angina pectoris is transient, lasting only 3 to 5 minutes. If blood flow is restored, no permanent myocardial damage occurs.
- Patterns of angina:

- stable angina (classic angina) —chest pain triggered by a predictable degree of exertion or emotion
- unstable angina (crescendo angina) — chest pain triggered by an unpredictable degree of exertion or emotion, which may occur at night. Attacks characteristically increase in number, duration, and intensity over time.
- variant angina (Prinzmetal's angina) — chest pain similar to classic angina but of longer duration that may occur at rest and tends to occur in the early hours of the day; may result from coronary artery spasm
- nocturnal angina - occurs only during the night
- angina decubitus — chest pain that occurs when client reclines and lessens when client sits or stands up
- intractable angina — chronic, incapacitating angina unresponsive to intervention
- postinfarction angina — occurs after a myocardial infarction (MI), secondary to residual ischemia
- Risk factors for angina are similar to those for CAD. Primary prevention is achieved through a lifelong commitment to decreasing these risk factors.

CLINICAL MANIFESTATIONS

- transient paroxysmal attacks of substernal or precordial pain with the following characteristics:
  - sensation — squeezing, burning, choking, or pressing
  - severity — mild to moderate in intensity
  - location - retrosternal or slightly to the left of the sternum
  - radiation — to the left shoulder and upper arm and travels down the inner aspect of the left arm to the elbow, wrist and fourth and fifth fingers. Pain may also radiate to right shoulder, neck, jaw, or epigastric region.
  - duration - usually less than 5 minutes
  - relief — quickly subsides with the administration of nitroglycerin and rest
- dyspnea
- pallor
- sweating

53

- faintness
- palpitations

MEDICAL MANAGEMENT

- vasodilators — [nitrates/nitrites: nitroglycerin, isosorbide dinitrate (Isordil)] — relax smooth muscle of coronary and peripheral blood vessels, decreasing workload of heart and improving oxygen demand to supply ratio
- beta-blocking agents — [propranolol (Inderal), atenolol (Tenormin), metoprolol (Lopressor)] — decrease myocardial workload and oxygen demand by decreasing contractility, heart rate
- calcium channel blockers — [diltiazem (Cardizem), nifedipine (Procardia), verapamil (Calan)] — reduce vascular smooth muscle tone decreasing afterload and myocardial oxygen demand
- analgesics — morphine sulfate is most commonly used as it also reduces venous return (preload), thereby decreasing myocardial workload
- dietary modifications—low fat, low cholesterol, low calorie, high fiber (lowers triglyceride and cholesterol levels)

NURSING MANAGEMENT

Medical

Until the angina is controlled and coronary blood flow reestablished, the client is at risk for myocardial damage due to myocardial ischemia
- Monitor cardiac rhythm.
- Provide restful environment.
- For episodes of angina:
  — maintain bedrest
  — assess pain characteristics and associated symptoms
  — administer PRN nitroglycerin
  — monitor vital signs
  — administer PRN analgesic
  — administer supplemental oxygen
  — obtain 12-lead EKG
  — monitor blood pressure during nitroglycerin administration

— notify physician for chest pain not relieved by three nitroglycerin tablets or ordered analgesic

FOCUSED DISCHARGE CARE

MEDICAL

Instruct the client regarding:
- disease process and treatment regime
- management of anginal episodes
  - avoid known activities that precipitate angina (i.e., eating large meals, strenuous exercise, cold weather)
  - lie or sit down
  - take nitroglycerin tablets sublingually 5 minutes apart
  - if pain not relieved after three nitroglycerin, the client should be taken to an emergency department
- modification of risk factors
  - hypertension management
  - dietary restrictions
  - weight control
  - smoking cessation
  - stress management
  - regular program of daily exercise

(For more information, see pp. 679-684 of Polaski and Tatro, *Luckmann's Core Principles and Practice of Medical-Surgical Nursing.*)

Anorexia Nervosa

OVERVIEW

- Anorexia nervosa is a loss of 15-25 per cent of ideal body weight due to voluntary restriction of food intake.
- Clients with this disorder experience:
  (1) severe weight loss
  (2) physiologic changes associated with starvation
  (3) distorted mental perceptions (weight phobia, alterations in body image, fear of being fat).

- The highest risk group is girls between the ages of 12 and 18 with low self esteem.

CLINICAL MANIFESTATIONS

The changes seen are physiologic, but the real disorder is psychologic:
- weight loss (as above)
- amenorrhea
- cachexia
- constipation
- fine hair over the body
- dry, sandpaper-like skin
- bradycardia, hypotension, hypothermia
- facial puffiness (from parotid hypertrophy)
- bizarre rituals associated with food
- fluid and electrolyte imbalances

MEDICAL MANAGEMENT

- improving the nutritional status through eating (if possible) or tube feeding
- improving self image through psychotherapy and behavior modification

NURSING MANAGEMENT

- Assist to select food from all food groups.
- Allow to refuse two to three foods.
- Remain with client for at least one hour after meals.
- Maintain accurate calorie count.
- Obtain weights at regular intervals.
- Monitor serum potassium and for signs/symptoms of hypokalemia.
- Assist to develop improved self esteem.

FOCUSED DISCHARGE CARE

- Instruct client regarding:
  — reinforcement of nutritional plan (as above)
  — signs/symptoms to report to physician
- Refer to outpatient therapy program.

(For more information, see pp. 1034-1035 of Polaski and Tatro, *Luckmann's Core Principles and Practice of Medical-Surgical Nursing.*)

Anterior Cruciate Ligament Injury

OVERVIEW

- The ligaments of the knee stabilize the joint and control motion. The anterior cruciate ligament is the most frequent completely torn ligament of the knee.

CLINICAL MANIFESTATIONS

- snapping sensation at the time of injury
- tense, swollen, stiff and painful knee
- knee gives way leading to falls

SURGICAL MANAGEMENT

- autograft or artificial ligament placement with application of leg brace

NURSING MANAGEMENT

In addition to routine postoperative care:
- Collaborate with physical therapy for prescribed exercises and adaptive devices.
- Apply continuous motion machine (supports the limb and puts the knee through preset degrees of passive range of motion) if prescribed. Usually used at least three hours per day.

FOCUSED DISCHARGE CARE

Instruct client regarding:
- prescribed exercises
- use of leg splint

(For more information, see p. 1321 of Polaski and Tatro, *Luckmann's Core Principles and Practice of Medical-Surgical Nursing.*)

Appendicitis

OVERVIEW

- Appendicitis is an inflammation of the vermiform appendix. It develops most commonly in adolescents and young adults.
- The appendix becomes obstructed, and the intraluminal pressure increases, leading to decreased venous drainage, thrombosis, edema and bacterial invasion of the bowel wall. Perforation will result if untreated.

CLINICAL MANIFESTATIONS

- acute wavelike abdominal pain
- pain in epigastrium or periumbilical region
- pain eventually shifts to the right lower quadrant and becomes steady
- loss of appetite, vomiting, low grade fever, coated tongue, bad breath

SURGICAL MANAGEMENT

- appendectomy (removal of the appendix) within 24 to 48 hours of onset of the symptoms
- delay in treatment can result in rupture and peritonitis

NURSING MANAGEMENT

MEDICAL

- Assess quality of pain.
- Monitor for signs/symptoms of ruptured appendix and notify physician immediately if these occur:
  — rigid boardlike abdomen
  — generalized abdominal pain.
- Administer pain medication as prescribed and assess effectiveness.
- *Never* give enemas, laxatives or apply heat to the abdomen (may cause perforation).
- Monitor intake and output.
- Maintain nasogastric tube to suction.

- Monitor vital signs, assessing for increased temperature or a change in pulse or blood pressure (signifying a ruptured appendix).

SURGICAL

In addition to routine postoperative care:
- Maintain wound packing and patency of drain if appendix ruptured.
- Monitor vital signs, urine output and level of consciousness.
- Assess wound drainage.

FOCUSED DISCHARGE CARE

- Instruct client regarding:
  — resumption of normal activity in 2 to 4 weeks
  — signs/symptoms of infection
  — wound care if appendix ruptured — irrigation with sterile saline and sterile dressing change several times daily
- Assess need for home health care referral for assistance with wound care.

(For more information, see pp. 1058-1059 of Polaski and Tatro, *Luckmann's Core Principles and Practice of Medical-Surgical Nursing.*)

Arterial Occlusion, Acute

OVERVIEW

- Acute occlusion of a limb's main artery may be caused by trauma, embolism or thrombosis and may occur in a healthy or diseased artery. About 90 per cent are in the lower limbs.
- Arterial thrombosis is usually due to arterial obstruction by a blood clot that forms in an artery damaged by atherosclerosis.
- In arterial embolism, the wall of the artery is often healthy; the obstruction arises most frequently from

a thrombus within the heart. In the lower extremities, the emboli lodge in either the superficial femoral or the popliteal artery. Causes include: arterial fibrillation, myocardial infarction, prosthetic heart valves.

CLINICAL MANIFESTATIONS

- pain
- paresthesia
- loss of position sense
- coldness
- paralysis
- pallor progressing to mottled cyanosis
- pulselessness

MEDICAL MANAGEMENT

- anticoagulant therapy
- thrombolytic therapy

SURGICAL MANAGEMENT

- embolectomy — removal of the embolus through an incision
- for thrombus, a reconstructive procedure for revascularization of the limb may be performed. See "Arterial Occlusion,Chronic", p. 61.

NURSING MANAGEMENT

MEDICAL

- Administer anticoagulant or thrombolytic therapy as prescribed. See "Arterial Occlusion,Chronic", p. 61.

SURGICAL

- See Surgical Management, "Arterial Occlusion, Chronic", p. 61.

(For more information, see pp. 803-806 of Polaski and Tatro, *Luckmann's Core Principles and Practice of Medical-Surgical Nursing.*)

Arterial Occlusion, Chronic

OVERVIEW

- Peripheral arterial occlusive disorders are conditions that involve narrowing of the arterial lumen or damage to the endothelial lining.
- Most of the pathologic changes that occur in peripheral arterial occlusive disease are due to atherosclerosis. Other causes include embolism, thrombosis, trauma, vasospasm and inflammation.
- The clinical manifestations of chronic arterial occlusion due to peripheral vascular disease do not appear for twenty to forty years. The most common locations for stenosis in a lower extremity are the aortoiliac bifurcation and the femoral bifurcation. These lesions cause narrowing of the blood flow, possibly producing thrombosis or aneurysm.

CLINICAL MANIFESTATIONS

Onset of clinical manifestations is gradual as plaques encroach progressively into the lumen.
- tightening pressure in the calves or buttocks or a sharp, cramplike sensation that occurs during walking and disappears quickly with rest (intermittent claudication)
  — symptoms are constant and reproducible
  — as disease progresses, episodes occur more frequently with less exertion
- pain at rest, usually at night when client is supine
  — described as a dull aching in the toes or forefoot
  — hanging the legs over the side of the bed or walking around brings relief
- dependent rubor of affected foot
- weak or absent peripheral pulses
- hypertrophied toenails
- paresthesias with exertion
- cramping and numbness
- inability to sense temperature changes
- edema
- lesions, poor healing

MEDICAL MANAGEMENT

Medical management is recommended for clients with intermittent claudication and, in general, mild to moderate disease. Surgical intervention is reserved for clients who develop rest pain, non-healing ulcers or disabling claudication.

- smoking cessation — clients who have quit smoking have been shown to improve their treadmill walking distance
- vascular rehabilitation — daily walking exercise
- dietary management — weight reduction, low cholesterol, low fat, high fiber (beneficial effect on lipid levels)
- pharmacologic management
  - nicotinic acid, fibrin acid derivatives, bile acid resins, meglutol and probucol — decrease lipid levels
  - vasodilators — Trental
- endovascular interventions
  - percutaneous transluminal angioplasty (PTA, balloon angioplasty) — a catheter with a distal inflatable balloon is used to mechanically dilate vessel stenosis
  - laser-assisted balloon angioplasty (LABA) — uses laser energy and balloon catheter to reverse ischemia by reforming the diseased artery
  - peripheral atherectomy — uses a catheter with high speed rotating drill, circular cutters or blades to pulverize the plaque into small particles which are suctioned back through the catheter
  - intravascular stents — generally placed after balloon angioplasty, stents are designed to provide a scaffold to maintain the intraluminal structure of the artery
  - following endovascular interventions, clients will take aspirin or dipyridamole as antiplatelet therapy on a long-term basis
- thrombolytic therapy — thrombolytic agents, such as streptokinase and urokinase, are given through a peripheral vein or intra-arterial catheter

SURGICAL MANAGEMENT

- axillofemoral grafting - graft starts at the axillary artery and travels subcutaneously along the lateral chest wall to the femoral artery

- reserved for clients who have increased operative risk
- higher incidence of occlusion than aortofemoral grafts
- aortofemoral bypass grafting — use of client's own saphenous vein or synthetic graft to bypass femoral artery and anastomose to the popliteal artery (for above the knee occlusion) or to the posterior tibial, anterior tibial or peroneal arteries (for below the knee occlusion)
- arterial reconstruction — use of the client's saphenous vein that is stripped of its valves and anastomosed proximally and distally in area of occlusion

NURSING MANAGEMENT

MEDICAL

- Assess area distal to occlusion for pulses, skin changes or sensory changes.
- Position the client to maintain tissue perfusion to affected extremity.
  - Place in reverse Trendelenburg position.
  - Encourage to sit with feet flat on floor.
- Provide warm environment (chilling can cause vasoconstriction).
  - The use of hot water bottles, heating pads or hot foot soaks is contraindicated because heat increases tissue metabolism, and if arteries are unable to dilate, blood flow is inadequate and tissues become necrotic.
- Encourage nicotine and caffeine restriction (cause vasoconstriction).
- Provide restful environment and instruct on relaxation techniques (high emotional levels cause vasoconstriction).
- Keep areas of ulceration clean and free from pressure and irritation.
  - Debridement and/or whirlpool treatments may be standard interventions.
- Provide meticulous skin and foot care.
- Administer PRN analgesics.
- Implement prescribed exercise program and monitor tolerance.
  - When assisting with a walking program, make it clear that pain should be the guide to amount of

activity. (Intermittent claudication signals that muscles and tissues are not receiving enough oxygen).

- Maintain bedrest as ordered for clients with ulcers, pain at rest, cellulitis or deep vein thrombosis (even minimal activity can raise oxygen requirements above what damaged arteries can provide).

POST ENDOVASCULAR INTERVENTION

- Assess arterial puncture sites for swelling, bleeding, ecchymosis or hematoma formation (clients are anticoagulated during procedure).
- Assess peripheral pulses as ordered.
- Maintain bedrest and limb movement restriction as ordered.
- Monitor for signs/symptoms of circulatory compromise, such as sudden change in limb color or temperature, increasing muscle discomfort, pain at rest and motor or sensory paresthesias.

THROMBOLYTIC THERAPY

- Obtain baseline values for partial thromboplastin time, prothrombin time, thrombin time, platelet count, hematocrit and white blood count (a recent streptococcal infection may diminish the drug's effectiveness).
- Obtain baseline pulses and assessment of affected extremity.
- Assess vital signs, pulses, skin color, movement and sensation during infusion as ordered.
- Assess for signs of bleeding or hematoma formation at infusion site.
- Assess for clinical manifestations of bleeding from gastrointestinal or genitourinary tracts or into intracerebral or retroperitoneal areas.
- Monitor serial laboratory tests (see above).
- Position affected extremity in straight alignment to facilitate perfusion.
- Avoid intramuscular injections for 24 hours after infusion.

SURGICAL

PREOPERATIVE CARE

In addition to routine preoperative care:

- Obtain baseline peripheral pulses and mark area where found to assist in postoperative assessment.
- Administer prescribed preoperative broad spectrum antibiotics (usually for 48 hours) — all infections must be resolved, especially if using a synthetic graft.
- Protect the limb from pressure or trauma and position level or slightly dependent.
- Administer preoperative IV fluids to ensure adequate circulating blood volume to perfuse the graft.

POSTOPERATIVE CARE

In addition to routine postoperative care:
- Monitor anticoagulation therapy (heparin infusion).
- Maintain bedrest with leg flat in bed.
  — Leg is usually wrapped with light dressings or a vascular boot.
  — Leg swelling is commonly related to reperfusion of ischemic muscles and surgical dissection around lymphatic drainage systems.
- Monitor for signs/symptoms of fluid volume deficit related to hemorrhage, hematoma or third spacing of fluid:
  — Observe for increase in pulse, decrease in blood pressure, anxiety, restlessness, pallor, thirst, oliguria and change in level of consciousness.
  — Check dressings for excessive drainage.
  — Assess pulmonary artery pressures and/or cardiac output.
  — Monitor daily weights.
  — Monitor intake and output.
- Monitor patency of graft by checking pedal pulses, skin color, movement and sensation of extremity as ordered.
- Monitor oxygen saturations.
- Monitor laboratory findings — arterial blood gases, partial thromboplastin time, hemoglobin, hematocrit, white blood count.
- Monitor for signs of bleeding from anticoagulation therapy (gastrointestinal, retroperitoneal, intracerebral, operative site, etc.).
- Avoid raising knee gatch or placing pillow under the knees.
- Administer broad spectrum antibiotics and monitor for clinical manifestations of infection.

- Assess for signs/symptoms of compartment syndrome — pain, paresthesia, diminished or absent pulses, coolness.
- Administer PRN analgesics.
- Encourage range of motion exercises while on bedrest and progressive ambulation when out of bed activities are permitted.
- Facilitate physical therapy consult.
- Monitor response to increased activity.

FOCUSED DISCHARGE CARE

MEDICAL

Instruct client regarding:
- disease process and treatment regime
- foot care:
  - do not soak feet
  - dry well between toes
  - check bath temperature with thermometer or elbow to prevent burns
  - gently rub corns or calluses, avoid cutting or home surgery
  - use clippers (not scissors) to cut toenails and trim straight across
  - never go barefoot
  - wear well-fitted shoes
- skin care:
  - inspect affected extremity daily
  - report ulcerations, redness, blisters or cracks
  - use lotion (non-perfumed) to prevent dryness
  - avoid sunburn
  - do not use heating pads, hot water bottles, etc.
  - do not cross legs
- dietary modifications — low fat, low cholesterol, low calorie, no caffeine
- prescribed exercise regime
  - walking is most often prescribed
    - rest if pain occurs and then begin again
    - walk indoors in the winter to prevent injury from falls and avoid vasoconstriction from cold temperatures
  - exercise instruction
- smoking cessation programs
- importance of long-term antiplatelet therapy (aspirin or dipyridamole)

- relaxation techniques
- importance of check-ups (usually every three months) to assess progress of disease

SURGICAL

Instruct client regarding:
- wound care
- exercise regime
- avoidance of constrictive clothing
- foot and skin care (see "Focused Discharge Care," Medical section)
- long-term antiplatelet or anticoagulation therapy
- importance of follow-up visits

(For more information, see pp. 795-803 of Polaski and Tatro, *Luckmann's Core Principles and Practice of Medical-Surgical Nursing.*)

Arteriovenous Malformation

- Arteriovenous malformations (AVMs) are congenital malformations consisting of tangles of thin-walled blood vessels without intervening capillaries located in the cerebrovascular system. Arterial and venous blood shunt together, and hence, brain perfusion cannot occur through them.
- The vessels may leak small amounts of blood or rupture, causing hemorrhage into the subarachnoid space or brain.
- Bleeding vessels usually produce focal neurological symptoms.
- Ruptured vessels produce clinical manifestations similar to those of subarachnoid hemorrhage. Aneurysm precautions may be prescribed (see "Aneurysm and Subarachnoid Hemorrhage, p. 50).
- About one-half of AVMs can be completely removed surgically. Other interventions that may be used to reduce the size of the aneurysm are:
  — laser therapy

- radiation
- detachable balloon procedures
- artificially embolizing (clotting) the arteriovenous malformation
- ligating the feeding arteries of the arteriovenous malformation

(For more information, see pp. 332-333 of Polaski and Tatro, *Luckmann's Core Principles and Practice of Medical-Surgical Nursing.*)

Ascites

OVERVIEW

- Ascites is the accumulation of fluid in the peritoneal cavity. It results from the interaction of several pathophysiologic changes: portal hypertension, lowered plasma colloidal osmotic pressure and sodium retention.
- Three mechanisms that underly the development of ascites are :
  - portal hypertension resulting in increased plasma and lymphatic hydrostatic pressures
  - hypoalbuminemia resulting in decreased colloid osmotic pressure
  - hyperaldosteronism resulting in renal sodium and water retention.
  Diseases that may lead to these events include cirrhosis of the liver, right-sided heart failure, cancer, and complications of pancreatitis.

CLINICAL MANIFESTATIONS

- abdominal distention
- bulging flanks
- protruding, downward umbilicus
- shortness of breath, dyspnea

MEDICAL MANAGEMENT

- correction of fluid and electrolyte imbalance

- discontinuation of medications that inhibit prostaglandin synthesis (such as aspirin or indomethacin) and thus renal sodium excretion
- paracentesis — repeated paracenteses have fallen into disfavor because of the repeated removal of fluid protein and electrolytes that disrupts homeostasis
- diuretics
- intravenous albumin
- low sodium diet with fluid restriction (protein in the diet is allowed, unless the client is encephalopathic)

SURGICAL MANAGEMENT

- insertion of a peritoneovenous shunt (such as a LeVeen or Denver shunt) for refractory and disabling chronic ascites — moves fluid from the peritoneal (abdominal) cavity into the venous blood of the superior vena cava.

NURSING MANAGEMENT

- Assess whether ascites is interfering with eating, sleeping and breathing.
- Discuss diet and plan fluid restriction with the client.
- Measure abdominal girth daily or twice daily (mark spot on abdomen for consistency in measurements).
- Daily weights.
- Monitor intake and output.
- Discuss avoidance of aspirin and indomethacin.
- Monitor client after paracentesis:
  — check vital signs frequently.
  — assess dressing over site for excessive fluid drainage.
- Position in high-Fowler's to facilitate breathing.
- Assist to cough and deep breathe and use incentive spirometer hourly.
- Monitor respiratory status for development of atelectasis or pneumonia.
- Encourage small, frequent meals if gastric reflux is present.
- Administer antacids and place bed in reverse Trendelenburg to reduce gastric reflux.
- Provide support for distended abdomen and good skin care.
- Position in high Fowler's for sleeping, if needed.

FOCUSED DISCHARGE CARE

* Instruct client regarding:
  — causes/treatment of ascites
  — need for dietary modifications and fluid restrictions
  — need to stop alcohol intake
  — measures to improve sleeping
  — measures to reduce gastric reflux
* Refer to chemical dependency programs or support groups such as Alcoholics Anonymous as appropriate.

Also see "Cirrhosis", p. 164, and "Portal Hypertension", p. 529

(For more information, see pp. 1128-1130 of Polaski and Tatro, *Luckmann's Core Principles and Practice of Medical-Surgical Nursing*.)

Asthma

OVERVIEW

* Asthma is a complex disorder of the bronchial airways characterized by periods of bronchospasm. It may be extrinsic (allergic) or intrinsic (non-allergic). Extrinsic asthma usually begins in childhood. The client is allergic to dust, lint, pollen, insects, mold spores, smoke, medications and foods. Intrinsic asthma is triggered by internal disorders such as common colds, upper respiratory infection or exercise. There are no easily identified allergens, and it usually occurs over age 35.
* Asthma is believed to be an inherited disorder that interacts with environmental factors to cause the disease.
* Asthmatic symptoms usually worsen at night.
* A severe, life-threatening complication of asthma is status asthmaticus. It is an acute episode of bronchospasm that can increase the workload of breathing 5 to 10 times, which can lead to acute cor

pulmonale. Pneumothorax, cardiac arrest or respiratory arrest can occur if untreated.
- Risk factors include air pollution and cigarette smoking.

CLINICAL MANIFESTATIONS

Asthma Attack

- use of accessory muscles
- marked respiratory effort
- inspiratory and expiratory wheezing
- non-productive coughing
- tachycardia
- pursed lip breathing
- nasal flaring

MEDICAL MANAGEMENT

Emergency Management

- inhaled beta-adrenergics
- intravenous theophylline
- intravenous steroids
- oxygen, if needed

Status Asthmaticus

- intravenous corticosteroids
- inhaled beta-adrenergics
- oxygen, if needed
- intubation and mechanical ventilation, if needed

NURSING MANAGEMENT

- Assess respiratory status every hour during acute phase:
  — lung sounds
  — respiratory rate and depth
  — presence and severity of wheezing (the inability to auscultate wheezing in an asthmatic with acute respiratory distress may indicate that the small airways are too constricted to allow any airflow. The client may require immediate medical intervention).
  — breathing pattern

— presence of pursed lip breathing, nasal flaring, shortness of breath, sternal and intercostal retractions, prolonged expiratory phase
- Monitor arterial blood gases.
- Monitor results of pulmonary function tests.
- Monitor color, consistency and amount of sputum production (client may have upper respiratory infection).
- Place client in Fowler's position.
- Encourage fluids to thin secretions.
- Reposition frequently.
- Administer oral care every 2 to 4 hours.
- Assess effectiveness of therapy.
- Monitor for side effects of bronchodilator therapy (tachycardia/tremors).
- Monitor for therapeutic levels of theophylline (8 to 20 ug/mL).

FOCUSED DISCHARGE CARE

Instruct client regarding:
- prescribed bronchodilators and steroids, including side effects
- taking bronchodilators at bedtime (to alleviate asthma symptoms during the night)
- taking steroids with food to avoid gastric upset
- importance of follow-up serum theophylline levels and signs/symptoms of theophylline toxicity
- use of inhalers and nebulizers
- early symptoms of asthma and when to seek medical attention
- avoidance of known allergens
- avoidance of stress
- avoidance of outdoor activities when pollen counts and pollution indexes high

(For more information, see pp. 570-574 of Polaski and Tatro, *Luckmann's Core Principles and Practice of Medical-Surgical Nursing.*)

Atrophic (Senile) Vaginitis

- Atrophic vaginitis refers to thinning and atrophy of the vaginal mucosa that occurs in postmenopausal women. Vaginal secretions become more watery and alkaline.
- The vaginal mucosa is susceptible to infection due to the changes that occur.
- Clinical manifestations include: discharge that may be blood-flecked, a burning sensation, itching of the vagina and vulva, and dyspareunia.
- Treatment is short term use of diethylstilbestrol suppositories or estrogen creams and antibiotic therapy if needed.

(For more information, see p. 1493 of Polaski and Tatro, *Luckmann's Core Principles and Practice of Medical-Surgical Nursing.*)

Balance Disorders

OVERVIEW

- Disorders of balance and coordination result from problems of the vestibular system and righting reflexes. More than 90 million Americans have experienced vertigo or a balance problem.
- Causes of balance problems or vertigo are:
  - viral neuronitis — self limiting disorder, sometimes associated with influenza and characterized by a sudden onset of vertigo without a hearing loss.
  - viral labyrinthitis — disorder affecting hearing and balance. Balance usually is recovered, but the hearing loss may be permanent.
  - presbyastasis — a balance disorder of aging.
  - Meniere's disease — recurring episodic, inca–pacitating bouts of vertigo, hearing loss and tinnitus . It is thought that this disorder occurs from an abnormality in the formation or absorption of endolymph.

CLINICAL MANIFESTATIONS

- spinning vertigo
- sensation of falling
- imbalance
- staggering
- lightheadedness
- veering in one direction while walking
- faintness
- clumsiness
- feeling of floating
- nausea, vomiting

MEDICAL MANAGEMENT

- vasodilators for chronic vertigo
- vestibular rehabilitation — head and total body exercises performed by the client to compensate for the disorder
- low sodium diet, diuretics and balance exercises for Meniere's disease

SURGICAL MANAGEMENT

- labyrinthectomy — removal of the membranous labyrinth
- vestibular nerve resection

NURSING MANAGEMENT

- Discuss ways to prevent injury when dizzy.
- Provide desired foods and fluids and small frequent meals if nausea and vomiting are present.
- Assist with ambulation.
- Discuss nature of disorder and planned tests.

FOCUSED DISCHARGE CARE

Clients with vertigo usually are managed as outpatients.

(For more information, see pp. 471-473 of Polaski and Tatro, *Luckmann's Core Principles and Practice of Medical-Surgical Nursing.*)

Bell's Palsy

OVERVIEW

- Bell's palsy (facial paralysis) is the most common type of peripheral facial paralysis.

- Bell's palsy is an acute, unilateral paralysis of the facial muscles of expression with no evidence of a pathologic cause. Most clients recover from Bell's palsy within a few weeks without residual symptoms.
- Bell's palsy affects both women and men in all age groups. It is most common between the ages of 20 and 40 years.

CLINICAL MANIFESTATIONS

- upward movement of the eyeball on closing the eye (Bell's phenomenon)
- drooping of the mouth
- pain behind the face or ear
- inability to wrinkle forehead, smile, whistle, grimace or close eyelid
- difficulty eating

MEDICAL MANAGEMENT

No known cure—symptoms are treated with:
- analgesics
- cortisone therapy
- physiotherapy — moist heat, gentle massage
- corneal protection — artificial tears, eye patch at night, sunglasses, etc.

NURSING MANAGEMENT

- Administer medications and assess effectiveness.
- Apply moist heat PRN to affected area of the face.
- Provide measures to protect cornea - patch, artificial tears, etc.

(For more information, see p. 416 of Polaski and Tatro, *Luckmann's Core Principles and Practice of Medical-Surgical Nursing.*)

Benign Prostatic Hyperplasia

OVERVIEW

- Prostatic tissue undergoes benign hyperplasia with aging. The periurethral glands undergo hyperplasia and compress surrounding normal prostatic tissue, pushing it toward the gland periphery.
- Potential complications of prostatic enlargement include (1) impeded urinary outflow and (2) urinary reflux because of decompensation of the uretero-vesical junction.
- By age 50, it is estimated that 50 per cent of men have some degree of benign prostatic hyperplasia (BPH); the incidence increases to more than 75 per cent in men over age 80.

CLINICAL MANIFESTATIONS

- frequent urination
- reduction in size and force of urinary stream
- hematuria
- feeling of not emptying the bladder
- urinary retention

MEDICAL MANAGEMENT

- conservative interventions to treat symptoms— advise client to;
  - void whenever the urge is present
  - avoid taking large amounts of fluid over a short time
  - avoid alcohol because of its diuretic effect
- antibiotic therapy for prostatitis that may be associated with BPH
- pharmacological agents:
  - testosterone-ablating agents — decrease amount of circulating testosterone leading to suppression of prostatic tissue growth — diethylstilbestrol (DES), flutamide (Eulexin)
  - testosterone-sparing agents — decrease prostatic tissue without side effects of antitestosterones — finasteride (Proscar)

— alpha-adrenergic blocking agents — block alpha receptors improving urination by decreasing outlet obstruction — prozasin (Minipress), phenoxybenzamine (Dibenzylene)

SURGICAL MANAGEMENT

- Enlarged prostate tissue may be removed by various approaches, depending upon the size of the prostate and general health of the client. They include:
  - transurethral resection (TUR) — most widely used
  - suprapubic prostatectomy — approach made through lower abdominal incision into the bladder
  - retropubic prostatectomy — lower abdominal incision approaching the prostate without entering the bladder
  - perineal prostatectomy — incision made into the perineum between the anus and scrotum
- Other newer surgical procedures:
  - balloon dilation of the prostate
  - microwave/hyperthermia of the prostate
  - transurethral laser incision
  - insertion of prostatic stents

NURSING MANAGEMENT

MEDICAL

- Monitor intake and output.
- Palpate bladder post-voiding to assess for urinary retention.
- Maintain a fluid intake of 2500-3000 ml/day unless otherwise contraindicated.

SURGICAL

In addition to routine postoperative care:
- Assess wound drains, wound packing and catheter drainage for excessive bleeding.
- Avoid overdistention of the bladder because it can precipitate secondary hemorrhage — keep catheter from kinking or obstructing secondary to clot formation, mucous plug, sediment, etc.

- Maintain indwelling catheter (urethral or suprapubic) system:
  — monitor continuous bladder irrigation (CBI) (closed irrigation permits constant or intermittent irrigation without breaking aseptic technique)
  — frequently assess catheter patency
  — maintain clear, slightly pink outflow
- Strict intake and output.
- Administer PRN antispasmodics to control bladder spasms.
- Administer stool softeners to prevent straining at stool which could precipitate bleeding.
- Observe for local or systemic indications of infection.
- Prevent wound infection after perineal surgery by avoiding the use of enemas, rectal tubes, or rectal thermometers. Cleanse the wound thoroughly after each bowel movement.
- Assess for urinary retention (inability to pass urine and bladder overdistention) and urethral stricture (small urinary stream and dysuria) after urinary catheter removal.
- Monitor electrolytes and renal function tests.
- Encourage fluids.

FOCUSED DISCHARGE CARE

Instruct the client regarding:
- driving, activity, and weight-lifting restrictions
- need to avoid straining during defecation — use of stool softeners, juice, etc.
- perineal exercises to help client regain urinary sphincter control
- importance of urinating when the client first feels the urge
- the possibility of urinary incontinence or frequency occurring for up to three months postoperatively
- when to seek medical attention:
  — bleeding
  — signs of infection
  — symptoms of obstructed urine flow
- need to maintain high fluid intake (2000-3000 ml/day)
- catheter care, if discharged with catheter in place

(For more information, see pp. 1447-1457 of Polaski and Tatro, *Luckmann's Core Principles and Practice of Medical-Surgical Nursing.*)

Biologic Response Modifiers

OVERVIEW

- Biologic response modifiers (BRMs) are agents that are capable of modifying the relationship between the tumor and the host by strengthening the host's immune function.
- The classifications of BRMs include:
  — interleukins
  — interferons
  — monoclonal antibodies
  — colony-stimulating factors
- Most BRMs are still investigational.

NURSING MANAGEMENT

- Administer ordered BRM therapy according to hospital protocol.
- Monitor for potential side effects:
  — interleukins
    — hypotension, pulmonary edema, and weight gain due to increased capillary permeability
    — generalized rash and pruritus
  — interferons
    — flu-like syndrome
  — monoclonal antibodies — to date clinical trials have shown limited success as a therapeutic option
  — colony-stimulating factors
    — bone pain in pelvis, sternum and long bones
- Monitor laboratory findings — CBC, platelet count.

FOCUSED DISCHARGE CARE

- Instruct client regarding:
  — disease process and treatment regime
  — signs/symptoms to report to physician
  — care of venous access device
  — importance of follow-up clinic and laboratory appointments
- Refer to available community resources.

(For more information, see pp. 19-20 of Polaski and Tatro, *Luckmann's Core Principles and Practice of Medical-Surgical Nursing.*)

Bladder Neoplasms (Cancer)

OVERVIEW

- Bladder cancer occurs most frequently in the fifth to seventh decades of life. It occurs in men two to three times more often than in women.
- Common sites for metastasis include liver, bone, and lungs.
- Risk factors include:
  — cigarette smoking
  — industrial exposure to certain substances, such as aniline dyes, aromatic amines, and leather finishings. Processing petroleum products and industrial exposure to metal machinery also increase risk.
  — pelvic radiation
  — use of cyclophosphamide
  — chronic cystitis
  — bladder calculus disease
  — large phenacetin intake

CLINICAL MANIFESTATIONS

- painless, intermittent hematuria (early sign)
- bladder irritability, dysuria, gross hematuria, obstruction, or fistula formation (late signs)

MEDICAL MANAGEMENT

To determine the depth of penetration into the bladder wall and the degree of metastasis, staging is done before selection of treatment.

- intravesical installation of an alkylating chemotherapeutic agent, such as thio-TEPA, mitomycin C, doxorubicin, or cyclophosphamide.

- intracavity radiation — involves radiation to the bladder malignancy while adjacent tissues are protected — radium seeds are inserted through a cystoscope or through a suprapubic opening in the bladder and placed directly in the tumor
- external supervoltage radiation in combination with surgery or chemotherapy
- systemic chemotherapy with cisplatin, doxorubicin, methotrexate, cyclophosphamide or pyridoxine

SURGICAL MANAGEMENT

- transurethral resection of the tumor and fulguration (destruction of tissue by electrical current through electrodes placed in direct contact with the growth) — for very early superficial tumors or for palliation of inoperable tumors
- segmental or partial cystectomy (removal of up to one-half the bladder). Over several months the bladder tissue regenerates, increasing its capacity to 200 to 400 ml.
- total or radical cystectomy with urinary diversion for advanced potentially curable disease:
  - total cystectomy involves removal of the bladder and urethra in women and the bladder, urethra, prostate and seminal vesicles in men
  - radical cystectomy includes the above plus dissection of the pelvic lymph nodes and possibly the uterus, fallopian tubes, and ovaries in women
- permanent urinary diversion is necessary after total or radical cystectomy:
  - cutaneous ureterostomy — the ureter is brought to the surface of the abdomen where urine flows into a drainage appliance.
  - nephrostomy (temporary or permanent) — insertion of catheters into the renal pelvis by surgical incision or a percutaneous puncture procedure. The catheters are attached to an external drainage system.
  - ileal conduit (also called ureteroileostomy or Bricker's procedure)—the most common urinary diversion. A segment of the intestine is used as a conduit with the proximal end being closed and the distal end being brought out through a hole in

the abdominal wall. It is sutured to the skin to form a stoma. The ureters are implanted into the ileal segment and urine flows by peristalsis out through the stoma into an appliance the client wears.
— Kock pouch (continent internal ileal reservoir) — a reservoir made from a segment of ileum. Ureters are implanted into the side of the reservoir. A nipple valve is used to attach the reservoir to the skin. The client uses a catheter to drain the pouch rather than wearing a permanent drainage bag.
— Indiana pouch — a new procedure, similar to the Kock pouch, but a larger reservoir is created from the ascending colon and terminal ileum. Clients use a catheter to drain the pouch every 4-6 hours.

NURSING MANAGEMENT

MEDICAL

- Radiation therapy
  — Administer antispasmodics as prescribed.
  — Encourage fluid intake.
  — Administer urinary tract antiseptics for cystitis as prescribed.
  — For patients with proctitis, instruct on low-residue diet and administer agents to decrease intestinal motility.
  — See also, "Radiation Therapy", p. 543.
- Chemotherapy
  — See "Chemotherapy", p. 145.
  — Monitor for side effects of chemotherapy including hemorrhagic cystitis and bladder irritation.

SURGICAL

- TUR
In addition to routine postoperative care:
  — Maintain urethral catheter and bladder irrigation as appropriate.
  — See "Benign Prostatic Hyperplasia", p. 77.
- Segmental/Partial Cystectomy

In addition to routine postoperative care:

> —Maintain continuous urinary drainage from the urethral and suprapubic catheters to prevent any strain on the suture line due to bladder distention.
>
> —Instruct the client on care of the suprapubic catheter (it is usually left in place for two weeks).

- Kock or Indiana Pouch

In addition to routine postoperative care:

> — Maintain Medena catheter to continuously drain the urine (catheter will be removed 3-4 weeks after surgery).
>
> — Irrigate the catheter with normal saline as needed.
>
> — Instruct the client on the self catheterization procedure (will be done after the Medena catheter is removed).

- Urinary Diversion
  - Preoperative Care

    In addition to routine preoperative care:

    - Instruct that diversion results in elimination of urine through the skin or stoma and not through the urethral meatus.
    - Instruct on/perform bowel preparation: low residue diet; bowel cleansing with cathartics or enemas; sterilization of the bowel with neomycin.
    - Instruct on role of the enterostomal therapist.
    - Instruct on selection of the stoma site by enterostomal therapist.
    - Provide emotional support and allow to verbalize feelings concerning change in body image.

  - Postoperative Care

    In addition to routine postoperative care:

    - Measure urine output every hour for the first 24 hours and then at least every 8 hours. Monitor for blocking of ureteral catheters (urine will contain mucous from the bowel).
    - Keep drainage tubing patent, if nephrostomy tubes were placed.
    - Assess stoma site every hour for the first 24 hours postoperatively. Note the stoma's size, shape, and color. An edematous stoma is expected in the immediate postoperative period. A dusky or cyanotic color of the stoma may

indicate an insufficient blood supply or the onset of necrosis — this is an emergency. Other complications may include prolapse or retraction into the skin.
— Check the ostomy bag for leaks and the skin under it for irritation every 4 hours initially and then every 8 hours.
— Assess for signs/symptoms of peritonitis, bleeding, and urinary tract infection.
— Maintain nasogastric tube to prevent paralytic ileus.
— Assess skin integrity.
— Ensure proper fit of appliance as stoma shrinks.

FOCUSED DISCHARGE CARE

- Instruct client regarding:
    - suprapubic catheter or Medena catheter, if present
    - catheterization procedure for Kock or Indiana pouch once Medena catheter is removed
    - adequate fluid intake
    - signs/symptoms to report to physician
    - need for follow-up to ensure cancer has not recurred
- In males, refer to support groups as appropriate for impotence, which may develop after radical cystectomy.

Ileal Conduit/Urinary Diversion
- Instruct client regarding
    - stoma skin care
    - where to purchase stomal supplies
    - how to apply, remove, and empty the system appliance and attach it to the night drainage system
    - control of odor
    - need for fluid intake of 2000 ml/daily
    - selection of clothing that will not constrict the pouch
    - signs/symptoms to report to physician:
        - changes in color or quantity of urine output
        - cloudy or foul-smelling urine
        - stoma color changes
- Discuss concerns regarding work/leisure/sexual activity.

(For more information, see pp. 933-940 of Polaski and Tatro, *Luckmann's Core Principles and Practice of Medical-Surgical Nursing*.)

Bladder Trauma

OVERVIEW

- Bladder trauma is a blunt or penetrating injury to the bladder that may or may not cause bladder rupture.
- This injury may occur from a seat belt in an automobile accident; a fractured pelvis; bullet or knife wounds; or internal instruments, such as a catheter or cystoscope.

CLINICAL MANIFESTATIONS

- abdominal pain, which may be referred to the shoulder
- hematuria
- difficulty voiding

MEDICAL MANAGEMENT

- placement of a Foley or suprapubic catheter unless blood is coming from the urethral meatus

SURGICAL MANAGEMENT

- repair of the bladder wall and drainage of extravasated urine in the perivesical space

NURSING MANAGEMENT

MEDICAL

- Monitor intake and output.
- Monitor for hematuria.
- Report anuria to physician immediately.

In addition to routine postoperative care:
- Maintain patent urinary drainage system to prevent tension on the sutures in the bladder.
- Change dressings around Penrose drain as needed.

FOCUSED DISCHARGE CARE

- Instruct client regarding:
  — care of suprapubic or indwelling catheter as appropriate
  — signs/symptoms of urinary tract infection.
- Assess need for follow-up by home health care agency.

(For more information, see pp. 943-944 of Polaski and Tatro, *Luckmann's Core Principles and Practice of Medical-Surgical Nursing.*)

Blepharoplasty

- Blepharoplasty is the surgical removal of excess tissue from the upper or lower eyelid. It may be cosmetic, or, if eyelid tissue is obstructing vision, reconstructive.
- Excess eyelid tissue may occur due to aging, heredity, allergic reaction or as a result of cardiovascular or thyroid disease.
- Blepharoplasty usually is performed on a day surgery basis with local or general anesthesia.
- Postoperatively, the nurse instructs the client to:
  — apply cold compresses to the eyes, usually for 24 to 48 hours after surgery
  — sleep supine with the head elevated for the first 48 hours
  — avoid bending over from the waist for 48 hours
  — avoid vigorous activity for one month
  — report to the surgeon changing vision or eye pain not relieved by prescribed analgesics

— wear sunglasses, if desired, to cover initial bruising and swelling around the eyes

(For more information, see pp. 1397-1398 of Polaski and Tatro, *Luckmann's Core Principles and Practice of Medical-Surgical Nursing.*)

Blood Component Transfusion

OVERVIEW

- Blood component transfusion may be required for the following conditions:
  — hematologic disorders
  — hematologic diseases requiring aggressive ablative therapy
  — chronic or acute blood loss
- Two alternatives to homologous (random) blood transfusion should be considered:
(1) Autologous donation
  — clients who do not have leukemia or bacteremia may donate their own blood before a scheduled surgical procedure
    — donations may be made every 3 days if the donor's hemoglobin remains at or above 11 g/ 100 ml
  — intraoperative, postoperative or post-traumatic blood salvage
    — suctioning of blood from body cavities, joint spaces and other closed operative or trauma sites for reinfusion
(2) Directed (designated) donation
  — transfusion recipients designate their donors
- Irradiated blood components — clients with Hodgkin's or non-Hodgkin's lymphoma, acute leukemia or congenital immunodeficiency disorders and bone marrow transplant recipients may develop post-transfusion graft vs. host disease (GVHD) if lymphocytes containing cellular components engraft and divide. A small dose of radiation delivered to the unit renders the lymphocytes incapable of division.

NURSING MANAGEMENT

- Ensure that informed consent has been obtained (not required in all institutions).
- Obtain blood sample for type and crossmatch if central line is in place.
- Obtain venous access with large-bore cannula.
- Flush IV set-up with normal saline (no solution other than normal saline should be added to blood components).
- Obtain and record vital signs.
  — Fever may be a cause for delaying the transfusion— in addition to masking an acute transfusion reaction, fever can compromise the efficacy of platelet transfusions.
- Premedicate before transfusion as prescribed for the client who has a history of adverse reactions:
  — acetaminophen or diphenhydramine hydrochloride (Benadryl) to help prevent febrile reactions
  — steroids to avoid fever, rigors and chills that accompany granulocyte transfusions
  — antihistamines for a history of allergic reactions

BEGINNING THE TRANSFUSION

- Blood banking regulations state that refrigerated components may not be returned to inventory if they have been warmed more than 10°C (50°F). Most consider 30 minutes to be the maximal allowable time out of monitored storage.
- Confirm product compatibility and verify client identity.
- Inspect the unit for leaks, abnormal color, clots, excessive air and bubbles.
- Administer blood component through administration set as outlined in institutional policy.
  — A filter is used to trap fibrin, clots and other debris that accumulate during blood storage.
  — Blood warmers may be used to prevent hypothermia which can be induced by rapid infusion of large volumes of refrigerated blood.

- Initiate transfusion at a rate to infuse 50 ml over 10 to 15 minutes.
  — The first 10 to 15 minutes of any transfusion are the most critical. If a major ABO incompatibility exists or a severe allergic reaction (such as anaphylaxis) occurs, it is usually evident within the first 50 ml of the transfusion.
- Increase flow to prescribed rate if no reaction is noted in the first 15 minutes.
- Instruct client to report anything unusual immediately.
- Obtain and record vital signs per institutional policy.
- Monitor for signs/symptoms of a transfusion reaction:
  — immunologic:
    — allergic reaction
      - urticaria
      - hives
      - flushing
      - itching
      - no fever
    — sensitivity reaction
      - sudden chills and fever
      - headache
      - flushing
      - anxiety
      - muscle pain
    — acute hemolytic reaction (ABO incompatibility)
      - chills
      - fever
      - low back pain
      - flushing
      - tachycardia
      - hemoglobinuria
      - hypotension
      - shock
      - cardiac arrest
    — anaphylactic reaction
      - anxiety
      - urticaria
      - wheezing
      - cyanosis
      - shock
  — nonimmunologic

　　　　— circulatory overload (due to pre-transfusion
　　　　cardiac status or too rapid infusion)
　　　　　• cough
　　　　　• dyspnea
　　　　　• pulmonary congestion
　　　　　• hypertension
　　　　　• tachycardia
　　　　　• distended neck veins
　　　— septicemia (contaminated blood component)
　　　　— rapid onset of chills
　　　　— high fever
　　　　— vomiting
　　　　— diarrhea
　　　　— hypotension (marked)
　　　　— shock
- Stop the transfusion and keep the line open with normal saline if a reaction is suspected (remove blood infusion tubing and infuse normal saline through separate infusion set).
- Follow institution's standard procedure for suspected blood reaction.
- Administer prescribed therapies if reaction occurs.

FOCUSED DISCHARGE CARE

Instruct client regarding:
- signs/symptoms of delayed transfusion reactions (3 days to several months following a transfusion):
　— fever
　— mild jaundice
- signs/symptoms of iron overload (may occur in clients receiving more than 100 units over a period of time):
　— congestive heart failure (shortness of breath, ankle edema)
　— palpitations
- signs/symptoms of post-transfusion graft-vs.-host disease:
　— fever
　— rash
　— diarrhea
　— signs/symptoms of hepatitis
- signs/symptoms of hepatitis:
　— anorexia
　— malaise
　— nausea and vomiting

— dark urine
— jaundice

(For more information, see pp. 876-883 of Polaski and Tatro, *Luckmann's Core Principles and Practice of Medical-Surgical Nursing.*)

Bone Marrow Transplantation

OVERVIEW

- In the last 25 years, bone marrow transplantation has progressed from a treatment of last resort to a viable therapeutic modality for a variety of hematologic, malignant and non-malignant disorders.
- BMT allows the client to receive lethal and potentially more effective doses of chemotherapy without regard to hematopoietic toxicity. The damaged bone marrow is replaced by healthy donor marrow.
- Indications for bone marrow transplant include:
  — aplastic anemia
  — leukemia (certain types of acute and chronic)
  — lymphoma
  — multiple myeloma
  — neuroblastoma
  — selected solid tumors (metastatic breast cancer, small cell lung cancer, advanced ovarian cancer)
  — thalassemia, sickle cell anemia

BONE MARROW HARVESTING

- There are three classifications of bone marrow donors:
  — allogeneic:
    — obtained from a relative or unrelated donor having identical HLA type (HLA system antigens are a complex set of protein structures found on the surface membrane of all human nucleated cells, solid tissues and circulating blood cells except red cells. This genetically

92

inherited mixture of antigens is considered representative of the tissue type of each client.)
— siblings have a one in four chance of having identical sets of HLA antigens and would provide the optimal match. Non-related clients have less than a 1 in 5000 chance of matching.
— most common type of marrow transplant, but highest rate of morbidity and mortality
— syngeneic:
— donated by identical twin
— perfect HLA match eliminating the risk of rejection, but the risk of leukemic relapse is higher
— autologous:
— removed from the intended recipient during a remission phase
— eliminates risk of rejection, but relapse is frequent due to contamination of marrow cells by malignant cells
• Another type of bone marrow transplant is peripheral blood stem cell harvest. The peripheral stem cells are harvested by leukopheresis and stored. After the client receives lethal doses of chemotherapy and radiation therapy, the stem cells are reinfused.

Donor Preparation

• extensive work-up to insure compatibility and mental and physical well-being
• syngeneic and allogenic donors are required to donate autologous blood before the procedure because of the significant red blood cell loss

Marrow Collection

• general or spinal anesthesia is used
• marrow is obtained from the marrow spaces of the posterior and, occasionally, anterior iliac crests and sternum
• a total of 400 to 800 ml is obtained
• blood is placed in heparinized tissue culture media and filtered for removal of fat and bone particles
• marrow can be infused immediately or frozen

- physical and psychological work-up
- central line placement
- receives immunoablative therapy before transplant
  — common protocols combine total body irradiation with high doses of chemotherapy

BONE MARROW INFUSION

- marrow is infused from a large blood infusion bag through a standard blood filter
- potential immediate adverse reactions are allergic, volume overload and pulmonary complications secondary to fat emboli
- delayed reaction—graft-versus-host disease (GVHD)
  — the most common and potentially disastrous complication of bone marrow transplant
  — no therapy to prevent or treat
  — may occur acutely 7 to 30 days after infusion
  — probable cause— T lymphocytes from donor attack and destroy vulnerable host cells
  — the most likely organs to be affected are skin, gut, and liver
  — chronic GVHD
    — appears approximately 100 days after transplant
    — diagnosis of chronic GVHD is confirmed by skin and oral mucosal biopsy
    — may affect the liver, gastrointestinal system, oral mucosa, lungs, and skin

NURSING MANAGEMENT

PRE-TRANSPLANT

- Administer ablative chemotherapy as ordered. See "Chemotherapy", p. 145. See "Radiation Therapy", p. 543.
- Maintain protective isolation precautions.
- Assess for any signs/symptoms of infection.
- Monitor temperature.
- Monitor laboratory findings — CBC, platelet count, culture reports.
- Assess for any signs of bleeding and institute appropriate safety measures.

- Monitor vital signs for indication of altered tissue perfusion.
- Encourage well-balanced diet (no raw fruits or vegetables).
- Provide emotional support to client, family and donor (if present).

TRANSPLANT

- Infuse marrow per hospital procedure.
- Monitor for immediate adverse reaction:
  — allergic
  — volume overload
  — pulmonary complications (secondary to fat emboli)

POST-TRANSPLANT

- Maintain protective isolation and bleeding precautions.
- Assess for potential side effects of marrow infusion
  — fluid overload, micropulmonary emboli and hypersensitivity reaction to the white cells in the marrow.
- Assess for signs of GVHD.
- Monitor laboratory findings — indication of successful engraftment is an increase in platelets and red blood cells in the peripheral blood count.
- Assess for any signs of bleeding or infection.

FOCUSED DISCHARGE CARE

- Instruct client regarding:
  — treatment regime
  — measures to prevent infection:
    — good personal hygiene
    — avoidance of crowds and people with infectious disease
    — need to wear a mask in public
    — no fresh fruits or vegetables, no raw meat
  — measures to prevent bleeding:
    — soft toothbrush
    — electric razor
    — care when doing yardwork
    — safety precautions

- — signs/symptoms to report to physician
- — signs/symptoms of GVHD
- — importance of balancing activity and rest
- — importance of a well-balanced diet
- — central line care
- — see "Chemotherapy", p. 145, and "Radiation Therapy", p. 543
- — importance of follow-up clinic and laboratory visits
- Refer to available community resources.

(For more information, see pp. 19 and 859-861 of Polaski and Tatro, *Luckmann's Core Principles and Practice of Medical-Surgical Nursing.*)

Bone Tumors, Benign

OVERVIEW

- Benign bone tumors are often asymptomatic and may not be discovered until they are found on radiographic studies or when a pathologic fracture occurs.
- Benign tumors usually have well defined borders, grow slowly and seldom metastasize.
- Types of benign tumors:
  - — Chondrogenic tumors (from cartilage)
    - — Osteochondroma
      - • most common benign tumor
      - • 10 per cent become sarcomas
      - • femur and tibia are most common sites
    - — Endachondroma
      - • occurs in mature hyaline cartilage in the hands, feet, ribs, spine, sternum or long bones
      - • found at any age
    - — Chondroma
      - • slow growing
      - • frequently cause pathologic fractures
      - • found at any age
  - — Osteogenic tumor (from bone)
    - — Osteoid osteoma
      - • small, osteoblastic (bone forming) lesion with clearly defined borders

- male predominance, most occur in the second decade of life
- occurs in the femur, tibia, wrist or foot
- often causes night pain
— Osteoblastoma (giant osteoid osteoma)
  - grows more rapidly and is larger than osteoid osteoma
  - male predominance, onset in the first three decades of life
  - occurs in the vertebrae, femur, hands and long bones
— Osteoclastoma (Giant Cell tumor)
  - aggressive and extensive
  - has a tendency for local recurrence and can metastasize to lung tissue
  - affects women older than 20 years
  - occurs in the femur, tibia, radius, sacrum and humerus

CLINICAL MANIFESTATIONS

- may be asymptomatic
- bone pain
- fracture pain

MEDICAL MANAGEMENT

- pain management
- management of fracture

SURGICAL MANAGEMENT

- repair of fracture
- removal of tumor

NURSING MANAGEMENT

MEDICAL

- Administer analgesics as ordered.

SURGICAL

Routine postoperative care is dependent upon size and location of tumor.

FOCUSED DISCHARGE CARE

Instruct client regarding:
- use of PRN analgesics
- care of the incision
- cast care (if fracture repaired)

(For more information, see pp. 1299-1300 of Polaski and Tatro, *Luckmann's Core Principles and Practice of Medical-Surgical Nursing*.)

Bone Tumors, Malignant

OVERVIEW

- Primary malignant bone tumors originate in the bone. The vertebrae, pelvis, ribs and proximal long bones are the most common sites.
- Secondary (metastatic) malignant bone tumors originate in other tissues and metastasize to the bone. Skeletal metastases are the most common form of malignant bone tumors and virtually every malignant tumor can metastasize to bone. The most common sites of origin are the breast, lung, prostate, kidney, thyroid and ovary. Pathologic fractures are common, especially in the acetabulum and proximal femur.
- Malignant bone tumors may metastasize to the lungs or other bone sites.
- Types of primary malignant bone tumors:
  — Osteosarcoma
    — most common malignant bone tumor
    — is usually situated in the metaphyseal region of long bones
    — male predominance, onset in adolescents in second decade of life during maximal growth
    — common sites are femur, proximal tibia and proximal humerus
    — elevated serum alkaline phosphatase levels are present at diagnosis
  — Ewing's Sarcoma

- — most malignant of primary tumors
- — male predominance, onset between the ages of 5 and 20 years
- — common sites are pelvis and lower extremities
- — metastasizes quickly to the lungs and other bones
- — Chondrosarcoma
  - — male predominance, occurs in middle-aged and older individuals
  - — common sites are the pelvis, ribs, proximal femur and proximal humerus
- — Fibrosarcoma
  - — onset in individuals between 20 and 60 years of age
  - — sites include the femur and tibia
- Characteristics of metastatic bone tumors (secondary bone tumors):
  - — develop from tumor seed cells that travel through the lymphatic system, blood vessels and surrounding tissue
  - — the femur, pelvis, ribs and vertebrae are the most commonly affected bone sites
  - — pathologic fractures are common

CLINICAL MANIFESTATIONS

- bone pain
- local swelling
- guarded or restricted movement
- tender palpable mass
- lymph node enlargement
- elevated alkaline phosphatase
- elevated calcium and ESR (erythrocyte sedimentation rate)

MEDICAL MANAGEMENT

- pain management
- radical surgery combined with radiation and chemotherapy
- chemotherapy — used preoperatively to shrink the tumor and destroy pulmonary cells. Postoperatively, chemotherapy is aimed at destroying malignant seed cells that may have entered the blood stream.
- radiation therapy for inoperable tumors

SURGICAL MANAGEMENT

- radical excision of the tumor
- amputation
- disarticulation of the limb
- total joint replacement
- allografts from the iliac crest, rib or fibula after resection

NURSING MANAGEMENT

MEDICAL

- Administer analgesics as prescribed.
- Administer chemotherapy as prescribed and monitor/intervene for side effects. See "Chemotherapy", p. 145.
- See "Radiation Therapy", p. 543.
- Offer emotional support and facilitate referrals.

SURGICAL

Nursing management is dependent upon type of procedure performed.

FOCUSED DISCHARGE CARE

- Instruct client regarding:
  — disease process and treatment regime
  — management of chemotherapy and radiation therapy side effects (See "Chemotherapy", p. 145 and "Radiation Therapy", p. 543)
  — use of PRN analgesics
  — postoperative incision care and use of adaptive devices
  — importance of follow-up visits
- Refer to available community resources.

(For more information, see pp. 1299-1300 of Polaski and Tatro, *Luckmann's Core Principles and Practice of Medical-Surgical Nursing.*)

Breast Cancer

OVERVIEW

- One in every nine women is expected to develop breast cancer. Early detection and new treatment modalities have improved the 5-year survival rate. Breast cancer is the second leading cause of cancer deaths in women. Breast cancer in men is rare.
- Histopathologic types of breast cancer include:
  — intraductal carcinoma
    — a precancerous lesion
    — usually an incidental finding with removal of a benign breast lesion
    — axillary metastases are uncommon
    — excellent prognosis
  — infiltrating ductal carcinoma
    — found in 70 per cent of breast cancers
    — palpated as stony, hard lump
    — axillary metastases are common
    — poor prognosis
  — medullary carcinoma
    — 5 to 7 per cent of breast cancers
    — often reaches a large size but prognosis is better than for many other types of breast cancer
    — good prognosis
  — mucinous (colloid) carcinoma
    — frequently occurs with other types of cancer
    — good prognosis
  — tubular carcinoma
    — frequently occurs with other types of cancer
    — axillary metastases are uncommon
    — excellent prognosis
  — lobular carcinoma in situ
    — a precancerous marker that indicates a higher risk for invasive breast cancer
    — usually an incidental finding with removal of a benign breast lesion
    — excellent prognosis
  — infiltrating lobular carcinoma
    — found in 5 to 10 per cent of breast cancers
    — presents as an area of ill-defined thickening
    — axillary lymph node metastasis is frequently present

- — fair prognosis
- — inflammatory breast cancer
  - — edema, warmth, induration
  - — distant metastasis common
  - — poor prognosis
- Staging of breast cancer is based on the (1) size of the primary lesion, (2) extent of the cancer's spread to regional lymph nodes, and (3) presence or absence of metastases.
- Risk factors for development of breast cancer include (1) advancing age, (2) female gender, (3) mother or sister with history of breast cancer, (4) high socioeconomic status, (5) previous radiation to the chest, and (6) early menarche and late menopause.

CLINICAL MANIFESTATIONS

- unilateral, single mass or thickening most often in a breast's upper outer quadrant
- mass is usually painless, non-tender, hard, irregular in shape and non-mobile

MEDICAL MANAGEMENT

- radiation therapy in combination with lumpectomy or quadrantectomy is an accepted treatment for early stage breast cancer. May be administered via:
  - — external beam radiation
  - — interstitial implant therapy using iridium (^{192}Ir)
- adjuvant chemotherapy (given after surgical removal of any measurable cancer) — cyclophosphamide (Cytoxan), 5-fluorouracil (5-FU), methotrexate, doxorubicin
- high-dose chemotherapy with autologous bone marrow transplantation
- neoadjuvant chemotherapy (given before surgical removal of breast lesion to shrink local disease and reduce the risk of systemic spread) — methotrexate, 5-FU, cyclophosphamide
- systemic therapy for metastatic breast cancer
- hormonal therapy (breast cancer with a high level of estrogen receptor-positive (ER+) or progesterone receptor-positive (PR+) cells may respond to hormonal therapy) — tamoxifen, estrogen, androgen, progestin

SURGICAL MANAGEMENT

- lumpectomy — removal of cancerous mass and some normal tissue for clean margins
- quadrantectomy — removal of the quadrant of the breast where tumor is located; a greater portion of normal tissue surrounding the cancer with some overlying skin and underlying muscular fascia is removed to provide a clean margin
- modified radical mastectomy—removal of the breast, axillary lymph nodes, and overlying skin
  — most commonly performed mastectomy
- axillary node dissection — removal of ipsilateral lymph nodes
  — dissection is not done to treat the disease but to stage the disease and determine the need for more chemotherapy
  — may be the only additional surgery needed by a woman who had an excisional biopsy for removal of a small breast cancer
- total (simple) mastectomy — resection of breast tissue and some skin from clavicle to costal margin and from midline to the latissimus dorsi
  — rarely used to treat diagnosed cancer, more frequently done to prevent breast cancer in women at high risk
  — axillary nodes are not removed
- standard radical mastectomy — removal of the breast, overlying skin, pectoral muscles, and axillary nodes
- extended radical mastectomy — removal of internal mammary nodes in addition to structures removed during a standard radical mastectomy
- surgical hormonal manipulation — removal of the ovaries (bilateral oophorectomy) in premenopausal women with advanced breast cancer
- breast reconstruction—option for post mastectomy clients, with use of tissue expanders, implants, or autografts of latissimus dorsi muscle, transverse rectus abdominal muscle, or gluteus maximus muscle. See "Breast Reconstruction (Post Mastectomy),", p. 107.

NURSING MANAGEMENT

MEDICAL

- Administer chemotherapy or hormonal agents as prescribed and monitor side effects. See "Chemotherapy", p. 145.
- Monitor for side effects of radiation therapy. See "Radiation Therapy", p. 543.
- Provide emotional support to client and family.

SURGICAL (POST MODIFIED RADICAL MASTECTOMY)

In addition to routine postoperative care:
- Monitor incisional dressing and surgical drains.
- Elevate the arm on the affected side to promote drainage and prevent infection.
- Apply elastic bandage or custom-fitted pressure gradient elastic sleeve as prescribed.
- Encourage arm exercises as prescribed.
- Ensure that no blood pressure readings, injections, intravenous lines, or blood draws are done on the arm of the operative side.
- Encourage self-care activities (e.g., feeding, combing hair, washing face) and other activities that use the arm, with care taken not to abduct the arm or raise the arm or elbow above shoulder height until the drains are removed.
- Begin teaching wound care at the first dressing change; prepare the client to look at the incision.
- Facilitate Reach for Recovery consult if authorized by physician.
- Begin progressive full range of motion of upper arm after drains are removed.
- Administer pain medication as needed to allow exercise without pain hindrance.
- Prepare client for adjuvant chemotherapy, radiation therapy, or hormonal therapy.
- Facilitate/provide counsel and support regarding the issues of body image change, self esteem, fear of death, coping strategies, and fear of metastases.

FOCUSED DISCHARGE CARE

Instruct the client regarding:
- wound management

- arm exercises
- precautions after axillary lymph node dissection (the affected arm may swell and is less able to fight infection)
  — avoid any kind of trauma to the arm
  — avoid sunburn or insect bites
  — use an electric razor for underarm shaving
  — assess arm regularly for redness, soreness, pus, or other signs of infection
  — avoid strong detergents, harsh chemicals, and abrasive compounds
  — avoid injections, vaccinations, blood samples, and blood pressure measurements on the affected arm whenever possible
  — wear a medical alert identification that cautions no injections or blood pressure readings on affected arm
  — carry handbag and other heavy objects on the other arm
  — avoid elastic cuffs on blouses and nightgowns
  — elevate arm on pillow when lying or sitting
- delayed grieving, which commonly occurs 2 to 3 months after mastectomy
- available temporary and permanent prosthetic devices
- monthly self breast examination and annual mammogram and breast examination by a physician
- importance of laboratory and clinic visit follow-up
- Refer to available community resources.

(For more information, see pp. 1518-1530 of Polaski and Tatro, *Luckmann's Core Principles and Practice of Medical-Surgical Nursing.*)

Breast Cancer, Metastatic

OVERVIEW

- Breast cancer metastases usually develop in one or more of the following sites: lymph nodes, skin, remaining breast tissue, bones, lung, pleura, peritoneum, liver, and central nervous system. Women with metastases to the liver or central nervous system have a poorer prognosis.

- Metastases have been known to occur up to 25 years after initial diagnosis of breast cancer.

CLINICAL MANIFESTATIONS

- dependent upon site of metastasis

MEDICAL MANAGEMENT

- radiation therapy
- hormonal therapy
- chemotherapy
- management of hypercalcemia (common complication of metastatic breast cancer due to bone involvement or hormonal therapy)
  — hydration
  — diuretics
  — mithramycin C (calcium binder)

SURGICAL MANAGEMENT

- dependent upon site of metastasis

NURSING MANAGEMENT

- Administer chemotherapy and hormonal therapy. Assess for side effects and institute appropriate interventions. See "Chemotherapy", p. 145
- Assess for side effects of radiation therapy and institute interventions. See "Radiation Therapy", p.543.
- Assess for signs of hypercalcemia (muscle weakness, increased heart rate and blood pressure, disorientation, anorexia, and abdominal cramping).
- Administer diuretics, fluid, and calcium binders and monitor response.
- Provide emotional support.

FOCUSED DISCHARGE CARE

Instruct the client regarding:
- chemotherapy, hormonal therapy, or radiation therapy regime
- signs/symptoms of hypercalcemia

- importance of follow-up laboratory and clinic visits

(For more information, see pp. 1530-1531 of Polaski and Tatro, *Luckmann's Core Principles and Practice of Medical-Surgical Nursing.*)

Breast Reconstruction (Post-Mastectomy)

- Breast reconstruction may be performed immediately after mastectomy (during the same operation) or many years later.
- Several approaches are available:
  - insertion of a tissue expander. A tissue expander is inserted under the chest tissues and expanded slowly via percutaneous fluid injection. Eventually the expander is removed and an implant inserted.
  - rotation of the latissimus dorsi muscle and formation of a breast mound on the chest. An implant then is inserted.
  - transrectus abdominal musculocutaneous (TRAM) flap — breast reconstruction using abdominal muscle and skin
  - free flap — tissue is harvested from one area of the body to reconstruct the breast
- The nipple-areola area may also be reconstructed.
- In addition to routine postoperative nursing care:
  - Assess the breast or flap area including color, temperature and capillary refill.
  - Assess the nipple-areolar area — report to physician any dusky, deep-red, purple or black-edged color, as this indicates circulatory impairment.
  - Monitor effect of analgesics — if epidural analgesia is used, assess the respiratory rate, presence of numbness or paralysis in lower extremities and degree of pain relief.
  - Instruct the client that the implant will feel very firm and high initially. It will soften and drop with time.

— Reinforce that the reconstructed breast will not exactly match the opposite breast.

(For more information, see pp. 1399-1400 of Polaski and Tatro, *Luckmann's Core Principles and Practice of Medical-Surgical Nursing*.)

Bulimia Nervosa

OVERVIEW

- Bulimia nervosa is an eating disorder characterized by compulsive eating of large quantities of food followed by purging through vomiting or laxative use. It may overlap with anorexia nervosa. Clients binge after some psychological-emotional event, such as depression, anxiety, anger or boredom.
- Weight is essentially maintained but may be less for the client's age and height.
- Bulimia is a common problem among young women during late adolescence and early adulthood.
- Clients generally have a history of poor family relationships with low self esteem and poor impulse control.

CLINICAL MANIFESTATIONS

- history of repeated binge-eating (rapid consumption of a large amount of food in 2 hours or less) followed by purging
- awareness of abnormality of eating patterns with fear of being unable to stop eating
- depressed mood, self-deprecating thoughts following the eating binge
- inconspicuous eating
- frequent weight fluctuations of 10 pounds or more
- use of amphetamines, diuretics, laxatives, fasting and excessive exercise to avoid gaining weight
- psychological symptoms:
  — impaired impulse control
  — fear of obesity

- low self esteem
- depression, gloom, suicidal thoughts, irritability, impaired concentration
- rectal bleeding (from laxative abuse)
- irritation of the throat and esophagus, swelling of the salivary glands, fluid and electrolyte imbalances and erosion of tooth enamel from chronic vomiting

MEDICAL MANAGEMENT

- psychotherapy and self-help groups
- family therapy
- pharmacotherapy (a monoamine oxidase inhibitor may be used to decrease the urge to binge)

All interventions attempt to help the clients gain control of their eating habits and to change attitudes toward food, eating, body size and self.

NURSING MANAGEMENT

- Instruct on healthy diet with correct portions.
- Encourage to eat slowly.
- Assist to develop a regular exercise pattern.
- Provide emotional support for stressful periods.
- Monitor weight.
- Monitor serum potassium and for signs/symptoms of hypokalemia.
- Assist to develop improved self esteem.
- Assist to find ways to deal with stress, boredom, and anxiety other than bingeing-purging.

FOCUSED DISCHARGE CARE

- Instruct client regarding:
  - reinforcement of diet/exercise as above
  - signs/symptoms to report to physician
- Refer to outpatient therapy program.

(For more information, see p. 1035 of Polaski and Tatro, *Luckmann's Core Principles and Practice of Medical-Surgical Nursing*.)

Burn Injury

OVERVIEW

- Burns are injuries that result from direct contact or exposure to any thermal, chemical, electrical or radiation source.
    (1) Thermal burns are caused by exposure to or contact with flames, hot liquids, steam, semisolids (e.g., tar) or hot objects.
    (2) Chemical burns are caused by tissue contact with strong acids, alkalis or organic compounds.
    (3) Electrical burns are caused by heat that is generated by electrical energy as it passes through the body. Injury may result from contact with exposed or faulty electrical wiring or from being struck by lightning.
    (4) Radiation burns are caused by exposure to radiation sources in industry or medicine. A sunburn also is considered a radiation injury.
- Two million people in the United States suffer burn injuries each year; of these, 70,000 are hospitalized with severe injuries.
- Adults over age seventy are at high risk for burn injury.
- Risk factors include contact with scalding liquids, clothing ignition during meal preparation, and residential fires.
- Safety practices in the home are important and include: installation and maintenance of smoke detectors and availability of and instruction on use of fire extinguishers.
- Factors that determine the severity of the burn are:
    (1) burn depth
        — may be superficial (first degree) — epidermis only
        — partial-thickness (second degree) — epithelium and into the dermis

  — full-thickness (third degree) — epidermis, dermis and possibly subcutaneous tissue; produces eschar (devitalized tissue)
  — fourth-degree — full thickness burn involving subcutaneous fat, fascia, muscle or bone
 (2) burn size—determined by rule of nines (body divided into anatomical sections, each representing nine per cent or a multiple of nine) or Lund and Browder method (modifies percentage according to age and is more accurate)
 (3) burn location
 (4) age
 (5) general health
 (6) mechanism of injury

MEDICAL MANAGEMENT

MAJOR BURNS

Emergent Phase - begins at the time of injury and ends with restoration of capillary permeability (usually at 48 to 72 hours following injury).

With the exception of chemical burns, the burn wound should not take precedence over other life-threatening trauma or complications. The primary goal during the emergent phase of recovery is to prevent hypovolemic shock and to preserve vital organ functioning.

- ensurance of adequate airway, breathing and circulation
- treatment of any associated trauma
- initiation of fluid resuscitation
- placement of an indwelling urinary catheter
- placement of a nasogastric tube
- vital signs
- pain management
- tetanus prophylaxis
- wound care

Acute Phase - begins when the client is hemodynamically stable, capillary permeability is restored and diuresis has begun (usually at 48 to 72 hours after the time of injury)

- control of infection
- wound care (e.g., hydrotherapy, debridement)
- specialized wound coverings
- autografting (surgical removal of a thin layer of the client's own unburned skin and application of it to the excised burn wound)

- nutritional support
- pain management
- physical therapy

NURSING MANAGEMENT

Emergent Phase (time of injury until 48 to 72 hours following injury)
- Assess for signs/symptoms of hypovolemia every hour for 36 hours.
- Monitor and document hourly intake and output.
- Daily weights.
- Administer intravenous fluid and electrolyte replacement as prescribed.
- Monitor serum electrolytes and hematocrit.
- Maintain nasogastric tube to low suction (ileus may occur with burn injury).
- Monitor amount, color, heme content and pH of gastric output.
- Ensure patency of urinary catheter.
- Monitor urine color (urine is red or dark brown when hemachromagens are present due to deep burn or crushing injury).
- Send urine samples for urine myoglobin/hemoglobin levels per physician order.
- Assess for signs/symptoms of respiratory distress (secondary to carbon monoxide poisoning, smoke poisoning or heat damage to the lungs).
- Monitor arterial blood gas and carboxyhemoglobin levels.
- Elevate head of bed.
- Assist with turning, coughing, deep breathing every one to two hours for 24 hours, then every two to four hours while awake.
- Instruct on use of incentive spirometer.
- Perform endo- or nasotracheal suctioning PRN.
- Monitor need for ventilatory support and endotracheal intubation.

Emergent and Acute Phase
- Prior to family's/significant other's initial visit, communicate extent of burn and changes in appearance.
- Explain basis of burn care, rationale and interventions.
- Discuss fluid resuscitation, wound care, physical therapy and nutritional needs.

- Maintain normothermia:
  - Monitor rectal or core temperature.
  - Limit the amount of body surface area exposed during wound care.
  - Limit hydrotherapy treatment sessions to 30 minutes or less with water temperature 98° to 102° F.
  - Maintain appropriate environmental temperature.
  - Use external sources of heat to maintain body temperature.
- Promote adequate tissue perfusion:
  - Remove all constricting jewelry and clothing.
  - Limit use of blood pressure cuffs on affected extremity.
  - Monitor strength of arterial pulses (by doppler if needed).
  - Assess capillary refill of unburned skin.
  - Elevate affected extremities above the level of the heart.
  - Anticipate and prepare client for escharotomy.
- Prevent gastric ulcer development:
  - Monitor gastric pH values and administer antacids as prescribed.
  - Administer hydrogen receptor antagonists as prescribed.
  - Hematest all stools and nasogastric drainage.
- Provide pain control:
  - Medicate prior to painful procedures.
  - Explore non-pharmacologic pain management techniques: relaxation technique, music therapy, guided imagery, distraction and hypnosis.
  - Document and evaluate response to pain management techniques.
- Prevent infection:
  - Administer tetanus prophylaxis as prescribed.
  - Cover burn wound with clean sheet during client transfer.
  - Instruct family on infection control measures.
  - Use strict, aseptic technique for all procedures.
  - Assess for and report any signs/symptoms of infection.
  - Debride wound of loose, non-viable tissue.
  - Shave or cut body hair in and around wound margins (exception: eyebrows and eyelashes).
  - Administer systemic and/or topical antibiotics as prescribed.

- Provide adequate nutrition:
  - Consult dietician for assessment of caloric and protein needs.
  - Provide oral hygiene every shift and PRN.
  - Administer oral, enteral and/or parenteral nutrition as prescribed.
  - If a feeding tube is in place, use twill tape tied around the head and above the ears to secure the tube. Ensure that it does not rub the ears.
  - For clients taking an oral diet:
    - Determine food/fluid preferences.
    - Schedule treatments to provide for uninterrupted mealtimes.
    - Allow rest periods before meals.
- Prevent impaired physical mobility:
  - Assess range of motion and muscle strength every day.
  - Maintain burned areas in functional position within limits imposed by associated injuries, grafting, etc.
  - Consult physical and occupational therapy for an individualized rehabilitation schedule.
  - Instruct on use of overhead trapeze.
  - If client is susceptible to neck contractures, sleeping with a pillow is contraindicated.
  - Encourage active range of motion every two to four hours unless contraindicated due to a recent grafting procedure.
  - Provide passive exercise and stretching if client unable to participate.
- Provide emotional support and assist with coping strategies.
  - Be consistent with treatment schedule.
  - Arrange for client to talk with others who have had similar injuries.
  - Assess effective coping strategies used in the past.
  - Explore coping strategies.
  - Provide emotional support.
  - Facilitate consults with psychologist, psychiatrist, or social worker.
  - Encourage client/significant other attendance at support group meetings.

Acute and Rehabilitation Phases
- Promote independence in self care.

— Assess ability to provide self care in grooming, bathing, eating and elimination.
— Obtain consult to occupational therapy for assistive devices.
— Encourage client participation in self care tasks and provide positive reinforcement for efforts.
• Assist to accept changes in body image.
— Explain and reinforce projected appearance of burns and grafts during the various phases.
— Encourage realistic perceptions of changes in body image.
— Allow to progress at own pace through stages of denial, grief and acceptance of injury and recovery.
— Provide encouragement by discussing progress made.
— Assist with coping strategies and help prepare for social interactions after discharge.

FOCUSED DISCHARGE CARE

Care after discharge will vary greatly depending upon many factors. In general:
• Arrange for transfer to long-term care facility and ensure continuity of care.
• If client returns home, make home health care referrals as needed to assist with needed therapy, further teaching and care requirements.
• In addition, instruct client/family on following as appropriate:
— ongoing need for physical therapy
— high caloric, high protein diet to facilitate healing
— use of Eucerine cream, Nivea oil, Keri lotion, or any lanolin-rich lotion to relieve itching and pain to areas that feel tight and dry (cover with loose gauze)
— skin care
— course of rehabilitation
— need to change or adapt to a new lifestyle and new goals in life and how this will affect the client and family
— coping strategies for emotions such as frustration, anger, and depression
— need to seek out and participate in mental health counseling when usual coping strategies are ineffective

- — challenges faced by client and family as they leave security and acceptance of hospital environment
- — coping with public appearances if visible, disfiguring effects remain after healing is complete.

(For more information, see pp. 1366-1386 of Polaski and Tatro, *Luckmann's Core Principles and Practice of Medical-Surgical Nursing.*)

Candidiasis, Oral (Moniliasis, Thrush)

OVERVIEW

- Candidiasis is an overgrowth of the normal flora, candida albicans, in the oral cavity.
- It commonly is seen in clients who are immunosuppressed, such as those receiving chemotherapy or those infected with human immunodeficiency virus (HIV). There is also a higher incidence in clients who are pregnant, under stress, on high doses of prolonged antibiotics, on prolonged tube feedings, or who have diabetes mellitus.
- Major risk factors include immunosuppression and the prolonged use of antibiotics.

CLINICAL MANIFESTATIONS

- white patches on the tongue, palate and buccal mucosa (often described as "milk curds")
- subjective complaints of lesions as dry and hot

MEDICAL MANAGEMENT

- oral nystatin swish and swallow
- mycelex troches

NURSING MANAGEMENT

- Administer oral analgesics, topical agents or swishes to relieve pain.
- Provide soft, pureed or liquid bland diet. Avoid spicy, citrus or hot foods.
- Provide solution of 1:1 warm water and hydrogen peroxide for oral rinses (avoid commercial mouthwashes because of their high alcohol content).
- Provide gauze pads or foam toothettes for oral care.

- Administer antifungals as prescribed.
- Administer oral antibiotics as prescribed to prevent secondary infection.

FOCUSED DISCHARGE CARE

Instruct client regarding:
- oral hygiene regimen
- diet
- medications
- signs/symptoms of complications and to report to physician

(For more information, see pp. 1011-1012 of Polaski and Tatro, *Luckmann's Core Principles and Practice of Medical-Surgical Nursing*.)

Carcinoma of the Gallbladder

OVERVIEW

- Cancer of the gallbladder accounts for only 5 per cent of all cancers.
- At least 70 per cent of these clients have gallstones.
- Of all clients who develop this malignancy, 91 per cent are over the age of 50 years and the incidence in women is three to four times that of men.
- The prognosis of gallbladder cancer is poor. About 88 per cent die within the first year, and only about 4 per cent are alive within 5 years.

CLINICAL MANIFESTATIONS

- abdominal pain
- weight loss, anorexia
- jaundice
- right upper quadrant mass

MEDICAL MANAGEMENT

Treatment modalities are widely debated and are generally palliative.

- chemotherapy
- radiation therapy
- measures to relieve duct obstruction
  - retrograde endoscopy (endoscope is passed into the duodenum, where a wire is passed into the common bile duct to remove stones, if present)
  - endoscopic papillotomy (endoscope is passed orally and the ampulla of Vater is enlarged)

SURGICAL MANAGEMENT

- radical resection of the gallbladder — widely debated

NURSING MANAGEMENT

- See "Chemotherapy", p. 145.
- See "Radiation Therapy", p. 543.

FOCUSED DISCHARGE CARE

See references in Nursing Management as listed above.

(For more information, see p. 1149 of Polaski and Tatro, *Luckmann's Core Principles and Practice of Medical-Surgical Nursing.*)

Cardiac Surgery

OVERVIEW

- There are three types of cardiac surgery: reparative, reconstructive, and substitional.
  - *Reparative surgeries* are likely to produce cure or prolonged improvement. These operations include closure of a patent ductus arteriosus; atrial septal defect and ventricular septal defect, repair of mitral stenosis; and simple repair of tetralogy of Fallot.
  - *Reconstructive procedures* are not always curative and reoperation may be needed. These procedures include coronary artery bypass graft and

reconstruction of an incompetent mitral, tricuspid, or aortic valve.

— *Substitional surgeries* are not curative because of the preoperative condition of the client. Examples include valve replacement, cardiac transplant, ventricular replacement or assistance, and cardiac replacement by a mechanical device.

- Cardiac transplantation is now a standard and effective treatment for clients with end stage cardiac disease. The current orthotopic technique retains a large portion of the recipient's right and left atria and implants the donor heart to the atria. Cardiopulmonary bypass is used during the surgery. Another type of heart transplant is the heterotopic transplant. In this form, the donor heart is placed parallel to the recipient's heart and the right side can continue to function while the dysfunctional left side is bypassed.

- The artificial heart is a commercially made device attached surgically in an operation similar to that described in the heart transplant procedure. Permanent use of this device is not recommended but it may serve as a bridge to transplantation for the client waiting for a donor heart.

NURSING MANAGEMENT

POSTOPERATIVE CARE

In addition to routine postoperative care:
- Monitor cardiovascular function and tissue perfusion by assessing vital signs, pulses, arterial blood pressures, venous and left heart filling pressures, and cardiac rhythm.
- Assess heart sounds for presence of pericardial rubs, murmurs, or gallops indicating possible complications.
- Monitor ECG rhythm for heart block, ventricular tachycardia, and atrial fibrillation, which commonly complicate open heart surgery.
  — Temporary pacing wires often are implanted during surgery and can be connected to an external pacemaker should bradycardia or heart block occur.

- Assess respiratory status: rate, depth, effort, presence of rales or rhonchi, skin color, and sputum production.
  - Ventilator and supplemental oxygen adjustments are determined by physical assessment and arterial blood gas analysis.
  - Sedate as needed for maximal ventilator benefit.
  - Encourage to cough, deep breathe, and use incentive spirometer every 1-2 hours after extubation.
  - Suction PRN to maintain patent airway.
- Assess for presence of pain and medicate as needed.
- Measure and observe chest/mediastinal tube drainage.
- Strict intake and output.
- Daily weights.
- Monitor laboratory values—electrolytes, hemoglobin, hematocrit, prothrombin time, and renal function.
- Administer inotropic and vasoactive agents as ordered.
- Monitor for hypertension—in the client who has undergone a coronary artery bypass graft, an elevated blood pressure may cause the graft to leak or loosen.
- Assess neurologic response: level of consciousness, orientation, ability to move extremities, and pupil size and reaction.
- Monitor for cardiac tamponade: sudden cessation of chest drainage, dyspnea, paradoxical pulse greater than 10 mm Hg (see glossary), distant heart sounds, distended neck veins, hypotension, narrowed pulse pressure.
- Initiate progressive activity schedule after extubation and monitor cardiopulmonary response.

Post Cardiac Transplantation

In addition to the above interventions:
- Monitor for clinical manifestations of rejection
  - decrease in oxygenation
  - fever
  - malaise
  - anxiety
  - infiltrates on chest film
- Administer immunosuppressive therapy as ordered (Cyclosporine)

- Monitor for toxic effects of immunosuppressives
  — renal failure
  — hypertension
  — liver toxic effects
  — neurologic disturbances
- Administer antibiotics as ordered
- Monitor for signs of infection
- Maintain aseptic technique and isolation precautions
- Be mindful that clients will demonstrate the following as a result of the severing of nerves (denervation) during surgery
  — lack of chest pain with ischemia
  — loss of sympathetic stimulation
  — orthostatic hypotension
  — resting heart rate of 90–110 beats/minute

FOCUSED DISCHARGE CARE

Instruct the client regarding:
- activity/rest schedule
- weight-lifting restrictions
- do not use arms to push out of bed or chair
- driving restrictions
- dietary restrictions
- need to monitor pulse daily for rate and regularity and when to call physician
- incision care
- notification of physician for:
  — signs and symptoms of infection
  — palpitations, tachycardia, or irregular pulse
  — dizziness
  — sudden weight gain or peripheral edema
  — shortness of breath
- need to monitor character of stools and take prescribed stool softeners to avoid straining
- need for lifelong anticoagulant therapy following valve replacement

POST CARDIAC TRANSPLANTATION

In addition to above, instruct regarding:
- life-long immunosuppressive therapy and monitoring for toxicity

(For more information, see pp. 759-768 of Polaski and Tatro, *Luckmann's Core Principles and Practice of Medical-Surgical Nursing.*)

Cardiac Tamponade

OVERVIEW

- Cardiac tamponade is a life-threatening complication. It exists when accumulated fluid or air in the pericardial sac restricts ventricular filling.
- Large or rapidly accumulating effusions raise the intrapericardial pressure to a point at which venous blood cannot flow into the heart, which decreases ventricular filling. As a result, venous pressure rises, and cardiac output and arterial blood pressure fall.

CLINICAL MANIFESTATIONS

- narrowing pulse pressure
- tachycardia
- hypotension
- jugular venous distention
- cyanosis of lips and nails
- dyspnea
- muffled heart sounds
- diaphoresis
- paradoxical pulse greater than 10 mm Hg
- feeling of impending doom

MEDICAL MANAGEMENT

- pericardiocentesis - needle aspiration of fluid or air from the pericardial sac

(For more information, see p. 743 of Polaski and Tatro, *Luckmann's Core Principles and Practice of Medical-Surgical Nursing.*)

Cardiomyopathy

OVERVIEW

- Cardiomyopathy is a heart muscle disorder of unknown etiology (idiopathic). The dominant feature is the involvement of the heart muscle itself.
- Possible etiologic factors include: inflammatory diseases, infections, toxins, endocrine disorders, hypersensitivities, etc.
- The three major classes are:
    — idiopathic dilated (congestive) cardiomyopathy
        — characterized by ventricular enlargement followed by impaired ventricular contractility leading to congestive heart failure.
    — idiopathic hypertrophic cardiomyopathy (also known as idiopathic hypertrophic subaortic stenosis (IHSS)
        — appears to be a genetically transmitted disease of the heart muscle
        — disproportionate thickening of the interventricular septum compared to the free wall of the ventricle.
    — idiopathic restrictive cardiomyopathy — an infiltrative process that results in fibrosis and thickening of the heart muscle.
- Four conditions lower the threshold for the development of cardiomyopathy:
    — chronic alcohol ingestion
    — pregnancy
    — systemic hypertension
    — a variety of infections.

CLINICAL MANIFESTATIONS

- Dilated cardiomyopathy:
    — fatigue and weakness
    — chest pain
    — symptoms of right-sided failure (dyspnea, orthopnea, tachycardia, peripheral edema)
    — S_3, S_4, and murmurs
- Hypertrophic cardiomyopathy:
    — sudden death may be first clinical manifestation
    — dyspnea, angina pectoris, fatigue, and syncope

— cardiac dysrhythmias
- Restrictive cardiomyopathy:
  — exercise intolerance, fatigue
  —neck vein distention, peripheral edema, and ascites

MEDICAL MANAGEMENT

- Dilated cardiomyopathy:
  —digitalis preparations, vasodilators, diuretics, and sodium restricted diet
  — prescribed rest and activity limitations
  — antiarrhythmic agents
  — anticoagulant therapy to decrease risk of clot formation from pooled blood within the heart
- Hypertrophic cardiomyopathy:
  —beta-adrenergic blocking agents to decrease myocardial contractility and heart rate (reduces myocardial workload)
  — calcium-channel blocking agents to improve activity tolerance
- Restrictive cardiomyopathy:
  — diuretics, vasodilators, and salt restriction

SURGICAL MANAGEMENT

- excision of a portion of the hypertrophied septum (myotomy or myectomy) in hypertrophic cardiomyopathy
- cardiac transplantation is becoming increasingly common

NURSING MANAGEMENT

MEDICAL

- Assess for signs/symptoms of increasing congestive heart failure.
- Maintain strict intake and output.
- Restrict fluids as ordered.
- Monitor BUN and creatinine.
- Daily weights.
- Monitor for signs/symptoms of decreasing cardiac output.
- Encourage adequate rest periods.
- Monitor pulses, respirations, color, and ECG during activity.

FOCUSED DISCHARGE CARE

Instruct client regarding:
- disease process and treatment regimen
- need to avoid strenuous physical exercise or competitive sports as syncope or sudden death may follow exertion
- prophylactic antibiotics before and after dental or surgical procedures due to high risk of infective endocarditis
- need to abstain from alcohol which depresses myocardial contractility
- signs and symptoms of worsening heart failure
- signs and symptoms of digitalis toxicity
- importance of adequate rest
- avoidance of emotional stress that may exacerbate the symptoms
- importance of CPR instruction for household members
- need for follow-up clinic appointments

(For more information, see pp. 744-748 of Polaski and Tatro, *Luckmann's Core Principles and Practice of Medical-Surgical Nursing.*)

Carpal Tunnel Syndrome

OVERVIEW

- Carpal tunnel syndrome is a frequently seen, painful disorder caused by pressure on the median nerve at the wrist.
- The exact cause is not known.
- Etiologic factors include:
  — recent fracture
  — arthritis
  — lipomas
  — ganglion
  — strenuous or repetitious use of the hands

- Occurs in women five times more often than men and in clients between 40 and 50 years of age.

CLINICAL MANIFESTATIONS

- burning or tingling pain in thumb, index or middle finger
  — may radiate to upper extremity, shoulder, neck or chest
  — may be episodic or constant with exacerbation at night and by movement
- presence of Tinel's sign (tingling or shocklike pain elicited by light percussion over the median nerve)
- presence of Phalen's sign (hand tingling with acute wrist flexion)

MEDICAL MANAGEMENT

- pain management
- wrist immobilization

SURGICAL MANAGEMENT

- relieve compression of median nerve

NURSING MANAGEMENT

MEDICAL

- Administer analgesics.

SURGICAL

- Routine postoperative care.

FOCUSED DISCHARGE CARE

Instruct client regarding:
- use of PRN analgesics
- use of wrist splint
- incisional care

(For more information, see p. 1300 of Polaski and Tatro, *Luckmann's Core Principles and Practice of Medical-Surgical Nursing.*)

Casts

OVERVIEW

- Casts are temporary devices of plaster or fiberglass that immobilize a body part, usually an extremity. Before the cast is applied, the skin is cleansed thoroughly and covered with stockinette or padding.
- Casts are used for (1) immobilization, (2) prevention or correction of deformity, (3) maintenance, support and protection to realign bone, and (4) promotion of healing which allows early weight bearing.
- Types of casts include:
  — arm or leg casts
  — cast brace —consists of two parts, one above and one below the knee, with a hinge at the knee to allow range of motion (used for distal femur fractures)
- Windowing casts is the cutting of windows into a dried cast to allow visualization of certain areas, to assess a pulse, or to remove drains or care for wounds.
- Bivalving a cast means splitting it along both sides to (1) allow for tissue swelling, (2) allow removal of one-half of the cast to facilitate care and x-rays, and (3) make a half-cast for use as an intermittent splint.

NURSING MANAGEMENT

- Assess the following in the casted extremity: color, warmth, sensation, swelling, pulses distal to cast, and movement of distal fingers or toes . Compare to opposite extremity.
- Promote the circulation of warm, dry air around the cast to speed the drying process.
- Cover non-casted areas to provide adequate warmth (the client may feel cold while the cast is drying).
- Instruct the client that there may be a sensation of heat under the cast during its early setting.
- Turn the client in a new cast periodically to expose more of the cast to air (unless contraindicated).
- A casted extremity should be elevated to minimize swelling and promote drainage. This is especially important in the first 24–48 hours.
- Avoid overhandling, use palms of hands to move cast until dry.

- Place new plaster casts on pillows protected by plastic until they are dry.
- Monitor for signs/symptoms of complications:
  Impaired Blood Flow
  — Assess for:
    — pulselessness, diminished capillary refill
    — skin pallor, prolonged blanching time, cyanosis (a late indication of impaired circulation), coolness
    — paresthesias, numbness
  Nerve damage from pressure where a nerve passes over a bony prominence:
    — increasing, persistent, localized pain
    — diminished sensitivity, numbness, motor weakness or paralysis not previously present
  Infection, necrosis due to skin breakdown:
    — musty, unpleasant odor
    — drainage
    — "hot spot" on cast
    — fever
  Compartment syndrome (which compromises circulation, viability and function of tissues within the compartment):
    — dramatic increase in pain, no longer controlled with analgesics
    — loss of movement or sensation
    — pain with passive motion
    — pulselessness
  Cast syndrome — occurs with body casts — may be fatal if untreated:
    — prolonged nausea and vomiting
    — abdominal distention and pain
- Assess skin around cast edges for skin damage or swelling.
- Smell for odors indicative of tissue necrosis and infection.
- Assess the cast surface for wound drainage or bleeding. Assess for wet spots, which may indicate drainage beneath the cast. Feel the surface of the cast. "Hot spots" (areas that feel warmer) may indicate tissue necrosis or infection under the cast.
- Prevent swelling by elevating the casted extremity above the level of the heart (especially in the first 24 to 48 hours), exercising fingers or toes, and placing ice bags around the cast.

- Ensure that the foot is supported in a 90-degree flexion angle to prevent foot drop if a leg is casted.
- Encourage the client to exercise joints above and below the cast to prevent complications of disuse (especially the shoulder if the arm is casted).
- Change position frequently to prevent complications of immobility.
- Instruct client on isometric exercises for the casted extremity.
- Instruct on gluteal sitting, abdominal tightening and deep breathing if client is confined to bed.
- Encourage dietary fiber and fluids to maintain normal elimination.

FOCUSED DISCHARGE CARE

Instruct client/significant other regarding:
- skin care and how to prevent skin damage
- how to assess skin condition
- assessment and reporting of: swelling or discoloration of the extremity distal to the cast; areas of friction; skin irritation; and change in movement or sensation of the distal extremity
- cast care
  — keep the cast dry
  — protect the cast with plastic when bathing
  — do not insert objects inside the cast
  — do not use powder inside the cast
  — use of slings/crutches to enhance comfort, safety, and ambulation.
- need to report signs and symptoms of infection
  — increased swelling
  — tingling or burning sensation
  — inability to move muscle around the cast
  — foul odor around cast edges
  — drainage, especially that which shows through the cast
  — warmth beneath the cast after it has dried
- reporting loose, cracked, molded, soft or broken casts to physician
- follow-up with physical therapy
- when to return for cast removal and care after cast is removed
  — soften and condition skin
  — use dampened cloth and gentle soap or detergent

— rinse well and pat dry
— elevate limb to reduce swelling
— it will take 1 to 4 weeks to regain limb strength

(For more information, see pp. 1278-1285 of Polaski and Tatro, *Luckmann's Core Principles and Practice of Medical-Surgical Nursing.*)

Cataracts

OVERVIEW

- A cataract is an opacity of the lens of the eye.
- Cataract formation is characterized by a reduction in oxygen uptake and an initial increase in water content followed by dehydration of the lens. The protein in the lens undergoes numerous changes, including yellowing.
- Types of cataracts:
  — age-related (senile)
    — most common
    — onset — around the age of fifty
  — related to other disorders, such as:
    — diabetes
    — Down's syndrome
    — trauma
    — chronic corticosteroid use
    — exposure to infrared light

CLINICAL MANIFESTATIONS

- blurred vision
- monocular diplopia
- photophobia and glare
- ability to see better in low-lighted conditions when the pupil is dilated, which allows vision around a central opacity
- cloudy lens
- absence of pain

MEDICAL MANAGEMENT

No measures can prevent or reduce cataract formation

SURGICAL MANAGEMENT

- cataract extraction— excision of the lens
- phacoemulsification — use of ultrasound vibrations to break up the lens into particles which are then removed by suction
- intraocular lens implementation — following cataract extraction, a new lens is inserted (or the client may be left without a lens and corrected by use of eyeglasses or contact lenses)

NURSING MANAGEMENT

Surgical

Preoperative

- Administer preoperative eye drops —mydriatic tropicamide (Mydriacyl) — to dilate the pupil and cycloplegic, cyclopentolate (Cyclogyl) — to paralyze ciliary muscles.
- Administer preoperative sedative and medications to decrease intraocular pressure.

Postoperative

In addition to routine postoperative care:
- Maintain eye patch in place.
- Monitor for signs of increased intraocular pressure (pain, nausea).
- Assist with ambulation and activities of daily living.
- Instruct not to lie on operative side.
- Instruct on measures to prevent increased intraocular pressure (see Focused Discharge Care).

FOCUSED DISCHARGE CARE

Instruct client regarding:
- measures to avoid increasing intraocular pressure:
  — no lifting heavy objects
  — no bending from the waist
  — no straining with stool

— avoidance of coughing and vomiting
— no sleeping on the operative side
- eye care
- technique for instilling eye drops, antibiotics and/or corticosteroids
- signs/symptoms of increased intraocular pressure (pain, decreased vision, nausea)
- signs/symptoms of infection (redness, swelling, drainage, blurred vision or pain)
- need to wear eye protection (shield or glasses)
- safety in the home environment
- importance of clinic follow-up visits

(For more information, see pp. 440-443 of Polaski and Tatro, *Luckmann's Core Principles and Practice of Medical-Surgical Nursing*.)

Cellulitis and Erysipelas

- Cellulitis is a suppurative inflammation of the dermis and subcutaneous tissues that spreads widely through tissue spaces. The skin is erythematous, edematous, tender and sometimes nodular. The areas of inflammation are without sharp, indurated borders. Lymphangitis may occur. If untreated, gangrene, metastatic abscesses and sepsis may result. Streptococcus pyogenes is the most common causative organism.
- Erysipelas is an acute, superficial, rapidly spreading inflammation of the dermis and lymphatics. The usual causative organism is beta-hemolytic streptococcus group A.
- With erysipelas, the organism enters tissue via a wound or abrasion. The skin is elevated, beginning with a small, bright red area. The involved area spreads peripherally to become a plaque with sharp, indurated borders. Lesions are common on the face and extremities.
- Clients at risk for cellulitis and erysipelas include the elderly and clients with lowered resistance due to

diabetes, malnutrition, steroid therapy or the presence of wounds or ulcers. There is a tendency for recurrence.
- Medical treatment is with systemic antibiotics; penicillin is the antibiotic of choice.

NURSING MANAGEMENT

- Monitor client's temperature and administer antipyretics as prescribed.
- Provide warm soaks as prescribed.
- Monitor for and report signs/symptoms of sepsis: high fever, tachycardia, confusion or hypotension.
- Instruct client on careful handwashing and careful disposal of linen, clothing and dressings to prevent spread of infection.
- Elevate edematous areas.
- Monitor infected areas for signs/symptoms of worsening infection, such as increasing redness or increasing edema.

(For more information, see p. 1354 of Polaski and Tatro, *Luckmann's Core Principles and Practice of Medical-Surgical Nursing.*)

Cerebrovascular Accident (CVA)

OVERVIEW

- A cerebrovascular accident (CVA) or stroke is infarction (death) of a specific portion of the brain due to insufficient blood supply. The blood vessel affected determines the area and extent of infarction.
- Stroke may occur from:
  — thrombosis—this is the most common cause and usually is due to atherosclerosis.
  — embolism — a cerebral vessel is occluded by emboli (fragments of clotted blood, tumor, fat, bacteria or air).

- intracerebral hemorrhage - rupture of a cerebral vessel that causes bleeding into the brain tissue.
- cerebral arterial spasm — usually due to some irritation of the outer part of the arterial wall, it reduces blood flow to the area of brain supplied by the vessel.
- compression of cerebral vessels due to tumor, large blood clot, or swollen brain tissue.
- Cerebrovascular disorders are the third most common cause of death in the United States. Stroke occurs equally in men and women with a higher incidence of death rate in blacks than in whites and in persons over age 75.
- Risk factors related to stroke are:
  - prior ischemic episodes
  - cardiac disease
  - diabetes mellitus
  - atherosclerotic disease of intracranial and extracranial vessels
  - hypertension
  - polycythemia
  - hypercholesterolemia
  - smoking
  - oral contraceptive use
  - emotional stress
  - obesity
  - family history of stroke
  - age (incidence increases with age)

CLINICAL MANIFESTATIONS

Warning signs that may precede CVA:
- paresthesias
- transient loss of speech
- hemiplegia
- severe occipital or nuchal headaches
- vertigo (dizziness) or syncope (fainting)
- motor or sensory disturbances (tingling, transient paralysis)
- epistaxis (nosebleed)

Other findings associated with stroke include:
- retinal hemorrhage
- vomiting
- seizures
- fever
- headache

- coma
- nuchal rigidity
- elevated blood pressure
- confusion
- disorientation
- memory impairment
- weakness
- paralysis
- language disorders
- reflex changes

Specific deficits that may occur after CVA

(Deficits depend upon the area of the brain damaged as well as the side of the brain, i.e., dominant vs. non-dominant.)

- hemiplegia — paralysis on one side of the body. Muscles of the thorax and abdomen are usually not paralyzed because they are innervated from both cerebral hemispheres.
- aphasia — a defect in using and interpreting the symbols of language — it may involve any or all aspects of language use (reading, writing, speaking or understanding spoken language). Aphasia may be sensory or motor (usually is a combination of both).
  — sensory aphasia (also called receptive aphasia)
    — loss of the ability to comprehend written, spoken or printed words
  — motor aphasia (also called expressive aphasia) — loss of the ability to write, make signs or speak (i.e., words may be recalled, but the client cannot combine speech sounds into words and syllables)
- apraxia — a condition in which a client can move the affected part but cannot use it for specific purposeful actions (walking, speaking or dressing)
- homonymous hemianopia — defective vision or visual loss in the same half of the visual field of each eye
- agnosia — a disturbance in interpreting visual, tactile or other sensory information. The client is unable to recognize objects.
- dysarthria — imperfect articulation that causes difficulty in speaking (client understands language, but has difficulty pronouncing and enunciating words). Clients with dysarthria often have difficulty chewing and swallowing food because of poor muscle control.

- kinesthesia — alterations in sensation — may include:
  - paresthesia (feelings of numbness, tingling, heaviness)
  - hemianesthesia (loss of sensation)
  - loss of muscle-joint sense
- incontinence — bowel/bladder
- shoulder pain
- Horner's syndrome — paralysis of the sympathetic nerves to the eye, causing sinking of the eyeball, ptosis of the upper eyelid, lack of tearing in the eye and slight elevation of the lower lid
- unilateral neglect — failure to attend to one side of the body, failure to report or respond to stimuli on one side of the body; or failure to use one extremity
- other problems with memory, spacial perception, and loss of direction

Emotional or Behavioral Reactions
- severe mood swings
- social withdrawal
- inappropriate sexual behavior
- outbursts of frustration/anger
- regression to earlier behavior

MEDICAL MANAGEMENT

- supportive care for infarctive stroke
- prevention of further emboli for embolic stroke
- management of increased intracranial pressure and hyperthermia with hemorrhagic stroke
- bedrest with head of the bed elevated 30 degrees
- external ventriculostomy drainage — may be used to reduce pressure from cerebrospinal fluid accumulation
- blood pressure management — prevent excessively high blood pressure but maintain adequate cerebral perfusion
- fluid volume management — avoidance of fluid volume excess
- tissue plasminogen activator (tPA) to dissolve the clot
- steroids or osmotic diuretics to reduce intracranial pressure
- antihypertensives and diuretics to control hypertension

- anticoagulants
- mild analgesics (codeine and acetaminophen) to treat headache and neck stiffness, yet prevent sedation which would make neurological assessment inaccurate
- phenytoin or phenobarbital, if the client develops seizures
- rehabilitation which begins during the acute period after the CVA.

SURGICAL MANAGEMENT

- rapid evacuation of the hematoma for select clients with hemorrhagic stroke or bleeding

NURSING MANAGEMENT

- Monitor intracranial pressure hourly, if intracranial pressure monitor is placed.
- Perform neurological assessments hourly using the Glasgow Coma scale. Monitor for changes in level of consciousness and for signs/symptoms of increased intracranial pressure.
- Prevent any increases in intracranial pressure:
  — Suction minimally.
  — Keep head of the bed elevated with neck straight.
  — Prevent excessive coughing, straining with stool, vomiting, lifting, or use of arms to change position.
  — Administer laxatives or stool softeners as prescribed.
  — Treat fever with antipyretics and cooling blanket (avoid inducing shivering).
  — Avoid restraints which may increase agitation.
  — Keep room quiet and dark.

After intracranial pressure is stabilized:
POSITIONING/ACTIVITY

- Change hemiplegic client's position every two hours (keep mainly on unaffected side).
- Avoid long periods of sitting (may contribute to hip flexion deformity).
- No pillows under the knee when client supine (contributes to flexion deformity and thrombus formation).

- Do not flex the upper thigh acutely when turning to side (contributes to hip flexion deformity).
- Position prone for 15 to 30 minutes several times daily with pillow under pelvis to hyperextend hip joints.
- Use trochanter roll (from crest of ilium to mid-thigh) to prevent external hip rotation.
- Prevent adduction of the affected shoulder by placing a pillow in the axilla between the upper arm and chest wall to keep the arm abducted 60 degrees. Periodically place the forearm on another pillow in a "Statue of Liberty" position (with the elbow above the shoulder and the wrist above the elbow). This will stretch the internal rotators of the shoulder.
- Place the hand in a splint or hand roll to prevent finger flexion and thumb adduction. The preferred position is slight supination with fingers slightly flexed and the thumb in opposition.
- Discuss exercises the client can do in bed (gluteal setting, quadriceps setting).
- Perform passive range of motion exercises four times daily and encourage active range of motion if client is able.
- Assist with progressive activity as prescribed (transferring to chair, wheelchair).
- Assist with progressive self care activities (washing, eating, grooming), encouraging use of paralyzed limb and instructing client to avoid tendency to do everything with the unaffected limb.

Prevention of Injury

- If eye is paralyzed, irrigate with physiologic saline, instill artificial tears and cover with eye patch as prescribed.
- Keep bed side-rails raised.
- Remind client to walk slowly, rest adequately between intervals of walking and to look ahead while walking.
- Inspect skin for any injury or breakdown — provide protective devices as needed.
- Inspect oral mucosa for any injuries (especially affected side of tongue and mouth). Provide oral care three to four times daily.

- Assess total intake and facilitate referral to dietician as needed.
- Monitor hemoglobin, lymphocytes and nutritional panel.
- Provide supplemental snacks or high calorie liquid supplements.
- Place patient in most upright position for meals.
- Assist with specific difficulties in feeding process as needed: mouth opening, mouth closing, sucking, tongue movement, swallowing or inadequate salivation.

COMMUNICATION

- Facilitate referral to speech therapy — reinforce lessons as appropriate.
- Repeat simple directions until they are understood.
- Do not shout — patient can hear.
- When a client cannot identify objects by name, give practice in receiving word images (point to an object and state its name).
- When a client has difficulty with verbal expression, give practice in repeating words after you.
- When working with an aphasic client, practice speech.
- When talking to a client with receptive difficulty, stand within six feet and face the client directly.
- Assist family with communication techniques.

MISCELLANEOUS

- Reorient the client and position a calendar and clock where the client can see them.
- If visual impairment is present, approach the side that is not visually impaired. Position needed items on that side.
- Minimize environmental stimuli if patient has perceptual defects.
- For clients with unilateral neglect, initially adapt environment by positioning items on unaffected side. Gradually move personal items, etc. to affected side. Encourage the client to groom the affected side first. Cue the client to scan the entire environment.
- Provide emotional support to the client and family and assist to identify coping strategies to deal with

loss of function, powerlessness, self esteem disturbance and social isolation. Make referrals as necessary.
- Encourage attempts at independence and praise all successes.
- Assist to become as independent as possible in activities of daily living.
- Reinforce techniques taught by physical therapy/occupational therapy.

FOCUSED DISCHARGE CARE

- If client returns home:
  — Instruct client/significant other regarding:
    — ways to prevent recurrence: dietary modification, stress reduction, smoking cessation, exercise program and prescribed medications
    — residual deficits and balancing realistic expectations while allowing maximal independence
    — equipment needed at home
    — special methods of feeding or enteral feedings
  — Make home health care referrals as appropriate.
- Provide continuity of care and emotional support to client and family if client is placed in a nursing home or rehabilitation facility.

(For more information, see pp. 312-327 of Polaski and Tatro, *Luckmann's Core Principles and Practice of Medical-Surgical Nursing.*)

Cervical Cancer

OVERVIEW

- Cervical cancer is the second most fatal cancer of the reproductive system, although death rates have dropped 50 per cent over the last twenty years.
- The cause is unknown, but seems to have a strong relationship with chronic irritation and human papillomavirus.

- All women with carcinoma in situ potentially can be cured. Ninety per cent of women with non-metastatic disease can be cured.
- The Pap smear is the primary diagnostic tool for cervical cancer.
- Spread occurs by direct extension to the vaginal mucosa, lower uterine segment, parametrium, pelvic wall, bladder and bowel. Distant metastasis may be to the liver, lungs or bone.
- Risk factors include:
  — lower socioeconomic class
  — prostitutes
  — blacks, native Americans
  — multiparity
  — early age of and frequent intercourse with multiple partners
  — early first pregnancy
  — untreated, chronic cervicitis
  — sexually transmitted disease
  — women whose partners have a history of penile or prostate cancer

CLINICAL MANIFESTATIONS

There are no early indications of carcinoma in situ or early cervical cancer.
  Late Assessment Findings:
- vaginal discharge and bleeding
- metrorrhagia (uterine bleeding between normal menses)
- postmenopausal bleeding
- polymenorrhea (increased frequency of menstrual bleeding)

MEDICAL MANAGEMENT

- irradiation (usually curative but induces menopause)

SURGICAL MANAGEMENT

- cryosurgery for local stage 0 tumors (involves the local freezing of abnormal cells and tissues with volatile gases, such as nitrous oxide, Freon or carbon dioxide — the dead tissue sloughs off)

- conization for local stage 0 tumors (involves the removal of a small cone of tissue with a sharp instrument)
- total abdominal hysterectomy (removal of the uterus and cervix) for carcinoma in situ, if the client is finished with childbearing
- total abdominal hysterectomy with bilateral salpingo-oophorectomy (TAH-BSO) — removal of the uterus, cervix, fallopian tubes and ovaries
- radical hysterectomy for invasive cancer (same as a TAH-BSO plus removal of the lymph nodes, upper one-third of the vagina and parametrium)
- pelvic exenteration (removal of all pelvic organs including the uterus, fallopian tubes, ovaries, vagina, bladder, rectum, colon) for invasive cancer. An ileostomy or ileal conduit also are formed.

NURSING MANAGEMENT

CRYOSURGERY OR LASER THERAPY

- Discuss that the procedure is performed with a vaginal speculum in place, much like a routine pelvic examination.
- Discuss that headaches, dizziness, flushing and some cramping may be felt during the procedure.
- Discuss use of slow deep breathing during the procedure.

For other nursing management:
- See "Uterine Tumors, Benign", p. 646, for care of the client after a hysterectomy.
- See "Radiation Therapy", p. 543, for care of the client with a radiation implant.
- See "Bladder Neoplasms (Cancer)", p. 81, for care of the client with an ileal conduit.
- See "Ulcerative Colitis", p.634, for care of the client with an ileostomy.

FOCUSED DISCHARGE CARE

Instruct client regarding:
- need for regular Pap smears and health examinations to detect possible recurrence as directed by physician

- use of mild analgesics for pain that may continue for several days
- presence of clear, watery drainage initially, which will change into a discharge containing dead cells that may be malodorous
- reporting discharge lasting longer than 8 weeks to physician
- meticulous perineal hygiene
- use of showers or sponge baths, avoidance of tub or sitz baths

IRRADIATION

- need for vaginal penetration to minimize vaginal adhesions and stenosis (may be accomplished by client's own fingers, a vaginal dilator or sexual partner's fingers or penis)
- need for vaginal lubrication

POST HYSTERECTOMY

- See "Uterine Tumors, Benign", p. 646, for discharge teaching following hysterectomy.
- If client had ovaries removed, see "Uterine Tumors, Benign", p. 646, for instructions on surgical menopause.

Also see sections listed under "Nursing Management" for discharge care for other procedures.

(For more information, see pp. 1485-1487 of Polaski and Tatro, *Luckmann's Core Principles and Practice of Medical-Surgical Nursing.*)

Chemotherapy

OVERVIEW

- Chemotherapy is the administration of cytotoxic drugs to kill or suppress tumor activity.
- The objective of cancer chemotherapy is to destroy all malignant tumor cells without excessive destruction of normal cells.
- Cancer cells reproduce in the same manner as normal cells. However, growth occurs in an uncontrolled manner. In general, cells that are actively dividing are the most sensitive to chemotherapy.
- Chemotherapy may be used as three types of treatment modalities:
  — primary treatment modality
    — chemotherapy is the only treatment used and leads to cure
  — adjuvant treatment modality
    — in conjunction with surgery
    — in conjunction with radiation therapy
  — palliative treatment modality
    — to relieve pain or obstruction
- Most types of chemotherapy do not kill all cancer cells during one exposure. Only a percentage of cancer cells will be killed with each course of chemotherapy. Repeated doses, therefore, must be used.
- Combination chemotherapy has been consistently superior to single-agent therapy. When combined, medications destroy malignant cells more effectively and produce fewer side effects.
- Chemotherapeutic agents are classified according to pharmacologic action and effect on cell generation cycle.
- Chemotherapy administration routes:
  Intravenous Routes
  — peripheral access
    • large veins in the forearm are the preferred sites
    • areas of impaired lymphatic drainage, phlebitis, impaired venous circulation, joints and sites distal to a recent venipuncture site need to be avoided

— vascular access
  - a catheter is inserted into one of the major veins of the upper chest and the distal tip advanced to the level of the superior vena cava at or above the junction of the right atrium

Intra-arterial Routes
— chemotherapy is administered into an artery of an involved organ (i.e., hepatic artery infusion for liver cancer)

Intrathecal Routes
— instillation of chemotherapy into the central nervous system through a reservoir placed in the ventricle of the brain(Omaya reservoir) or via a lumbar puncture

Intracavitary Routes
— instillation of chemotherapy directly into areas such as the abdomen, bladder or pleural space

Topical

- Antineoplastic agents are capable of damaging not only malignant cells but also certain normal cells. Normal cells most vulnerable are those that divide and proliferate rapidly, specifically cells of the bone marrow, hair and mucosa. In addition, these agents may exert organ specific toxicities resulting in cardiac, renal, hepatic, reproductive and neurologic dysfunction.

NURSING MANAGEMENT

- Check complete blood count and platelet count results before administration of chemotherapy and periodically after drug administration.
- Administer premedications (anti-emetics, sedatives) and hydration as prescribed.
- Administer chemotherapy according to institutional policy and safe handling guidelines.
- Monitor IV site for edema, redness and presence of a blood return at frequency outlined in institutional policy before, during and after infusion:
  — institutional guidelines for management of extravasation should be readily available
- Take precautions to ensure client safety when administering antineoplastics with anaphylactic potential (L-asparaginase, cisplatin, bleomycin).

— administer test dose as ordered
— stay with client the entire time the drug is administered
— have emergency drugs and equipment available
— establish a free-flowing IV line for administration of emergency drugs should the need arise
- Monitor for toxic effects of chemotherapy and implement appropriate interventions.

GASTROINTESTINAL EFFECTS:

- nausea and vomiting
- anorexia
- stomatitis, esophagitis
- taste alterations
- diarrhea
- weight loss

Management
- Administer PRN anti-emetics.
- Monitor laboratory findings — nutritional panel, electrolytes.
- Monitor intake and output.
- Daily weights.
- Perform frequent oral care and apply moisturizers and topical anesthetics.
- Encourage frequent, small, high-calorie, high-protein meals.
- Administer enteral or total parenteral nutrition as prescribed if nutritional requirements can not be met orally.
- Maintain calorie count.
- Administer PRN anti-diarrheals.

CUTANEOUS EFFECTS:

- dermatitis
- alopecia
- perianal ulcers
- hyperpigmentation

Management
- Provide meticulous skin/perineal care.
- Prepare the client for hair loss, if anticipated, and encourage the use of wigs, scarves, hats or turbans.

HEMATOPOIETIC EFFECTS:

- anemia
- thrombocytopenia
- neutropenia

Management

- Monitor temperature.
- Obtain cultures as ordered.
- Maintain protective isolation, if indicated.
- Institute bleeding precautions.
- Hematest urine, stool and NG contents.
- Do not administer rectal suppositories, enemas or perform rectal temperatures.
- Provide adequate rest.
- Administer blood component replacement therapy. See "Blood Component Therapy", p. 88.
- Monitor laboratory findings — WBC, RBC, platelet count, culture reports and absolute granulocyte count.

REPRODUCTIVE EFFECTS

- amenorrhea
- sterility
- azoospermia

Management

- Pretreatment sperm banking offers the possibility of retaining reproductive capacity for some clients

FOCUSED DISCHARGE CARE

- Instruct client regarding:
  - disease process and treatment regime
  - importance of clinic and laboratory follow-up
  - signs/symptoms to report to physician
  - care of venous access device, if in place
  - measures to protect against infection:
    - maintain adequate nutrition and fluid intake
    - avoidance of crowds, people with infections and those who have been recently vaccinated with live or attenuated vaccines
    - avoidance of contact with animal excrement
    - report fever over 100° F., cough, sore throat, chills, or painful urination immediately
    - maintain personal hygiene
    - obtain adequate rest and exercise
  - measures to reduce the risk of bleeding:

- soft toothbrush
- electric razor
- guard against falls
- report bleeding gums, increased bruising or petechiae, tarry stools, blood in urine, coffee-ground emesis, hemoptysis, epistaxis, or heavy menses immediately
- oral hygiene measures
- use of PRN anti-emetics and analgesics
- Refer to available community resources (cancer support groups).

(For more information, see pp. 9-19 of Polaski and Tatro, *Luckmann's Core Principles and Practice of Medical-Surgical Nursing.*)

Chest Trauma

- Chest injuries can result from falls, the use of certain types of machinery, or the employment of lethal weapons (guns, knives). Motor vehicle accidents are also a common cause.
- Chest injuries may be penetrating or non-penetrating.
  - Penetrating injuries are caused by bullets, knives or impaled objects. They may cause an open chest wound and permit air to enter the pleural space.
  - Non-penetrating injuries are caused by falls, blows to the chest or by deceleration injuries in motor vehicle accidents.
- General management includes:
  - initial assessment and treatment of life threatening conditions
  - maintenance of airway, breathing and circulation
  - thorough assessment and physical examination after initial emergencies are addressed
  - use of oxygen or mechanical ventilation
  - monitoring of respiratory status and arterial blood gases
  - frequent vital signs
  - monitoring for dysrhythmias

- — thoracentesis, chest tube insertion, bronchoscopic aspiration or thoracotomy as indicated
- — fluid replacement with blood, blood products or crystalloid intravenous solutions
- — monitoring for signs/symptoms of shock
- — use of analgesics to reduce pain and maximize effective breathing
- Possible complications of chest trauma include:
  - — pneumothorax
  - — tension pneumothorax and mediastinal shift
  - — open pneumothorax and mediastinal flutter
  - — hemothorax
  - — fractured ribs
  - — fractured sternum
  - — flail chest

These items are discussed individually - see index.

(For more information, see pp. 1573-1575 of Polaski and Tatro, *Luckmann's Core Principles and Practice of Medical-Surgical Nursing*.)

Chlamydial Infections

OVERVIEW

- Chlamydia trachomatis, the causative organism, is a gram-negative bacterium.
- The incidence of chlamydial infection is three times that of gonorrhea.
- The disease is always transmitted by intimate sexual contact, never casual contact.
- Infection does not cross the placenta, but exposure during delivery can cause conjunctivitis and pneumonia in newborns.
- The infection primarily affects the urethra, endocervix, and rectum.

CLINICAL MANIFESTATIONS

- Female:
  - — may be asymptomatic

- mucopurulent vaginal discharge
- friable, edematous cervix
- spotting at menstrual mid-cycle or with sexual intercourse
- dysuria
- Male:
  - may be asymptomatic
  - dysuria
  - white or clear urethral discharge

MEDICAL MANAGEMENT

All sexual contacts within 30 days before diagnosis should be treated.
- doxycycline twice daily or azithromycin given as a single dose
- repeat culture after therapy completed

NURSING MANAGEMENT

- Administer antibiotics as prescribed.
- Monitor temperature.

FOCUSED DISCHARGE CARE

Instruct client regarding:
- importance of completing the course of antibiotics and follow-up culture
- information about the disease, mode of transmission, and treatment regime
- the increased risk of infection with multiple sex partners
- importance of identifying and treating sex partners
- importance of avoiding all sexual activity until cured
- importance of the use of condoms thereafter to prevent reinfection
- medication administration:
  - take medication 1 to 2 hours after meals
  - avoid iron, dairy products, and antacids

(For more information, see pp. 1507-1508 of Polaski and Tatro, *Luckmann's Core Principles and Practice of Medical-Surgical Nursing.*)

Cholecystitis, Acute

OVERVIEW

- Acute cholecystitis refers to acute inflammation of the gallbladder wall.
- Gallstones are the major cause of acute cholecystitis. Stones obstruct the cystic duct, causing distention of the gallbladder. Subsequently, (1) venous and lymphatic drainage is impaired; (2) proliferation of bacteria occurs; (3) localized cellular irritation and/or infiltration takes place; and (4) areas of ischemia may develop. The inflamed gallbladder wall is edematous and thickened and may have areas of gangrene or necrosis.
- There is an increased incidence in clients who are overweight, especially those with sedentary lifestyles.

CLINICAL MANIFESTATIONS

- tenderness in right upper quadrant, epigastrium or both
- pain of sudden onset that steadily increases and reaches a peak in 30 minutes, located in epigastric, subscapular or right upper quadrant areas, sometimes referred to the right scapula
- positive Murphy's sign — while palpating the gallbladder, the client is asked to take a deep breath and experiences extreme tenderness and stops breathing on inspiration
- nausea and vomiting
- fever
- elevated white blood count
- mild jaundice

MEDICAL MANAGEMENT

- antibiotic therapy
- analgesics
- parenteral hydration
- nasogastric tube placement
- retrograde endoscopy, endoscopic papillotomy for stone removal (see Medical Management, "Cholelithiasis", p. 156)

SURGICAL MANAGEMENT

- cholecystectomy (removal of the gallbladder) — delayed until gallbladder inflammation has subsided with above medical management (see Surgical Management, "Cholelithiasis", p. 156)

NURSING MANAGEMENT

MEDICAL

- same as nursing management of clients with cholelithiasis except that these clients will receive a course of antibiotics (see "Cholelithiasis", p. 155)

SURGICAL

- same as nursing management for cholecystectomy (see "Cholelithiasis",   p. 156)

FOCUSED DISCHARGE CARE

(See Discharge Care, "Cholelithiasis", p. 157.)

(For more information, see pp. 1147-1149 of Polaski and Tatro, *Luckmann's Core Principles and Practice of Medical-Surgical Nursing.*)

Cholecystitis, Chronic

OVERVIEW

- Chronic cholecystitis refers to chronic inflammation of the gallbladder wall.
- Chronic cholecystitis sometimes arises as a sequelae to acute cholecystitis; however, it typically develops independently of acute cholecystitis and is almost always associated with gallstones.
- It affects middle-aged and older, obese women. The female-to-male ratio is 3:1.

CLINICAL MANIFESTATIONS

- pain — in epigastric, subscapular or right upper quadrant areas
- dyspepsia, dietary fat intolerance, flatulence

MEDICAL MANAGEMENT

- low fat diet
- weight reduction
- anticholinergics
- antacids
- analgesics

SURGICAL MANAGEMENT

- cholecystectomy — excision of the gallbladder (performed if medical management is ineffective)
  See "Cholelithiasis", p. 156.

NURSING MANAGEMENT

MEDICAL

- Administer medications as prescribed and assess effectiveness.
- Maintain low fat diet.

SURGICAL

- See "Cholelithiasis", p. 157.

FOCUSED DISCHARGE CARE

Instruct client regarding:
- medication regime
- dietary restrictions
- postoperative care for cholecystectomy, see "Cholelithiasis", p. 157.

(For more information, see p. 1149 of Polaski and Tatro, *Luckmann's Core Principles and Practice of Medical-Surgical Nursing.*)

Cholelithiasis (Gallstones)

OVERVIEW

- Cholelithiasis is the presence of gallstones in the biliary system, which is composed of the gallbladder, bile ducts and the cystic duct.
- Most gallstones form in the gallbladder but may also form in the common duct and hepatic ducts of the liver. Gallstones are divided into three groups: (1) cholesterol stones — the most common, (2) pigment stones — contain an excess of unconjugated bilirubin, and (3) mixed stones — a combination of cholesterol and pigment stones or either of these stones with another substance, i.e., calcium carbonate, phosphate, bile salts.
- It is estimated that 20 million people in the United States have gallstones. The incidence increases with age. Women account for nearly 70 per cent of those treated.
- Risk factors include:
    - diabetes mellitus
    - multiple pregnancies
    - vagotomy (removal of a section of the vagus nerve) — results in decreased gallbladder motility
    - long-term parenteral nutrition — decreases gallbladder motility
    - cirrhosis of the liver
    - obesity
    - pancreatitis

CLINICAL MANIFESTATIONS

- may be asymptomatic
- pain or biliary colic — starts in upper midline area, may radiate around to back and right shoulder blade or to the back and substernal area
- jaundice — when common bile obstruction is present
- nausea and vomiting
- bloating, dyspepsia
- intolerance to fatty foods

MEDICAL MANAGEMENT

- analgesics
- nasogastric tube placement
- intravenous therapy to maintain fluid and electrolyte balance
- retrograde endoscopy for stone removal — endoscope is passed orally through the throat into the duodenum, where a wire snare is passed into the common bile duct through the ampulla of Vater to secure and remove the stone
- oral administration of dissolution agents — urodeoxycholic acid (ursodiol)

SURGICAL MANAGEMENT

- cholecystectomy — excision of the gallbladder. The approach is usually through a right subcostal incision. Common bile duct exploration may also be performed with dilation of the common duct and stone removal by passing a fine instrument into the duct. Following exploration of the common duct, a T-tube is usually inserted to ensure adequate bile drainage during duct healing. It also provides a route for postoperative cholangiography or stone dissolution. Inserting a T-tube also prevents bile from spilling into the peritoneal cavity. The T-tube is attached to a gravity drainage system or to a collapsible bag.
- laparoscopic cholecystectomy
- extracorporeal shock wave lithotripsy — external application of shock waves to the area of stones to fragment them
- percutaneous cholecystolithotomy — use of cystoscopes, stone baskets, and instruments designed for nephrolithotomy. General anesthesia is not used.

NURSING MANAGEMENT

MEDICAL

- Administer analgesics as ordered and monitor effectiveness (Demerol is the medication most frequently ordered.)
- Administer oral dissolution agents.

- Provide a quiet, restful environment.
- Assess client for signs of dehydration - dry mucous membranes, decreased skin turgor, decreased urinary output.
- Maintain nasogastric tube — relieves distention and vomiting and removes gastric juices that stimulate cholecystokinin, which causes painful contractions of the gallbladder.
- Administer IV fluids as ordered.
- Monitor intake and output.

SURGICAL (POST CHOLECYSTECTOMY)

POSTOPERATIVE CARE

In addition to routine postoperative care:
- Provide frequent oral hygiene.
- Assess and monitor amount of T-tube drainage if placed during surgery.
  - T-tube usually drains 300-500 ml in the first 24 hours and decreases to 200 ml after 3 to 4 days
  - excessive drainage may indicate obstruction and may necessitate recycling the client's bile drainage through a nasogastric tube or orally in a medium such as fruit juice.
  - may be clamped after a few days during meals to aid fat digestion
- Assess pain, administer analgesics as ordered.

FOCUSED DISCHARGE CARE

MEDICAL

- importance of medication regime — analgesics and oral dissolution agents
- dietary restrictions — low fat, avoidance of greasy foods

SURGICAL

Post laparoscopic cholecystectomy
- wound care
- signs/symptoms of infection
- signs/symptoms to report — jaundice, dark-colored urine, pale-colored stools, and pruritus
- care of the T-tube (if in place)

- activity restrictions
- dietary restrictions
- importance of follow-up

Post-abdominal cholecystectomy
- all the above
- dressing changes and T-tube care if client discharged with T-tube in place

(For more information, see pp. 1142-1147 of Polaski and Tatro, *Luckmann's Core Principles and Practice of Medical-Surgical Nursing.*)

Chronic Airflow Limitations (CAL) or Chronic Obstructive Pulmonary Disease (COPD) (includes Chronic Obstructive Bronchitis, Emphysema)

OVERVIEW

- Chronic airflow limitation (CAL) is a term that encompasses the disorders of obstructive bronchitis, emphysema and asthma. Although the term COPD (chronic obstructive pulmonary disease) or COLD (chronic obstructive lung disease) is used commonly for this group of disorders, pulmonary specialists use the term CAL because it is more completely accurate.
- Chronic obstructive bronchitis and emphysema will be discussed in this section. Asthma is discussed under its own heading (p. 70).
- **Chronic obstructive bronchitis** is inflammation of the bronchi which causes increased mucous production and chronic cough. Thicker, more tenacious mucus and impaired ciliary function is present. The airways collapse, and air is trapped in the distal part of the lung. This obstruction leads to reduced alveolar ventilation, hypoxia and acidosis. There is

poor tissue oxygenation, a fall in PaO_2 and a rise in $PaCO_2$.

- **Emphysema** is a disorder in which the alveolar walls are destroyed, which leads to permanent overdistention of the air spaces. Air passages are obstructed due to these changes, rather than from mucous production as in chronic bronchitis. Expiration is difficult due to the destruction of the walls between the alveoli, partial airway collapse and loss of elastic recoil. As the walls collapse, pockets of air form between the alveolar spaces (called blebs) and within the lung parenchyma (bullae). There is increased ventilatory dead space.

- Cigarette smoking is the leading risk factor for this disorder. Chronic respiratory infections, aging, hereditary and genetic predisposition also may play a role.

CLINICAL MANIFESTATIONS

CHRONIC BRONCHITIS

- productive cough
- decreased exercise tolerance
- wheezing
- shortness of breath
- prolonged expiration
- elevated hematocrit, polycythemia
- cyanosis and peripheral edema
- signs/symptoms of cor pulmonale—right-sided heart failure

EMPHYSEMA

- dyspnea on exertion which progresses eventually to dyspnea at rest
- tachypnea with prolonged expiration
- use of accessory muscles
- enlarged anteroposterior diameter of the chest
- characteristic sitting position of learning forward with arms braced on knees to support the shoulders and chest for breathing
- thinness
- pink color (normal arterial oxygen levels) and dyspnea ("pink puffer")

- cor pulmonale (right-sided congestive heart failure)

MEDICAL MANAGEMENT

CHRONIC BRONCHITIS AND EMPHYSEMA

- bronchodilators, antihistamines
- steroids, antibiotics, expectorants
- mast cell membrane stabilizers
- oxygen for severe exertional or at rest hypoxemia
- nebulized bronchodilators
- positive-pressure airflow or positive end-expiratory pressure devices
- postural drainage and chest physiotherapy
- diuretics and digitalis for edema and cor pulmonale
- phlebotomy for elevations in hematocrit (>60%)

NURSING MANAGEMENT

- Assess respiratory status and report changes to physician:
  — respiratory rate, pattern, use of accessory muscles
  — arterial blood gas results
  — skin color
  — signs/symptoms of hypoxia/hypercapnia
- Maintain high-Fowler's position.
- Administer low flow oxygen — remember that the normal respiratory drive is obliterated by long-standing hypercapnia. Use caution as excessive oxygen may diminish respiratory drive.
- Monitor effectiveness of bronchodilators and assess for side effects.
- Monitor for therapeutic levels of bronchodilators.
- Encourage 8 to 10 glasses of fluid daily, if not contraindicated.
- Use caution when administering narcotics, sedatives and tranquilizers which are respiratory depressants.
- Instruct on:
  — proper coughing techniques
  — pursed lip breathing (performed during exhalation to prevent early airway collapse and to help the lungs empty more completely)
    — Encourage the client to relax and breathe in through the nose

— Next, instruct the client to exhale slowly and completely through pursed lips for a comfortable length of time. Expiration should take twice as long as inspiration.
— diaphragmatic breathing (abdominal breathing)
  — a technique that involves using the diaphragm more effectively, thereby reducing the use of accessory muscles for breathing.
    — Instruct the client to assume a comfortable semi-Fowler's position with the knees bent.
    — Place your thumbs in the client's epigastric notch, i.e., just below the xiphoid process. Comfortably spread your fingers around the lower ribs. Maintain this position.
  — Ask the client to inhale through the nose while relaxing the abdomen. The practitioner should provide gradual abdominal pressure during inspiration, pushing the thumbs "out" with the abdominal wall.
  — Instruct the client to pause naturally and briefly at the end of inspiration. This creates a smooth ventilation pattern and an even distribution of air in and out of the lungs.
  — Ask the client to exhale gently as you press inward and upward on the epigastric notch with your thumbs. Have the client contract the abdominal muscles and purse the lips during exhalation.
  — Ideally, the length of exhalation should be two to three times that of inhalation.
  — When performed properly, diaphragmatic breathing causes the abdomen to rise visibly during deep inhalation and contract during exhalation.
— program of progressive walking
— avoidance of conditions that increase oxygen demand, such as smoking, temperature extremes, excess weight and stress
— pacing activities throughout the day and energy conservation techniques
— performing active exercise after respiratory therapy or medication

- Assess for any changes in vital signs during activity and instruct client to stop if these occur.
- Remain with the client during acute episodes of dyspnea.
- During acute episodes, open doors and curtains and limit number of people in the room.
- Promote adequate nutrition:
  — encourage high-calorie liquid supplements
  — assist with oral care before meals
  — encourage 6 small meals per day
  — instruct to avoid gas producing foods (may cause abdominal bloating, distention and impair ventilation)
  — instruct to use oxygen via nasal cannula during mealtimes
  — monitor food intake, weight, serum hemoglobin and albumin levels
- Use/encourage relaxation techniques (massage, music, warm bath, warm beverage) to promote sleep.
  — Suggest patient sleep in recliner chair when dyspnea is severe.
  — Avoid caffeine and exercise in the evening.
- Provide emotional support to the family and client for coping with long-term illness.
- Facilitate discussion of changes in sexual function — suggest alternative positions, alternative forms of sexual expression (hugging, cuddling) and use of bronchodilators before sexual activity.

FOCUSED DISCHARGE CARE

- Instruct client/significant other regarding:
  — smoking cessation programs; use of nicotine patch
  — avoidance of known allergens, smoke, dust, mold, pollution and high altitudes
  — use of inhalers
  — prescribed medications, side effects and symptoms of toxicity and to report these to physician
  — importance of follow-up laboratory tests, arterial blood gases and pulmonary function tests
  — hazards of infection and ways to avoid (obtain immunizations against influenza and pneumococcal organisms, avoid crowds, cleanse respiratory equipment well)
  — signs/symptoms of impending respiratory problems (increased confusion, drowsiness) and right-

sided heart failure (peripheral edema, distended neck veins) and to report these to physician
— above information in "Nursing Management"

- Make arrangements for home oxygen therapy and instructions on use.
- Refer to Meals on Wheels if help with nutrition is needed.
- Encourage use of self-help or support groups, such as Better Breathers Club sponsored by the American Lung Association.
- Refer to a professional skilled in sexuality, if appropriate.

(For more information, see pp. 574-584 of Polaski and Tatro, *Luckmann's Core Principles and Practice of Medical-Surgical Nursing.*)

Chronic Venous Insufficiency

- Chronic venous insufficiency, also known as postphlebotic syndrome, is characterized by (1) chronic swollen limbs, (2) thick, coarse, brownish skin around the ankles (referred to as the "gaiter" area), and (3) venous stasis ulceration.
- Chronic venous insufficiency results from dysfunctional valves that reduce venous return, which increases venous pressure, causing venous stasis.
- Chronic venous insufficiency follows most severe cases of deep vein thrombosis (DVT) but may take as long as five to ten years to manifest. Therefore, clients with a history of DVT must be monitored periodically throughout their lives.
- Instruct the client regarding:
  — elevation of the legs above the heart level whenever possible when sitting or lying
  — not crossing legs
  — not using chairs that are too high for feet to touch the floor and thus apply pressure to the popliteal area
  — avoiding constrictive clothing
  — use of elastic stockings

- avoiding standing or sitting for prolonged periods of time
- importance of daily skin inspection for signs of skin cracking or ulceration
- risk factor modification

((For more information, see p. 818 of Polaski and Tatro, *Luckmann's Core Principles and Practice of Medical-Surgical Nursing.*)

Cirrhosis

OVERVIEW

- Cirrhosis of the liver is the disorganization of the liver architecture by widespread fibrosis and nodule formation. It occurs when the normal flow of blood, bile and hepatic metabolites is altered by fibrosis and changes in the hepatocytes, bile ductules, vascular channels and reticular cells.
- The two major clinical problems of cirrhosis are decreased liver function and portal hypertension.
- Risk factors include: alcohol abuse, viral hepatitis, biliary disorders, genetic predisposition with a familial tendency, congestive heart failure and exposure to industrial or chemical compounds.
- Progression of the cirrhotic process usually results in death due to hepatic encephalopathy, bacterial infection, peritonitis, liver tumor or complications of portal hypertension.
- More than 65 per cent of all cirrhosis cases are related to alcohol. Cirrhosis is the fourth leading cause of death in clients between 35 and 54 years of age. It is the ninth leading cause of death overall in the United States.

CLINICAL MANIFESTATIONS

EARLY STAGES

- hepatomegaly (enlarged liver)
- firm and nodular liver on palpation

- ascites
- prominent abdominal wall veins
- gastrointestinal bleeding (from esophageal varices)
- muscle wasting
- leg edema
- purpura/ecchymosis
- palmar erythema
- encephalopathy
- spider angiomata

MEDICAL MANAGEMENT

- adequate rest, nutritious diet high in protein (if not encephalopathic) and measures to prevent infection
- corticosteroids
- B vitamins and fat-soluble vitamins (vitamins A, D, E and K)
- control of complications (ascites, bleeding esophageal varices and hepatic encephalopathy)

NURSING MANAGEMENT

- Monitor for ascites and hepatic encephalopathy.
- Provide diet high in carbohydrates and calories with some protein, but not enough to precipitate hepatic encephalopathy.
- Maintain calorie count.
- Monitor nutritional panel.
- Restrict sodium and fluids as prescribed if ascites or edema present. (These may be admitted intravenously, in severe malabsorption.)
- Obtain daily weights.
- Measure abdominal girth daily.
- Monitor intake and output every shift.
- Provide small, frequent meals if anorexia is present.
- Administer oral fat soluble vitamins (vitamins A, D, E and K) if fat absorption present.
- Be aware that medications metabolized by the liver may require dosage adjustment or discontinuation.
- Ensure adequate rest to reduce metabolic demands on the liver.

- Assist client to plan reasonable activity with rest periods.
- Avoid administering sedatives and opiates.
- Monitor for signs/symptoms of bleeding:
  — bleeding gums
  — melena
  — purpura
  — hematuria
  — hematemesis
- Prevent bleeding:
  — maintain safety precautions
  — avoid intramuscular and subcutaneous injections, but if unavoidable, use small gauge needle
  — instruct the client to avoid vigorous nose blowing and straining with bowel movements.
  — discuss use of soft toothbrush or foam toothettes for oral care.

FOCUSED DISCHARGE CARE

- Instruct client/significant other regarding:
  — avoidance of ingesting hepatotoxins, especially alcohol
  — prevention of, and signs/symptoms of bleeding
  — need for nutritious diet high in calories, carbohydrates and protein (unless encephalopathy is present)
  — low sodium diet and fluid restriction, if needed due to edema or ascites.
  — need for potassium supplements if on a thiazide diuretic
  — signs/symptoms of fluid retention
  — signs/symptoms of progressive liver failure or complications (such as encephalopathy or bleeding varices) and when to call physician
- Refer to a substance abuse program or support groups such as Alcoholics Anonymous for assistance with abstinence from alcohol.
- Discuss importance of follow-up at regular intervals to follow progression of the disease.

Also see "Portal Hypertension", p. 529, "Ascites", p. 68, and "Hepatic Encephalopathy", p. 315 for further information.

(For more information, see pp. 1120-1125 of Polaski and Tatro, *Luckmann's Core Principles and Practice of Medical-Surgical Nursing.*)

Closed Chest Drainage

OVERVIEW

- Closed chest drainage is the use of a chest drainage system (closed to atmospheric pressure) connected to a chest catheter for the purpose of removing air or fluid from the pleural space.
- Closed chest drainage commonly is used after chest surgery and to treat pneumothorax or empyema.
- Closed chest drainage may be accomplished by glass bottle water-seal set-ups or with disposable single units (e.g., Pleur-evac). Most health care facilities now use the disposable single units.
- Three principles are used in all closed drainage systems: gravity, water seal and suction.
- (1) gravity — air and fluid flow from a higher level to a lower level
- (2) water seal — a water seal provides a barrier between atmospheric pressure (pressure on the outside of the body) and subatmospheric (negative) intrapleural pressure. On expiration, air and fluid from the pleural space travel through the drainage tubing into the first compartment. The air bubbles up through the chamber and enters atmospheric air. On inspiration, the water seal prevents atmospheric air from being sucked back into the pleural space.
- (3) suction — air or fluid moves from higher to lower pressure. A suction of 20 cm H_2O creates a subatmospheric pressure of 746 mm Hg.
- In a Pleur-evac system, the first chamber collects drainage from the pleural cavity, the second chamber acts as the water seal and the third chamber acts as the suction control.

NURSING MANAGEMENT

- Monitor the amount and type of chest tube drainage. Report abnormally large amounts of grossly bloody drainage. (Following surgery, 500 to 1000 ml may drain in the first 24 hours. Grossly bloody drainage is normal for the first few hours following surgery.)
- Monitor respiratory status and lung sounds.
- Encourage frequent coughing, deep breathing and incentive spirometry.
- Observe the water seal for tidaling (fluid in the water-seal compartment rises with inspiration and falls with expiration). If this is not present, the tubes may not be patent. (Tidaling may not occur or may be minimal in systems using suction.) If no tidaling is present:
  — check to be sure the tube is not kinked or compressed
  — milk or strip the tube (as prescribed)
  — change the client's position
  — ask the client to cough and deep breathe
- Observe for bubbling in the water-seal compartment (intermittent bubbling is normal, but constant bubbling represents an air leak and must be immediately reported to the physician).
- Maintain prescribed amount of suction and ensure continuous bubbling in suction control compartment.
- Check for air leaks in the system if the bubbling in the suction control chamber stops.
- Ensure that the atmospheric vent is not occluded.
- Ensure that all connections of the system are tight.
- Maintain patent tubing and ensure the tubing is correctly positioned, not kinked and has no dependent loops.
- Keep the drainage apparatus about two to three feet below the client's chest (if the apparatus is above the level of the client's chest, fluid from the drainage chamber is siphoned back into the pleural cavity).
- Position the client as prescribed. If turning to the side with chest tube catheters, be sure they are not compressed.
- Check the patency of drainage tubing and chest catheters frequently.
- "Milk" or "strip" chest tubes only as prescribed (routine milking or stripping is not performed because it creates excessive negative pressure).

- Maintain a clean, dry and intact dressing over the chest catheter site (a petroleum gauze pad should be placed directly over the insertion site).
- Encourage activity as prescribed, always keeping the drainage system two to three feet below the chest.
- Always keep rubber-shod clamps at the bedside — never clamp the catheter unless prescribed.
- Contact the surgeon immediately if the drainage system is accidently elevated above the client's chest.
- If a chest tube is accidently removed, cover the insertion site with sterile petroleum gauze and notify the surgeon.

(For more information, see pp. 607-613 of Polaski and Tatro, *Luckmann's Core Principles and Practice of Medical-Surgical Nursing.*)

Colon Cancer

OVERVIEW

- Cancer of the colon is the second most frequent cause of death from cancer in the United States.
- Some researchers propose that bulk in the stool and the rate of transit of fecal matter may influence the development of colon cancer. They theorize that metabolic and bacterial end products are carcinogenic and that constipation allows a longer contact with the bowel wall, thus increasing the probability of cancer developing.
- Early detection includes yearly digital rectal and stool guaiac examinations after age 40 and proctoscopic examination after age 50.
- Risk factors include:
  — family history of colon cancer
  — previous colon cancer
  — over age 40
  — ulcerative colitis
  — high fat, low residue diet that is high in refined foods
  — familial polyposis

— adenomatous polyps
— living in highly industrialized, urban societies.

CLINICAL MANIFESTATIONS

- rectal bleeding
- change in bowel habits
- intestinal obstruction
- abdominal pain
- weight loss
- anorexia
- nausea and vomiting
- anemia
- palpable mass

MEDICAL MANAGEMENT

The primary treatment for colon cancer is surgery, but medical treatment is used as an adjunct to improve survival, when the tumor cannot be completely removed.

- radiation therapy prior to surgery
- implantation of isotopes into the tumor area and electrocoagulation after surgery
- chemotherapy to reduce metastasis and control symptoms of metastasis

SURGICAL MANAGEMENT

Intervention depends upon the type of tumor, its location and stage, and on the client's general condition. A variety of surgical procedures may be performed.

- colon resection with end-to-end anastomosis:
  — removal of the tumor with several inches of colon on either side of the tumor excised — the two remaining ends are rejoined
- colon resection with a temporary or permanent colostomy
- abdominal-perineal resection with a permanent or end colostomy — removal of the entire rectum and affected colon and closure of the anus (performed for rectal tumors)

NURSING MANAGEMENT

Preoperative Care

In addition to routine preoperative care:
- Encourage diet high in calories, protein and carbohydrates but low in residue.
- Administer total parenteral nutrition as ordered.
- Perform bowel preparation as ordered:
  — low residue or liquid diet
  — administer cathartics (e.g., GoLYTELY) for 24 hours preoperatively
  — administer antibiotics for 24 to 48 hours preoperatively
  — administer enemas
  — administer blood transfusions to correct anemia.
- Consult and discuss role of enterostomal therapist and reinforce teaching done by enterostomal therapist:
  — enterostomal therapist selects site
  — enterostomal therapist instructs on ostomy care.

Postoperative Care

In addition to routine postoperative care:

Colon Resection with Temporary or Permanent Colostomy

- Monitor colostomy output.
- Use care to keep fecal contents away from the incisional site.
- Assess the stoma for ischemia. If the stoma becomes dark or dusky, notify the physician immediately.
- Ensure that the colostomy pouch is not applying any pressure to the stoma, interfering with its blood supply.
- Assess for return of bowel sounds.
- Maintain nasogastric suction.
- Assess for abdominal cramps or abdominal distention. Report to physician (a rectal tube may be needed).
- Provide emotional support and encourage discussion of feelings and concerns.
- Encourage participation in care.
- Instruct on ostomy care:
  — application of pouch

- — emptying pouch
- — stoma care
- — colostomy irrigation (if end colostomy was performed)
- — stoma dilation to prevent strictures.
- • Encourage discussion of concerns regarding sexuality .

Abdominal-Perineal Resection

- • Maintain perineal drains and assess the character, volume and odor of the drainage.
- • Change rectal dressings as needed.
- • Provide sitz baths 3 to 4 times daily.
- • Encourage side-lying position.
- • Prevent postoperative phlebitis (increased risk due to the high lithotomy position used during surgery).
  - — Assess for Homan's sign.
  - — Assess for any redness, swelling or cords in calf area.
  - — Administer subcutaneous Heparin as ordered.
  - — Assist with leg exercises.
  - — Apply sequential pressure boots as prescribed.
  - — Maintain thigh high antiembolism stockings.

FOCUSED DISCHARGE CARE

- • Instruct client regarding:
  - — dressing change
  - — signs/symptoms of infection to report to physician
  - — colostomy care, if applicable
  - — dietary or activity restrictions
  - — signs/symptoms of intestinal obstruction and perforation
  - — colostomy care (if applicable) including:
    - — management of diarrhea:
      - • medications to control
      - • prevention of electrolyte imbalance
      - • prevention of skin breakdown
    - — management of constipation
    - — management of flatus:
      - • holding purse, jacket, arm over colostomy
      - • use of odor proof pouches or charcoal filter discs
      - • avoidance of gas causing foods

— also see items listed in Nursing Management, Preoperative Care
- Assess need for home health referral.
- Discuss need for follow-up with enterostomal therapist.
- Refer to ostomy support groups/American Cancer Society.

(For more information, see pp. 1071-1087 of Polaski and Tatro, *Luckmann's Core Principles and Practice of Medical-Surgical Nursing.*)

Coma

OVERVIEW

- Coma is a state of sustained unconsciousness. The client in a coma does not respond to verbal stimuli, has varying responses to painful stimuli, may not move voluntarily, has altered respiratory patterns, may exhibit altered pupillary responses to light, and does not blink. In general, the longer the state of unconsciousness lasts, the more likely it is due to a permanent disorder in the structure of the brain (and irreversible), rather than a temporary alteration in function (and reversible).
- To produce unconsciousness, a disorder must (1) disrupt the ascending reticular activating system that is found in the center of the brain stem and thalamus; (2) significantly disrupt the function of both cerebral hemispheres; or (3) metabolically depress the cerebrum or reticular activity system.
- Three kinds of disorders produce sustained unconsciousness. They are:
  (1) structural lesions in the brain that place pressure on the brain stem or in the posterior fossa—brain tumors, concussion, head trauma and cerebral hemorrhage
  (2) metabolic disorders, which impair the usual functions of the cerebrum by decreasing the oxygen supply or by allowing waste products to accumu-

late. Common causes include hypoxia, blood loss, high altitudes, carbon monoxide poisoning, drug overdose, ischemia, disorders of the liver, lungs and kidneys, poisons, hypoglycemia, fever, infection, fluid, electrolyte or acid-base imbalance.

(3) psychogenic causes, in which the client looks comatose but self-awareness is usually intact, such as seen in catatonia.

- Some clients in a coma awaken slowly and begin to respond normally. They may require physical and speech therapy to regain previous levels of function. Irreversible coma, also called cerebral death, is due to damage to the cerebral hemispheres, leaving the client unable to respond to the environment. The brain stem and cerebellum remain intact, and vital functions, such as heart, lung, and gastrointestinal functions, exist. Clients may remain in irreversible coma for years.
- Brain damage is irreversible damage to the cerebrum, cerebellum and brain stem. There is no hope for recovery, and life is maintained with a respirator and vasoactive drugs.

CLINICAL MANIFESTATIONS

- no motor or verbal response to the environment or any stimuli, even deep pain or suctioning
- change in respiratory rate or rhythm
  — Cheyne-Stokes — respirations that become faster and deeper than normal, then slower, alternating with periods of apnea
  — central neurogenic hyperventilation — sustained, regular, rapid respirations with forced inspiration and expiration
  — apneustic breathing - prolonged, gasping inspirations followed by extremely short, inefficient expirations
  — cluster breathing — clusters of irregular respirations alternating with longer periods of apnea
  — ataxic breathing — completely irregular pattern with random deep and shallow respirations
- impaired eye movement
  — dysconjugate gaze (conjugate deviation) — eyes do not track together

- — doll's eye test — doll's eyes are present if the eyes move to the right when the head is rotated to the left and vice versa
- — abnormal caloric test — failure to produce nystagmus (involuntary oscillation of the eyes) when water is instilled in the ear canal
- — eyes appear to be slowly jumping up and down or roving
- • pupillary changes
  - — fixed and dilated
  - — pinpoint
  - — unequal
- • posturing
  - — decorticate — abnormal flexion of arms, wrists and fingers with arms abducted, legs fully extended and internally rotated ,with feet in plantar flexion
  - — decerebrate — arms are extended and abducted, and hands are hyperpronated
- • impaired motor function
  - — primitive sucking or snort reflexes
  - — strong reflexic hand grasp
  - — restlessness
  - — resistance to passive movement
  - — hemiplegia
  - — hemiparesis
  - — seizures
  - — flaccidity
- • decreased pulse
- • widened pulse pressure (the difference between systolic and diastolic pressure readings)
- • abnormal deep tendon reflexes
- • loss of corneal reflex (client does not blink when sterile gauze or cotton is touched to the sclera)

MEDICAL MANAGEMENT

The goal of medical management is to remove or correct the cause. In the interim, the brain must be protected from further injury.
- • respiratory support — airway, intubation, ventilation
- • circulatory support — blood pressure monitoring, vasoactive drugs
- • diazepam (Valium) to control seizures

- parenteral therapy to correct fluid, acid-base or electrolyte imbalances
- osmotic or loop diuretics (Mannitol, furosemide) or corticosteroids to relieve cerebral edema
  — overhydration and IV fluids with glucose are avoided because cerebral edema may follow
- drug antidotes and gastric lavage for drug overdose
- nutritional support
- prevention of complications — heparin administration, pulmonary hygiene, etc.

NURSING MANAGEMENT

- Perform complete neurologic and mental status assessments, compare with previous assessments and note trends.
  — The glasgow coma scale (GCS) is the most common neurologic assessment tool. The scale provides objective measurements of three essential components — eye opening, best motor response, and best verbal response. The three components are scored, totalled, and range from 3 to 15. The client who is unresponsive to painful stimuli, does not open the eyes, and is flaccid has a score of three.
- Monitor for signs of airway obstruction (the most common source of harm to patients with decreased consciousness), abnormal lung sounds, cyanosis, unequal lung expansion, and stridor.
- Maintain respiratory support — oral airway, intubation, tracheostomy.
- Position patient in a lateral position with head elevated 30 degrees to facilitate drainage of secretions and to prevent tongue from obstructing the airway.
- Perform tracheobronchial suctioning as needed. Never suction the nasal passages in patients who have had brain surgery or head injuries.
- Institute aspiration precautions.
- Monitor arterial blood gases and oxygen saturation results.
- Maintain NPO status.
- Reposition every 2 hours. Extreme rotation and flexion of the neck are avoided because these positions compress the jugular veins and increase ICP. Extreme hip flexion is avoided because this position

increases intra-abdominal and intrathoracic pressure which increases ICP.

- Monitor for signs of increased intracranial pressure— seizure activity, bradycardia, posturing, hypertension with widened pulse pressure.
- Administer loop diuretics and steroids.
- Frequent oral care.
- Monitor skin for areas of breakdown and implement preventive measures — foam mattress, low air loss bed, meticulous hygiene.
- Prevent corneal abrasion and irritation with moisturizing eye drops and eye shields.
- Maintain extremities in functional positions.
- Perform passive range of motion exercises.
- Daily weights.
- Monitor intake and output. Over hydration and IV fluids with glucose are avoided because cerebral edema may follow.
- Monitor laboratory results — hemoglobin, electrolytes, nutritional panel, white blood count.
- Administer nasogastric feedings. Monitor residual amounts and ensure correct placement.
- Institute appropriate safety measures.
- Monitor for signs of complications — deep vein thrombosis, pulmonary embolism, constipation.
- Offer support to significant others.

FOCUSED DISCHARGE CARE

The site for discharge placement is totally dependent upon the condition of the client and the cause of the coma. If the client is still in a coma and recovery is expected, placement in a rehabilitation center is planned. If client is in a coma but not expected to awaken, placement in a skilled nursing center is common.

(For more information, see pp. 284-299 of Polaski and Tatro, *Luckmann's Core Principles and Practice of Medical-Surgical Nursing.*)

Confusional States

OVERVIEW

- Confusion is a mental state marked by alterations in thought and attention deficit followed by problems in comprehension. Confusion is accompanied by a loss of short-term memory and often irritability alternating with drowsiness.
- Three mechanisms account for the development of acute confusion: (1) damage to the brain with swelling or loss of oxygen, blood or both; (2) impairment of the action of the nervous system by chemicals or other substances (metabolic disorder); and, (3) the rebound overactivity of a previously depressed center in the brain. Injury results in increased intracranial pressure. Chemicals that cross the blood-brain barrier impair the metabolism of the neuronal cells. When drug action wears off or a drug is withdrawn, the lower centers of the brain become over active.
- Chronic confusional states (dementia) are due to disorders that cause brain tissue destruction, biochemical imbalances or compression of the brain.
- Common causes of confusion include:
  — trauma
  — alcohol withdrawal
  — drug ingestion
  — fever
  — heart failure
  — hypoxia
  — hypoglycemia
  — severe fluid and electrolyte imbalance
  — sepsis
  — liver and renal failure
  — poisons
  — Alzheimer's disease
  — neoplasms
  — stroke
  — viruses (Creutzfeldt-Jakob disease)

CLINICAL MANIFESTATIONS

- attention deficit
- restlessness

- emotional lability
- insomnia and vivid nightmares
- anxiousness
- agitation
- fluctuations in cognition
- difficulty with immediate recall and ability to abstract
- hallucinations, illusions and delusions

MEDICAL MANAGEMENT

- determination and correction of the cause
- control of symptoms
- nutritional support

SURGICAL MANAGEMENT

There are no surgical interventions unless confusion is due to a structural disorder, such as a tumor or hematoma.

NURSING MANAGEMENT

- Assess mental and behavioral status, compare to previous assessments and note trends.
- Maintain consistency in environment and routine.
- Give simple instructions and explanations.
- Reorient as necessary. Clients with chronic untreatable confusion do not benefit from reorientation and may become more agitated at attempts to reorient.
- Provide clock and calendar in room.
- Keep room quiet and softly lit without producing shadows.
- Allow use of familiar objects from home.
- Implement safety measures:
  — room close to nursing station
  — bed in low position, side rails up
  — mechanical and chemical restraints as indicated
- Allow for uninterrupted sleep.
- Keep client active during the daytime hours to promote sleep.
- Encourage balanced diet.

See care of client, "Alzheimer's Disease", p. 28.

FOCUSED DISCHARGE CARE

- Instruct family regarding:

- — safety measures
- — measures to decrease confusion —
  - — frequent reorientation
  - — quiet environment
  - — simple instructions
- — use of hypnotics and sedatives
- — importance of balanced diet
- Refer to available community resources.

(For more information, see pp. 299-302 of Polaski and Tatro, *Luckmann's Core Principles and Practice of Medical-Surgical Nursing.*)

Congestive Heart Failure

OVERVIEW

- Congestive heart failure (CHF) is defined as a physiologic state in which the heart is unable to pump enough blood to meet the metabolic needs of the body (determined as oxygen consumption) at rest or during exercise, even though filling pressures are adequate. Heart failure is not a disease itself; instead, the term denotes a group of manifestations related to inadequate pump performance. Pump failure results in hypoperfused tissue, followed by pulmonary and systemic venous congestion.
- The myocardium of the left ventricle may either (1) be diseased and unable to meet normal circulatory demands or (2) be intrinsically normal but unable to meet increased circulatory needs. When failure first begins, the left ventricle fails to eject a sufficient amount of blood. At this point, the compensatory mechanisms of sympathetic nervous system activation (tachycardia, dilation, and hypertrophy) come into play. When these mechanisms fail, the amount of blood remaining in the left ventricle at the end of diastole increases. This increase in residual blood in turn decreases the ventricle's capacity to receive blood from the left atrium. The left atrium, having to work harder to eject blood, dilates and hypertrophies. It is unable to receive the full amount of

incoming blood from the pulmonary veins, and left atrial pressure increases. This leads to subsequent pulmonary congestion, pulmonary edema, and respiratory symptoms. The right ventricle, because of the increased pressure in the pulmonary vascular system, must now dilate and hypertrophy to meet the increase workload and it too eventually fails.

- The healthy heart can meet the demands of life though the use of cardiac reserve (the ability to increase output in response to stress). The failing heart, even at rest, is pumping near its capacity and has lost much of its reserve.

- Right ventricular failure usually follows left sided failure. Occasionally, right sided failure develops independently of left ventricular failure. Causes include: pulmonary diseases, constrictive pericarditis, tricuspid and pulmonic valve disorders.

- Causes of congestive heart failure include:
  — congenital heart defects
  — systemic hypertension
  — pulmonary hypertension
  — valvular stenosis or regurgitation
  — cardiac tamponade
  — cardiomyopathy
  — conditions that precipitate heart failure — dysrhythmias, physical or emotional stress, infection, anemia, thyroid disorders, pulmonary disease, pregnancy, myocardial infarction, hypervolemia, etc.

CLINICAL MANIFESTATIONS

LEFT VENTRICULAR FAILURE:

- dyspnea
- weakness, fatigue
- mental confusion
- insomnia
- anorexia
- diaphoresis
- anxiety
- edema (peripheral)
- orthopnea or paroxysmal nocturnal dyspnea (PND)
- tachycardia, premature atrial contractions
- S_3, S_4
- pulmonary crackles

- enlarged point of maximal impulse
- elevated pulmonary artery wedge pressure
- cough
- nocturia
- signs of acute pulmonary edema — severe dyspnea; orthopnea;pallor; tachycardia; frothy, blood-tinged sputum; and cyanosis

Right ventricular failure:

- weight gain
- ankle or pretibial swelling
- abdominal distention
- anorexia, nausea, gastric distress
- pitting edema in dependent areas
- ascites
- jugular vein distention
- hepatomegaly
- increased central venous pressure
- subcostal pain
- anxiety

MEDICAL MANAGEMENT

- oxygen administration
- digitalis therapy to improve contractility
- pre-load reduction:
  — diuretics — furosemide (Lasix), ethacrynic acid
  — sodium and fluid restriction
  — high Fowler's position
- afterload reduction:
  — vasodilators — nitroprusside, nitroglycerin, hydralazine, isosorbide dinitrate, prazosin
  — physical and emotional stress reduction
- inotropic agents (facilitate myocardial contractility and enhance stroke volume) — dopamine, dobutamine, amrinone)
- angiotensin-converting enzyme (ACE) inhibitors (suppresses renin - angiotensin - aldosterone system) - captopril. Ace inhibitors have been shown to prolong survival of clients with CHF.
- dietary modifications — low sodium, high potassium, water restriction

Refractory heart failure— heart failure is termed refractory or intractable when recommended diet, medications, and interventions fail to alleviate symptoms and restore partial cardiac reserve. Medical management includes:

- a prolonged period of complete bedrest
- severe sodium restriction
- severe fluid restriction
- diuretic therapy with several different medications

SURGICAL MANAGEMENT

- venoarterial bypass — diverts blood to a pump or counterpulsation device that returns the blood to the arterial tree allowing the heart to rest and recuperate
- cardiac transplantation or artificial heart

NURSING MANAGEMENT

MEDICAL

- Monitor intake and output.
- Maintain fluid restriction.
- Provide frequent oral care.
- Daily weights.
- Monitor laboratory results — electrolytes, digoxin level.
- Assess for signs/symptoms of decreased cardiac output.
- Assess heart rate and rhythm.
- Auscultate heart sounds.
- Assess for changes in mental status.
- Monitor blood pressure closely with diuretic and vasodilator therapy.
- Assess for jugular vein distention, peripheral or sacral edema, hepatic engorgement, or pain in right upper quadrant.
- Administer oxygen therapy and monitor arterial blood gas results and oxygen saturations.
- Assess lung sounds.
- Maintain high-Fowler's positioning with legs in a dependent position as much as possible.
- Monitor for digitalis toxicity — bradycardia, first-degree heart block, "colored vision", headache, fatigue, anorexia, etc.
- Maintain sodium restricted diet.

- Promote adequate rest, quiet environment.
- Monitor response to diuretic therapy — increased urinary output, decreased peripheral edema, clear lung sounds.
- Monitor for signs of hypokalemia due to diuretic therapy — lethargy, hypotension, muscle cramping. Hypokalemia, a particularly dangerous problem, potentiates digitalis toxicity and can cause myocardial weakness and cardiac arrhythmias.
- Monitor response to inotropic and vasodilator therapy — increased activity tolerance, increased urinary output, improved respiratory status.
- Monitor cardiopulmonary response to progressive exercise program.

FOCUSED DISCHARGE CARE

Instruct the client regarding:
- importance of medication regime
- dietary modifications — low sodium, high potassium and possible fluid restriction
- need to avoid salt substitutes, which are usually high in potassium
- importance of avoiding over-the-counter preparations, such as alkalizers, cough remedies, laxatives, and pain relievers that contain sodium
- importance of potassium supplement if taking non-potassium sparing diuretics (furosemide, thiazides, ethacrynic acid) to prevent dysrhythmias and digitalis toxicity
- signs/symptoms of increasing heart failure
- activity restrictions
- need for adequate rest
- importance of follow-up visits

(For more information, see pp. 691-706 of Polaski and Tatro, *Luckmann's Core Principles and Practice of Medical-Surgical Nursing.*)

Conn's Syndrome

OVERVIEW

- Conn's syndrome is a hypersecretion of aldosterone due to an adrenal tumor.
- Conn's syndrome affects females twice as often as males.
- Hypersecretion of aldosterone affects the tubular reabsorption of sodium and water and the excretion of potassium and hydrogen ions. Hypersecretion of aldosterone leads to hypokalemia, hypernatremia, hypervolemia, and metabolic alkalosis.

CLINICAL MANIFESTATIONS

- hypertension
- hypernatremia
- hypokalemia with muscle weakness and cardiac dysrhythmias
- metabolic alkalosis
- overt edema is rare because excess water is excreted with potassium ions

MEDICAL MANAGEMENT

- antihypertensive therapy
- potassium replacement
- renal support

SURGICAL MANAGEMENT

Surgical management is the treatment of choice.
- unilateral or bilateral adrenalectomy (removal of the adrenal gland(s))

NURSING MANAGEMENT

- See "Cushing's Syndrome", p. 194.

FOCUSED DISCHARGE CARE

Instruct client regarding:
- importance of daily hormonal replacement

- medication injection technique should client not tolerate oral medication
- signs of under and over-dosage
- need to call for dosage adjustment if experiencing physical or emotional stress
- dietary modifications
- need for Medic Alert bracelet and card

(For more information, see pp. 1241-1243 of Polaski and Tatro, *Luckmann's Core Principles and Practice of Medical-Surgical Nursing.*)

Corneal Dystrophies

OVERVIEW

- Corneal dystrophies are a group of hereditary and acquired disorders of unknown etiology, characterized by deposits in the layers of the cornea and alteration of corneal structure.
- Specific dystrophies characteristically appear at different ages. They may be stationary or slowly progressive. The most common, Fuch's dystrophy, usually begins in the third or fourth decade, affects women more than men and is slowly progressive.

CLINICAL MANIFESTATIONS

- cloudy cornea
- pain
- visual impairment

MEDICAL MANAGEMENT

None

SURGICAL MANAGEMENT

- keratoplasty (corneal transplantation) obtained from cadaver donors

NURSING MANAGEMENT

In addition to routine postoperative care:
- Maintain eye patch and shield in place.
- Administer PRN analgesics.
- Monitor for signs/symptoms of increased ocular pressure (pain, nausea).
- Assist with ambulation and activities of daily living.
- Administer antibiotic/steroid eye drops.

FOCUSED DISCHARGE CARE

Instruct client regarding:
- technique for instilling eye drops
- importance of eye protection (glasses, shields)
- eye care
- signs/symptoms of graft rejection:
  — redness
  — swelling
  — decreased vision
  — pain
- the need to evaluate the vision in the operative eye each day and if no improvement is noted or vision is worse, to notify physician
- signs/symptoms of increased intraocular pressure (pain, nausea, decreased vision)
- signs/symptoms of infection (redness, swelling, drainage, blurred vision or pain)
- safety measures for the home environment
- importance of follow-up clinic visits

(For more information, see pp. 447-448 of Polaski and Tatro, *Luckmann's Core Principles and Practice of Medical-Surgical Nursing*.)

Corneal Ulcers

OVERVIEW

- Corneal ulcers that severely damage the integrity of the eye are often caused by a corneal infection (keratitis). Sources of infection include staphylococcus aureus, Pseudomonas aeruginosa, streptococcus pneumoniae, candida and herpes zoster. Clients with a systemic collagen disease, such as rheumatoid arthritis, are susceptible to infection and ulceration.

CLINICAL MANIFESTATIONS

- tearing
- photophobia
- blurred vision
- pain that worsens with eye movement

MEDICAL MANAGEMENT

- topical antibiotic, antifungal or antiviral therapy (may need to be instilled every 15 minutes around the clock to prevent progression to perforation)
- analgesics

SURGICAL MANAGEMENT

- tarsorrhaphy (suturing the eyelid shut)

NURSING MANAGEMENT

MEDICAL

- Administer eye drops as ordered.
- Administer PRN analgesics.
- Promote effective rest and sleep.
- Cleanse the eyes to remove crustation.

FOCUSED DISCHARGE CARE

Instruct client regarding:
- technique for instilling eye drops
- signs/symptoms of increasing infection (redness, swelling, drainage, blurred vision or pain)
- eye care
- measures for a safe home environment
- importance of follow-up clinic appointments

(For more information, see p. 449 of Polaski and Tatro, *Luckmann's Core Principles and Practice of Medical-Surgical Nursing.*)

Coronary Artery Disease

OVERVIEW

- The heart muscle must have an adequate blood supply to contract properly. When a coronary artery is narrowed or blocked, the area of the heart muscle supplied by that artery becomes ischemic and injured, and infarction (tissue death) may result. The major disorders due to insufficient blood supply to the myocardium are: angina pectoris, congestive heart failure (CHF), and myocardial infarction (MI). These disorders are collectively known as coronary artery disease (CAD), also called ischemic heart disease (ISHD).
- CAD results from the development of obliterative artherosclerotic lesions within the coronary arteries that narrow and obstruct these vessels.
- Coronary artery disease is the leading cause of death in Americans today.
- Risk factors can be presented in three categories:
  (1) Nonmodifiable risk factors that cannot be changed:
  — heredity — hypertension, dyslipidemia, diabetes, and obesity
  — age —appears predominantly in clients over 40
  — gender — affects men more often than women
  — race — black men die more frequently from CAD than white men.
  (2) Modifiable risk factors that can be changed:
  — environment—urban, less affluent populations have a higher incidence
  — cigarette smoking — smokers have more than twice the risk of heart attack than do nonsmokers. Clients who quit smoking lose their increased risk in 24 months.
  — hypertension — hypertensive clients have a 50 per cent higher chance of mortality.
  — elevated serum cholesterol — clients with elevated serum cholesterol are 3 times more likely to develop coronary artery disease.
  — diabetes — frequently appears in middle-aged, overweight clients and contributes to increased risk for coronary artery disease.

(3) Contributing factors:
— obesity
— lack of exercise
— response to stress

- Coronary artery disease is a progressive disorder; if not prevented or treated in early stages, it will progress to more severe forms of cardiac disorders. Common sequelae include sudden cardiac death, angina pectoris, and myocardial infarction. In addition, clients may develop heart failure, chronic dysrhythmias, conduction disturbances, and unstable angina.

CLINICAL MANIFESTATIONS

Atherosclerosis, by itself, does not necessarily produce symptoms. For manifestations to develop, there must be a critical deficit in blood supply to the heart in proportion to the demands of the myocardium for oxygen and nutrients. When atherosclerosis progresses slowly, the collateral circulation that develops generally can meet the heart's demands.

- See "Angina Pectoris", p. 51.

MEDICAL MANAGEMENT

- reduction of cholesterol and fat intake
- smoking cessation
- diabetic management
- hypertension management
- cholestyramine (Questran) and colestipol (Colestid) to decrease serum cholesterol levels

SURGICAL MANAGEMENT

- percutaneous transluminal coronary angioplasty (PTCA)—ballon-tipped catheter is inserted and "floated" into a blocked artery. The balloon is then inflated to mechanically dilate the artery.
- atherectomy—uses a device with a balloon and motorized cutter. The cutter is positioned against the blockage and mechanically debrides the plaque.
- intravascular stent—a coilspring tube is placed in the coronary artery and acts as a mechanical scaffold to reopen the blocked artery.

- laser therapy—after initial balloon angioplasty, a brief burst of laser radiation vaporizes remaining plaque.
- coronary artery bypass graft (CABG) surgery—invloves the bypass of a blockage in one or more coronary arteries using saphenous or mammary veins as replacement vessels. A median sternotomy approach is used. The distal end of the vein is sutured to the aorta and the proximal end to the coronary vessel distal to the blockages.

NURSING MANAGEMENT

MEDICAL

- See "Angina Pectoris," pg. 51

SURGICAL

- Post PTCA/atherectomy
  - monitor vital signs and arterial line pressure readings.
  - monitor heparin infusion
  - monitor cardiac rhythm continuously
  - keep affected extremity straight
    - monitor catheter insertion site for bleeding and hematoma
    - check circulation, sensation and movement distal to insertion site
  - maintain bed rest
- See "Cardiac Surgery," pg. 119

FOCUSED DISCHARGE CARE

MEDICAL

- Instruct client regarding:
  - disease process and treatment regime
  - dietary modifications
  - establishing an exercise program
  - stress management
- Facilitate referral to smoking cessation and weight reduction programs.

(For more information, see pp. 674-679 of Polaski and Tatro, *Luckmann's Core Principles and Practice of Medical-Surgical Nursing.*)

Crohn's Disease (Regional Enteritis)

OVERVIEW

- Crohn's disease is a type of inflammatory bowel disease characterized by periods of exacerbation and remission. The disease usually is slow and unaggressive and involves the entire thickness of the bowel wall (transmural) and particularly the submucosa. Lesions typically develop in several separate segments of the bowel.
- The lesions ulcerate and fissures develop, which can lead to fistulas and abscesses. The small bowel wall becomes congested and thickened and the lumen narrows. In late disease, the intestinal wall becomes permanently fibrosed, thickened and narrowed.
- Transient arthritis develops in 20% of clients with Crohn's disease.
- The disease is considered autoimmune, and there may be a genetic or hereditary factor.
- It is most common in whites, Jewish people and people in their 30's. Both sexes are affected equally.

CLINICAL MANIFESTATIONS

- intermittent abdominal pain, weight loss
- steatorrhea
- soft or semi-liquid diarrheal stool
- anorexia, anemia, debility, fatigue
- nutritional deficits
- acute inflammatory symptoms:
  — right lower quadrant pain
  — cramping, tenderness
  — flatulence, nausea, diarrhea
  — borborygmus (stomach rumbling), increased peristalsis

MEDICAL MANAGEMENT

- anti-inflammatory therapy, including steroids
- fluid, electrolyte and blood replacement
- antidiarrheal preparations (Imodium)
- hydrophilic mucilloids (e.g., psyllium or methylcellulose)
- antispasmodics
- antibiotic agents and sulfonamides (e.g., sulfasalazine)
- bowel rest
- total parenteral nutrition
- antacids and histamine receptor antagonists
- anticholinergics during acute exacerbations
- diet high in protein and calories

SURGICAL MANAGEMENT

Surgery is used only to treat complications of Crohn's disease because there is a 50% chance of recurrence, even when the diseased portion is removed.

- ileotransverse colectomy, segmental colectomy or total colectomy with ileorectal anastomosis for colon disease

NURSING MANAGEMENT

- Administer antidiarrheals as prescribed.
- Monitor the number, color and consistency of stools — hematest all stools.
- Monitor intake and output; daily weights.
- Provide good perianal skin care — cleanse skin with warm water after each bowel movement and apply protective moisture barrier product.
- Administer total parenteral nutrition as prescribed.
- Monitor nutritional intake.
  — Monitor intake of fluids and food — encourage small servings of bland and easily digested foods.
  — Offer nutritional supplements.
- Assess quality of pain and note any changes, as this may signal the onset of complications.
- Administer pain medications as prescribed and assess effectiveness.
- Discuss stress management and relaxation techniques (stress may cause exacerbations).

FOCUSED DISCHARGE CARE

- Instruct client regarding:
  — diet high in calories and proteins
  — total parenteral nutrition administration and care of venous access device
  — perianal skin care
  — side effects of steroids
  — importance of follow-up physical examinations and colonoscopy every one to two years
  — signs/symptoms of fluid/electrolyte imbalance
  — exacerbating factors - dietary indiscretion, emotional upsets or illness
  — keeping a record of stools, their consistency and color and the presence of blood
  — reporting significant weight loss to physician
  — signs/symptoms of nutritional deficiency
- Make home health referral for total parenteral nutrition administration.
- Refer to Crohn's and Colitis Foundations of America for support groups and information.

(For more information, see pp. 1061-1071 of Polaski and Tatro, *Luckmann's Core Principles and Practice of Medical-Surgical Nursing.*)

Cushing's Syndrome

OVERVIEW

- Cushing's syndrome results from over-activity of the adrenal gland, resulting in hypersecretion of glucocorticoids.
- When Cushing's syndrome develops, the normal function of the glucocorticoids becomes exaggerated, causing persistent hyperglycemia and protein tissue wasting.
- Cushing's syndrome occurs mainly in women.
- Average age of onset is 20 to 40 years of age.
- Hypersecretion of cortisol can be caused by:
  — a cortisol-secreting tumor (most of which are benign)

— adrenal hyperplasia caused by overproduction of ACTH. The two sources of excessive ACTH secretion are (1) pituitary hypersecretion and benign pituitary tumors, and (2) ectopic ACTH secretion.
— administration of exogenous steroids

CLINICAL MANIFESTATIONS

- weakness
- ecchymosis (secondary to capillary fragility)
- osteoporosis (due to bone matrix wasting), compression fractures, stress fractures
- hypokalemia
- hypertension, edema (due to sodium and water retention)
- abnormal fat distribution:
  — moon-shaped face
  — dorsocervical fat pad (buffalo hump)
  — truncal obesity with slender limbs
- increased susceptibility to infection
- poor wound healing
- acne, thinning of scalp hair, and hirsutism
- memory loss, euphoria, and depression
- personality changes ("steroid psychosis")

MEDICAL MANAGEMENT

- radiation therapy for pituitary tumors and adenomas
  — external
  — internal — transphenoidal implant (approach through the inner aspect of the upper lip to implant radiation seeds)
- cytoxic antihormonal agents — interfere with ACTH production or adrenal hormone synthesis

SURGICAL MANAGEMENT

Surgical management is the treatment of choice.
- transphenoidal hypophysectomy (approach through the inner aspect of the upper lip for pituitary tumor removal)
- adrenalectomy (removal of adrenal glands)

NURSING MANAGEMENT

MEDICAL

- Monitor closely for signs/symptoms of infection. (Glucocorticoids suppress immune and inflammatory reactions. Cushing's syndrome clients may experience only mild symptoms even in the presence of severe infection.)
- Protect against falls and accidents.
- Monitor vital signs, assess for hypertension.
- Daily weights.
- Monitor intake and output.
- Monitor electrolytes and blood glucose.
- Test urine for acetone daily.
- Initiate a progressive activity schedule and assess client's response.
- Monitor skin for breakdown (extremely prone to breakdown secondary to tissue catabolism).
- Reassure client and significant others that mood swings and changes in appearance should gradually return to normal with treatment.

SURGICAL

In addition to routine postoperative care:
- Adrenalectomy:
  — Monitor for signs of shock (due to hemorrhage).
  — Administer corticosteroids as prescribed to protect from acute adrenal insufficiency. Even if only one adrenal gland is removed, temporary corticoid support may be needed until remaining gland begins to secrete sufficient amounts of cortisol.
  — Monitor for signs of Addisonian crisis:
    — sudden profound weakness
    — severe abdominal, back and leg pain
    — hyperpyrexia followed by hypothermia
    — coma
    — renal shutdown
  — Monitor for signs of wound or respiratory infection.
- Transphenoidal hypophysectomy
  — Assess for signs of cerebral edema and rising intracranial pressure (elevated blood pressure, widened pulse pressure, bradycardia, altered respiratory pattern).

— Monitor for signs of target gland deficiencies (pituitary no longer produces tropic hormones):
  — adrenal insufficiency
  — hypothyroidism
  — diabetes insipidus (ADH deficiency)
— Assess for signs of meningitis (elevated temperature, headache, irritability, nuchal rigidity).
— Provide frequent oral hygiene.
— Observe client for rhinorrhea after nasal packing removed — can indicate a cerebrospinal fluid (CSF) leak.

FOCUSED DISCHARGE CARE

Instruct client regarding:
- importance of taking daily replacement hormone
- medication injection technique if client not able to tolerate oral medications
- signs of under and over-dosage
- need to call for dosage adjustment if experiencing physical or emotional stress
- dietary modifications
- post-hypophysectomy
  — need to report persistent postnasal drainage
  — need to avoid sneezing, coughing, and bending from the waist for specified period of time
  — need for Medic Alert bracelet or card
- post-bilateral adrenalectomy
  — need for Medic Alert bracelet or card
  — need to carry prepared syringe of hydrocortisone in case of emergency.

(For more information, see pp. 1237-1241 of Polaski and Tatro, *Luckmann's Core Principles and Practice of Medical-Surgical Nursing.*)

Cystic Fibrosis

OVERVIEW

- Cystic Fibrosis (CF) is a hereditary, chronic disease characterized by abnormal secretion of the exocrine glands.
- Pancreatic exocrine function is affected by decreased lipase released into the bowel. This results in malabsorption of lipids and causes blockage of the pancreatic ducts with thick mucous. Pancreatic degeneration, fibrosis and atrophy of tissues follow, with eventual development of fatty infiltration and loss of function. The lack of pancreatic enzyme causes steatorrhea.
- Pulmonary symptoms are the most obvious complications and develop secondary to increased viscosity of bronchial secretions with subsequent obstruction of glandular ducts. These clients have respiratory compromise with frequent bronchopneumonia and chronic bronchitis.

CLINICAL MANIFESTATIONS

- small stature, appear emaciated
- barrel-chested
- clubbed fingers
- steatorrhea

MEDICAL MANAGEMENT

- dietary modifications
- pancreatic enzyme administration
- fat soluble vitamins
- respiratory complication management:
  — pulmonary hygiene
  — IV antibiotics

NURSING MANAGEMENT

- Assess respiratory status and implement pulmonary hygiene measures.
- Monitor arterial blood gas results.

- Administer supplemental oxygen and monitor oxygen saturations.
- Administer antibiotic therapy.
- Suction PRN and instruct on self-suctioning technique.
- Administer pancreatic enzyme replacement.
- Encourage dietary management—high protein, high calorie, high salt, low fat.

FOCUSED DISCHARGE CARE

- Instruct client regarding:
  — importance of pulmonary hygiene
  — pancreatic enzyme replacement therapy
  — dietary modifications
  — importance of follow-up visits
- Refer to available community resources.

(For more information, see pp. 1155-1156 of Polaski and Tatro, *Luckmann's Core Principles and Practice of Medical-Surgical Nursing.*)

Deep Vein Thrombosis

OVERVIEW

- Deep vein thrombosis (DVT) refers to thrombophlebitis of the deep veins. Veins damaged by deep vein thrombosis increase the risk for another DVT, pulmonary embolism and venous stasis ulcers.
- Thrombus development is a local process. It begins by platelet adherence to the endothelium. As the thrombi become larger in diameter and length, they obstruct the vein.
- Etiologic factors for thrombus formation include:
  (1) venous stasis—caused by any condition that results in immobility or absence of calf muscle pump action
  (2) hypercoagulability—caused by any condition that raises the platelet count, decreases fibrinolysis, increases clotting factors, or increases the viscosity of the blood
  (3) injury to the vein wall—caused by trauma or agents administered into the vein (certain antibiotics, sclerosing agents, etc.)
- DVT is more common in women than men. About one-third of clients over 40 years of age who have had major surgery or an acute myocardial infarction develop DVT.
- Risk factors associated with DVT include:
  — surgery
  — immobility
  — congestive heart failure
  — myocardial infarction
  — malignancy
  — history of DVT
  — pregnancy
  — trauma
  — estrogen therapy or oral contraceptives
  — obesity
  — varicose veins

- Pulmonary emboli, most of which start as thrombi in the large deep veins of the leg, are an acute and potentially lethal complication of DVT.
- Measures to prevent DVT include:
  — active and passive range of motion exercises if immobilized
  — early ambulation postoperatively
  — compression stockings
  — intermittent calf muscle compressors
  — pharmacologic prevention with warfarin, platelet antiaggregation agents, heparin and dextran

CLINICAL MANIFESTATIONS

- may be asymptomatic
- pain in the region of the thrombus
- unilateral swelling distal to the site
- redness and warmth of the leg
- dilated veins
- low grade fever
- the first manifestation may be signs/symptoms of a pulmonary embolism
- positive Homan's sign - pain in upper calf during forced dorsiflexion of the foot

MEDICAL MANAGEMENT

- bedrest with leg elevation
- anticoagulation therapy to prevent clot extension (does not induce thrombolysis) — IV heparin course followed by oral warfarin sodium (Coumadin)
- fibrinolytic agents — dissolve thrombi — streptokinase, urokinase

SURGICAL MANAGEMENT

- venous thrombectomy — direct removal of venous thrombi, now rarely performed
- umbrella procedure — under local anesthesia, a filter or an umbrella is inserted into the vena cava to trap emboli

NURSING MANAGEMENT

- Maintain bedrest and provide good skin care.

- Administer anticoagulant therapy and titrate as prescribed according to partial thromboplastin (PTT) levels.
- Administer thrombolytic therapy as ordered. See "Chronic Arterial Occlusion," p. 61.
- Encourage in-bed exercises for all but affected limb.
- Administer analgesics.
- Elevate legs above the level of the heart to facilitate blood flow. Apply elastic stockings/wraps.
- Administer warm packs around involved area.
- Initiate Coumadin as ordered (Coumadin takes 24 to 48 hours to take effect; therefore, heparin is continued until therapeutic level is reached).
- Monitor prothrombin time (PT) to determine Coumadin dose.
  — PT must be measured every day before Coumadin is administered.
- Monitor for manifestations of excess anticoagulation:
  — blood in urine, stool, nasogastric contents
  — bleeding gums
  — subcutaneous bruising
  — flank pain
  — epistaxis
- Apply pressure to puncture sites.
- Initiate appropriate bleeding precautions.
- Monitor for signs/symptoms of a pulmonary embolus:
  — pleuritic-type chest pain with sudden onset and aggravated by breathing
  — hemoptysis
  — cough
  — diaphoresis
  — dyspnea
  — apprehension
- Advance activity as ordered.

FOCUSED DISCHARGE CARE

Instruct client regarding:
- disease process and treatment regime
- the importance of long-term anticoagulation therapy (three to six months)
- signs of hypocoagulation and need to report to physician
  — bleeding gums
  — blood in urine or stool
  — nosebleed

- — inability to stop bleeding from a minor cut
- safety measures to prevent bleeding:
  - — soft toothbrush
  - — electric razor
  - — fall prevention
  - — gloves when doing yard work
- measures to prevent recurrence of DVT:
  - — avoid standing or sitting for long periods of time
  - — no crossing legs
  - — no constrictive clothing
  - — elevate legs when sitting
  - — elastic stockings
- rationale for frequent blood tests
- importance of wearing Medic-Alert identification
- need to alert dentist and physician of anticoagulation status

(For more information, see pp. 813-817 of Polaski and Tatro, *Luckmann's Core Principles and Practice of Medical-Surgical Nursing.*)

Dermatitis, Atopic

OVERVIEW

- Atopic dermatitis is a common, chronic, relapsing, pruritic type of eczema. The word "atopic" refers to a group of three associated allergic disorders: asthma, allergic rhinitis (hay fever) and atopic dermatitis.
- The exact cause of atopic dermatitis is unknown. However, 75 to 80 per cent of clients with this disorder have a personal or family history of allergic disorders.
- Atopic dermatitis affects 0.5 to 1 per cent of people around the world.
- Complications may include development of viral, bacterial and fungal skin infections.

CLINICAL MANIFESTATIONS

Atopic dermatitis begins in many clients during infancy. Also called acute dermatitis, it first appears as a red, oozing, crusting rash. As the child grows, the chronic form of dermatitis is exhibited, with the clinical manifestations listed below.

Chronic Form
- thickened, dry texture of the skin
- brownish-gray color and scales on the skin
- localized areas of rash as client ages; found on elbow bends, back of knees, neck, sides of face, eyelids and the back of hands and feet
- pruritus

MEDICAL MANAGEMENT

- daily skin care to hydrate and lubricate the skin (may be accomplished by soaks and wet wraps)
- identification and elimination of factors causing flare-ups
- topical corticosteroids, occlusives, moisturizers or tar preparations
- systemic antibiotics and antihistamines
- dietary restriction of known allergens (common allergens are eggs, cow's milk, soy, wheat, nuts and fish)

NURSING MANAGEMENT

- Instruct client to bathe at least once daily for 15 to 20 minutes. Apply prescribed emollient or topical within 2 to 4 minutes after the bath before drying.
- Use only warm water — never hot.
- Apply prescribed topical preparations 2 to 3 times per day.
- Instruct client not to scratch and to keep fingernails short, smooth and clean.
- Encourage client and significant others to share feelings with each other regarding the client's appearance and the chronic nature of eczema.
- Reinforce client's sense of identity and self esteem.
- Encourage client to teach others that eczema is not contagious unless severely infected.

FOCUSED DISCHARGE CARE

Instruct client regarding:
- use of superfatted soaps
- avoidance of bubble bath

- washing all clothes before wearing to remove form-aldehyde and other chemicals
- avoidance of fabric softeners
- using mild detergent and adding second rinse cycle
- wearing light cotton-blend clothing
- maintaining surroundings at 68 to 75 degrees and humidity at 45 to 55 per cent
- use of sunscreen
- signs of infection and to report these to physician
- importance of taking full course of antibiotic
- how to determine need for treatment modalities, e.g. when to initiate wet wraps
- avoidance of known allergens
- medications — use and side effects
- techniques for self care (e.g., use of topicals, wet wraps)

(For more information, see pp. 1346-1350 of Polaski and Tatro, *Luckmann's Core Principles and Practice of Medical-Surgical Nursing*.)

Dermatitis, Contact

- Contact dermatitis is an inflammatory response of the skin to chemical or physical allergens.
- Clinical manifestations range from mild erythema or vesicles to ulceration.
- Management includes determination of the causative agent and use of topical medications, wet dressings, antihistamines or steroids.

(For more information, see p. 1350 of Polaski and Tatro, *Luckmann's Core Principles and Practice of Medical-Surgical Nursing*.)

Dermatitis, Stasis

- Stasis dermatitis is the development of areas of very dry skin and sometimes shallow ulcers (stasis ulcers) on the lower legs primarily due to venous insufficiency.
- The process of dermatitis begins with edema of the leg due to slowed venous return (clients usually have a history of varicose veins or deep vein thrombosis). As venous stasis continues, the tissue becomes hypoxic from inadequate blood supply. As the blood pools, hemoglobin is released from the red blood cells and deposited in the tissues. The tissues begin to necrose and are very slow to heal because of the lack of oxygenated blood.
- Clinical manifestations are itching, brown-stained skin, a feeling of heaviness in the legs and open shallow lesions.
- Treatment includes wet to dry dressings for débridement of the area, Unna's boot and skin grafts.
- Nursing management includes instructing the client on ways to promote venous return: leg elevation, support hose and avoidance of standing or sitting in one position for long periods of time.

(For more information, see p. 1350 of Polaski and Tatro, *Luckmann's Core Principles and Practice of Medical-Surgical Nursing.*)

Diabetes Insipidus

OVERVIEW

- Diabetes insipidus is a deficiency of antidiuretic hormone (ADH) resulting in water imbalance.
- The major functions of ADH are to: (1) promote water reabsorption by the kidneys, and (2) control the osmotic pressure of the extracellular fluid. When ADH production decreases excessively, the kidney tubules fail to reabsorb water, and consequently, the

client excretes large amounts of dilute urine. Urine in diabetes mellitus contains large amounts of glucose, whereas urine in diabetes insipidus is highly dilute and contains no glucose.

- Causes of ADH deficiency are categorized as follows:
  — central or neurogenic due to:
    — abnormalities in the hypothalamus and pituitary from familial or idiopathic causes (primary diabetes insipidus);
    — destruction of the gland by tumors, trauma, infection, vascular accidents, or metastatic tumors (secondary diabetes insipidus);
    — medications, such as Dilantin and lithium.
    — consumption of alcohol
  — nephrogenic — because of an inherited defect, the kidney tubules cannot respond to ADH.

CLINICAL MANIFESTATIONS

- polyuria
- polydypsia - client must drink fluid almost continuously to avoid severe dehydration and hypovolemic shock
- excretion of urine with abnormally low specific gravity

MEDICAL MANAGEMENT

- vasopressin or synthetic ADH to control polydypsia and polyuria
- benzothiadiazine diuretics

SURGICAL MANAGEMENT

- If diabetes insipidus is secondary to a tumor, excision of the tumor may be curative.

NURSING MANAGEMENT

MEDICAL

- Strict intake and output.
- Monitor electrolyte levels.
- Maintain adequate hydration.
- Monitor for symptoms of drug-induced water intoxi-

cation which can lead to fluid overload, cerebral edema, and seizures:
— diarrhea
— non-pitting edema
— cardiac dysrhythmias
— projectile vomiting

SURGICAL

- If client undergoes surgical resection of a tumor of the pituitary, provide nursing care for the hypophysectomy patient.

FOCUSED DISCHARGE CARE

Instruct client regarding:
- importance of vasopressin therapy
- signs of under- or over-dosage
- when to seek medical attention

(For more information, see pp. 1250-1251 of Polaski and Tatro, *Luckmann's Core Principles and Practice of Medical-Surgical Nursing*.)

Diabetes Mellitus

OVERVIEW

- Diabetes mellitus is a heterogeneous group of disorders characterized by glucose intolerance. It is a disease caused by an imbalance between insulin supply and insulin demand.
- Insulin is produced by the pancreas and normally maintains the balance between high and low blood glucose levels. In diabetes mellitus, either there is not enough insulin or the insulin that is produced is ineffective, resulting in high blood glucose levels.
- Diabetes mellitus also causes disturbances of protein and fat metabolism which are associated with

microvascular, macrovascular, and neuropathic changes.

- There are two main types of diabetes mellitus:
  - (1) Insulin dependent diabetes mellitus (IDDM) — Type I — also called juvenile diabetes, labile or brittle diabetes. It usually occurs before 30 years of age, but may occur at any age. There is little or no endogenous insulin production and insulin injections are required. It is believed to be caused from:
    - — genetic predisposition
    - — autoimmune response causing the body to develop islet cell antibodies and anti-insulin antibodies. The antibodies attack the beta cells of the pancreas where insulin is produced and the insulin molecules themselves.
    - — certain viruses, such as Coxsackie B (and rarely mumps, rubella, and strep) are etiologic factors in clients who are predisposed.
  - (2) Non-insulin dependent diabetes mellitus (NIDDM) — Type II — also called adult onset or mild diabetes. Usually occurs in clients over 35 years of age but can occur in children. There is below normal, normal or above normal insulin production with insulin injections being required in only 20 to 30 per cent of clients. Hyperglycemia develops when the pancreas cannot secrete enough insulin to match the body's needs or when the number of insulin receptor sites is decreased or altered (as in obesity). It is believed to be caused from:
    - — genetic predisposition
    - — obesity
    - — increasing age (the pancreas becomes more sluggish)
- Metabolic effects of diabetes include:
  - — decreased utilization of glucose — since insulin is needed as a carrier for glucose to go into the cells, glucose remains in the blood, and glucose levels rise.
  - — increased mobilization of fat — the body breaks down fat for energy since glucose is not available. Fat metabolism produces ketones which can lead to metabolic acidosis. When fats are used as the primary source of energy, the lipid level can rise to five times normal. This elevated level can lead to atherosclerosis.

— increased protein utilization — without insulin to stimulate protein synthesis, there is increased catabolism and, therefore, protein wasting.

- Complications of diabetes include:
  — neuropathy — nerve fibers do not receive adequate nutrients and oxygen across the membrane, so transmission of nerve impulses slows. Also, sorbitol accumulates in the nerve tissue affecting sensory and motor function. Clients may experience pain or tingling in the extremities; inability to perceive pain (especially in the lower extremities); paresthesias; sensory loss; and decreased or absent reflexes. Autonomic neuropathy also can develop which may manifest itself as: gastroparesis (slowed digestion); inability to recognize hypoglycemic symptoms; urinary incontinence or retention; orthostatic hypotension; and impotence in males.
  — retinopathy — microangiopathy or vascular degeneration of the small vessels supplying the eyes eventually can lead to partial or total permanent blindness.
  — nephropathy — damage and eventual obliteration of the capillaries supplying the glomerulus leads to pathologic changes that cause renal disease and possibly chronic renal failure.
  — cataracts, glaucoma, pyelonephritis and infections — these are more common in diabetic clients.
  — peripheral vascular lesions, coronary artery disease, stroke and hypertension — may result from disorders of the macrocirculation.
- There are approximately 12 million Americans with diabetes and approximately 6 million of these individuals are undiagnosed. Eighty-five to ninety per cent of clients are non-insulin dependent (NIDDM).
- Diabetes with its complications is the fourth leading cause of death by disease in the United States.
- Risk factors include a family history of diabetes and obesity.

CLINICAL MANIFESTATIONS

- polyuria — frequent urination (glucose acts as an osmotic diuretic and pulls fluid with it when excreted through the kidneys)

- polydipsia — excessive thirst due to severe dehydration resulting from polyuria
- polyphagia — excessive hunger due to unavailability of glucose for energy
- weight loss — due to protein wasting

MEDICAL MANAGEMENT

Diabetes management must be individualized and take into account the client's age, maturity, lifestyle, nutritional needs, activity level, occupation and ability to independently perform the skills required by the treatment plan.

- dietary regulation, discouraging foods with high sugar and fat content and correction of or avoidance of obesity
- oral hypoglycemic agents (sulfonylureas) for some NIDDM clients
- insulin therapy — required for IDDM clients and may be required for some NIDDM clients if diet, exercise and oral hypoglycemic agents are ineffective

SURGICAL MANAGEMENT

- pancreas transplants — usually performed for clients who have IDDM and who have had a kidney transplant. The client's own pancreas is left intact and the new pancreas is usually anastamosed to the iliac artery and vein, where insulin can enter the systemic pathway.

NURSING MANAGEMENT

- Discuss the basic pathophysiologic mechanism of diabetes mellitus — monitor for responses of denial or anger in the newly diagnosed client.
- Monitor blood glucose levels by meter or laboratory as ordered. Ensure accuracy of meter results by performing controls and quality control measures as outlined by your health care institution.
- Monitor for signs/symptoms of hypoglycemia (especially at times of peak insulin action) or hyperglycemia and treat accordingly (see "Hypoglycemia", p. 370, and "Hyperglycemia and Diabetic Ketoacidosis", p. 344).
- Be aware that "feeding" a client for hypoglycemia may be ineffective in a client with gastroparesis and

subcutaneous or intravenous treatment may be necessary (instruct client and significant other also).

- Ensure that the client receives meals as ordered. If meals are missed due to NPO status, replace meals with IV $D_{10}W$ or adjust insulin doses as prescribed.
- Administer insulin injections and supplemental doses as needed for high blood glucose levels, according to physician orders.
- Be aware that a client with autonomic nervous system neuropathy may not demonstrate any signs/symptoms of hypoglycemia during a hypoglycemic reaction. (Instruct client and significant other also on this).
- Develop an individualized teaching plan, including client and significant others, that addresses the following (as appropriate to client's needs):
  — blood glucose monitoring — visually or with meter
    — include when to test, technique, goals for good control, how to read test results, what to do for abnormal results and quality control measures
  — urine ketone testing and dangers of ketones
  — normal blood glucose range
  — dietary management (obtain dietician consult)
    • If on oral hypoglycemic agents or insulin, discuss:
    — eating meals and snacks at regular times and in amounts prescribed
    — caloric intake:
      • 55 to 60 per cent from carbohydrates
      • 30 per cent from fat
      • 12 to 20 per cent from protein
    — increasing caloric intake to compensate for periods of prolonged exercise
  — sick day rules
  — insulin administration
    — times of peak action
    — insulin storage
    — preparation and injection
    — site selection and rotation
    — techniques for self-injection
  — use of oral hypoglycemic agents and side effects
  — exercise program, effects of exercise and ways to compensate
  — signs/symptoms of hypoglycemia/hyperglycemia and management (see "Hypoglycemia", p. 370,

212

and "Hyperglycemia and Diabetic Ketoacidosis",
p. 344)
— glucagon administration by significant other
— need to always carry fast-acting sugar for treatment of hypoglycemia
— complications of diabetes and when to call physician

FOCUSED DISCHARGE CARE

- Instruct client regarding information included under
  "Nursing Management". Be sure the regimen has
  been individualized to client's typical daily routine.
- Discuss need for follow-up care and to maintain log
  of daily glucose levels and insulin.
- Instruct to obtain a Medic-Alert bracelet, necklace or
  to carry an identification card.
- Assess need for follow-up with home health care
  agency.
- Refer to American Diabetes Association as appropriate.

See also "Hypoglycemia", p. 370; "Hyperglycemia and
Diabetic Ketoacidosis", p. 344; and "Hyperglycemic,
Hyperosmolar, Nonketotic Coma" p. 348.

(For more information, see pp. 1174-1188 and pp. 1199-1201
of Polaski and Tatro, *Luckmann's Core Principles and Practice of Medical-Surgical Nursing.*)

Diabetic Retinopathy

OVERVIEW

- Diabetic retinopathy is a progressive disorder of the
  retina characterized by microscopic damage to the
  retinal vessels, resulting in occlusion and hemorrhage of the vessels. Background retinopathy is the
  early phase of retinopathy. Microaneurysms develop
  and allow fluid to leak. In proliferative retinopathy,
  the weakened, damaged vessels may rupture, causing retinal hemorrhage and exudates. Hemorrhage is
  followed by the growth of new capillaries into the

vitreous, called neovascularization and by retinal scar tissue formation.
- Diabetic retinopathy is one of the leading causes of blindness in the United States. All diabetics are prone to develop retinopathy, with approximately 30 to 40 per cent of the diabetic population having some degree of retinopathy.

CLINICAL MANIFESTATIONS

- wide range of visual disturbances
- experience black spots or floaters (areas of ischemia become blind spots)
- decreased central vision

MEDICAL MANAGEMENT

None

SURGICAL MANAGEMENT

- argon laser treatment to photocoagulate blood vessels
- vitrectomy (removal of a portion of the vitreous)

NURSING MANAGEMENT

POSTOPERATIVE CARE

In addition to routine postoperative care:
- Monitor for signs of increased intraocular pressure (nausea, pain).
- Monitor blood glucose levels.
- Assist with ambulation and activities of daily living.
- Discuss measures to prevent increased intraocular pressure—see below.

FOCUSED DISCHARGE CARE

- Instruct client regarding:
  — progressive nature of disease
  — importance of maintaining stable blood glucose levels
  — measures to prevent increased intraocular pressure:
    — no lifting heavy objects
    — no straining with stool

- no bending from the waist
- avoidance of coughing and vomiting
- importance of follow-up clinic appointments
- safety measures for the home environment
- Refer to available community resources.

(For more information, see p. 1198 and pp. 445-446 of Polaski and Tatro, *Luckmann's Core Principles and Practice of Medical-Surgical Nursing.*)

Dialysis

OVERVIEW

- Dialysis is used to relieve symptoms of renal failure temporarily until the client regains kidney function, or to sustain life in the client with irreversible kidney disease.
- Goals of dialysis therapy are to:
  - remove the end products of protein metabolism from the blood
  - maintain a safe concentration of serum electrolytes
  - correct acidosis and replenish the blood's bicarbonate buffer system
  - remove excess fluid from the blood.
- There are two types of dialysis:
  - (1) **Peritoneal dialysis** involves repeated cycles of instilling dialysate into the peritoneal cavity through a catheter, allowing time for substance exchange and then removing the dialysate.
    - There are 3 types of peritoneal dialysis:
      (a) Continuous Ambulatory Peritoneal Dialysis (CAPD)— the dialysate is instilled into the abdomen and left in place for 4-8 hours. The empty bag is disconnected and carried with the client until it is time to drain the dialysate. The dialysate is drained into the bag, and the process usually is repeated four times in 24 hours.

(b) Continuous Cycle Peritoneal Dialysis (CCPD) — similar to CAPD but requires a peritoneal cycling machine.

(c) Intermittent Peritoneal Dialysis — dialysis is performed for 10-14 hours, 3-4 times weekly, with use of a peritoneal cycling machine.

— Complications of peritoneal dialysis include peritonitis, catheter displacement or plugging.

— Pain during peritoneal dialysis may result from rapid instillation, incorrect dialysate temperature or pH, dialysate accumulation under the diaphragm or excessive suction during outflow.

(2) **Hemodialysis** involves diverting toxic-laden blood from the client into a dialyzer and then returning clean blood to the client. Hemodialysis clears waste products from the body; restores fluid, electrolyte and acid base balance; and reverses some of the untoward manifestations of irreversible renal failure.

— The major routes of access are external arteriovenous shunts for acute dialysis and internal arteriovenous fistulas and grafts for chronic dialysis.

— Hemodialysis for irreversible renal failure must be done for the client's lifetime unless a transplant is performed.

— A typical schedule is 3 to 4 hours of treatment, 3 days per week.

— Complications include muscle cramps, infection, hepatitis B, dialysis disequilibrium syndrome (develops as a result of rapid changes in the composition of extracellular fluid and involves nausea, vomiting, mental confusion, deterioration of the level of consciousness, twitching, headache, and seizures).

NURSING MANAGEMENT

- Monitor for fluid volume excess or deficit:
  — intake and output
  — vital signs, including postural blood pressure
  — obtain weights pre- and post dialysis.

- Encourage client/family to discuss feelings regarding chronic illness, chronic dialysis, and changes in lifestyle and body image.
- Peritoneal Dialysis:
  — Assess for signs/symptoms of infection or peritonitis.
  — Maintain aseptic technique when accessing peritoneal catheter.
  — Keep dressing dry at all times.
  — Relieve discomfort by slowing the rate of flow, lowering the head of the bed, massaging the abdomen or repositioning the client.
  — Provide small frequent meals if abdominal distention is present.
  — Encourage turning, coughing, and deep breathing (the client is at increased risk for respiratory problems due to increased pressure and reduced excursion of the diaphragm).
- Hemodialysis:
  — Maintain a sterile dressing over the access site.
  — Protect the access site from trauma that may cause clotting, bleeding or physical disruption of the device.
  — No blood pressures or laboratory draws on affected side.
  — Wash fistula or graft site with warm soap and water between dialysis treatments.
- See also "Renal Failure, Chronic", p. 554, and "Renal Failure, Acute", p. 551.

FOCUSED DISCHARGE CARE

- Instruct client regarding:
  — set-up and maintenance of dialysis and signs/symptoms to report to physician
  — hemodialysis regimen and signs/symptoms to report to physician
  — care of catheters, fistula, or graft as appropriate
  — possible changes in lifestyle and activities
- Make referrals to support groups as needed.
- Make referral to home health care agency as needed.

See also "Renal Failure, Chronic", p. 554 and "Renal Failure, Acute", p. 551 for related information.

(For more information, see pp. 965-969 of Polaski and Tatro, *Luckmann's Core Principles and Practice of Medical-Surgical Nursing.*)

Dislocation and Subluxation

OVERVIEW

- Dislocation and subluxation are both displacements of a joint from its normal position. Dislocation is the separation of both articulating surfaces. Subluxation occurs when the articulating surfaces lose partial contact.
- The displaced bone may impede blood supply, tear ligaments, rupture blood vessels, damage nerves or rupture muscle attachments.

CLINICAL MANIFESTATIONS

- deformity of affected extremity
- altered length of extremity
- joint pain and loss of function

MEDICAL MANAGEMENT

- closed reduction followed by immobilization with a splint or cast. See "Fractures, General Information", p. 266.

SURGICAL MANAGEMENT

- open reduction — see "Fractures, General Information", p. 266

NURSING MANAGEMENT

- Administer analgesics.
- Monitor for signs/symptoms of nerve damage — paresthesias, numbness, paralysis.
- Monitor for signs of impeded blood supply — coolness, pain, pallor.
- Collaborate with physical therapy for prescribed exercises and adaptive devices.

- See "Casts", p. 128, for cast care.

FOCUSED DISCHARGE CARE

- Instruct client regarding:
  — prescribed exercises
  — signs/symptoms of complications
- See "Casts", p. 128.

(For more information, see p. 1319 of Polaski and Tatro, *Luckmann's Core Principles and Practice of Medical-Surgical Nursing.*)

Disseminated Intravascular Coagulation (DIC)

OVERVIEW

- Disseminated intravascular coagulation (DIC) is diffuse or widespread coagulation within arterioles and capillaries throughout the body.
- DIC is characterized by the following chain of events:
  (1) Certain disease states cause the release of thromboplastic substances that activate thrombin, which activates fibrinogen and results in deposition of fibrin throughout the microcirculation.
  (2) Platelet aggregation is increased forming microthrombi in the brain, kidneys, heart, etc.
  (3) Red blood cells become trapped in the fibrin strands and are destroyed (hemolysis).
  (4) Platelets, prothrombin and clotting factors are consumed in the process, which compromises coagulation and predisposes to bleeding.
  (5) Excessive clotting activates the fibrinolytic mechanism, which causes the production of fibrin split products that inhibit platelet clotting functions, which causes further bleeding.
  (6) With clots being lysed and clotting factors depleted, the blood loses its ability to clot.
- Conditions that precipitate DIC include:

- shock
- cirrhosis
- transfusion reaction
- glomerulonephritis
- hepatitis (acute fulminant)
- acute bacterial and viral infections
- tissue damage due to trauma, burns, transplant rejection, or surgery
- neoplasms
- The prognosis for DIC varies from self-limiting to death within days.

CLINICAL MANIFESTATIONS

Onset is usually acute.
- purpura
- petechiae
- ecchymosis
- prolonged bleeding from venipuncture sites
- oliguria and renal failure
- convulsions, coma
- prolonged prothrombin time, low platelet count

MEDICAL MANAGEMENT

- identification/treatment of underlying cause
- fresh frozen plasma and platelet infusions
- packed red blood cell administration
- cryoprecipitate infusion for depletion of factors V and VIII
- aminocaproic acid (Amicar)

NURSING MANAGEMENT

- Administer prescribed therapies.
- Assess all body systems for signs/symptoms of bleeding.
- Monitor laboratory results — prothrombin time, partial thromboplastin time, platelet count, CBC.
- Institute bleeding precautions:
  - no intramuscular or subcutaneous injections
  - apply pressure to venipuncture sites
  - reposition frequently and gently
  - no aspirin or nonsteroidal anti-inflammatory drugs.

FOCUSED DISCHARGE CARE

The condition will be resolved prior to discharge, and care will be based on underlying etiologic factor(s).

(For more information, see pp. 869-871`of Polaski and Tatro, *Luckmann's Core Principles and Practice of Medical-Surgical Nursing.*)

Diverticular Disease

OVERVIEW

- A diverticulum is a blind outpouching or herniation of intestinal mucosa through the muscular coat of the large intestine. Diverticular disease is a term used to describe diverticulosis and diverticulitis.
- Diverticulosis is the presence of non-inflamed outpouchings (diverticulum) in the intestine. It is caused by atrophy or weakness of the bowel muscle, increased intraluminal pressure, obesity or chronic constipation.
- Diverticulitis is inflammation of a diverticulum. It occurs when undigested food blocks the diverticulum, leading to a decrease in blood supply to the area, predisposing the bowel to invasion of bacteria into the diverticulum.
- Risk factors include:
  — chronic constipation (usually due to a low fiber diet) for diverticulosis
  — ingestion of indigestible roughage (e.g., corn, popcorn, vegetables with seeds) for diverticulitis.

CLINICAL MANIFESTATIONS

- episodic, dull or steady left quadrant or mid-abdominal pain
- constipation, diarrhea or both
- increased flatus
- mucous in the stools
- anorexia
- low grade fever

MEDICAL MANAGEMENT

- Asymptomatic Disease
  — high fiber diet
  — prevention of constipation
- Diverticulitis
  — NPO, nasogastric suctioning, antibiotics and parenteral fluids until inflammation decreases

SURGICAL MANAGEMENT

Surgery is indicated for clients who develop complications, such as hemorrhage, obstruction, abscesses, or perforation.

NURSING MANAGEMENT

Acute management:
- Keep client NPO.
- Maintain nasogastric tube to suction.
- Monitor WBC and differential.
- Administer IV antibiotics.
- Slowly progress prescribed diet as symptoms subside.

FOCUSED DISCHARGE CARE

Instruct client regarding:
- prescribed antibiotics
- high fiber diet and avoidance of popcorn, seeds or corn
- prevention of constipation with bran and bulk laxatives (hydrophilic colloids)
- drinking at least 8 glasses of water daily
- weight reduction (if obese)
- avoidance of activities that increase intra-abdominal pressure, such as bending, lifting, stooping, coughing or vomiting
- notification of physician of any changes in bowel patterns (constipation or diarrhea) or stools (presence of mucous or blood), or, if fever, abdominal pain or urinary symptoms develop

(For more information, see pp. 1078-1079 of Polaski and Tatro, *Luckmann's Core Principles and Practice of Medical-Surgical Nursing.*)

Dysrhythmias

OVERVIEW

- Dysrhythmias, also called arrhythmias, are disorders of the heart rate and rhythm caused by disturbances in the conduction system. Dysrhythmias can lead to dramatic changes in circulatory dynamics, such as hypotension, heart failure, and shock.
- Dysrhythmias are caused by (1) abnormal rhythmicity of the sinus node (the internal pacemaker) of the heart, (2) a shift of the pacemaker function from the sinus node to another part of the atrium, (3) a block in transmission of the impulse through the heart, (4) abnormal pathways of conduction through the heart, and (5) spontaneous generation of impulses from anywhere along the conduction system.
- Dysrhythmias may occur from a primary problem within the heart or as a secondary response to systemic disorders, electrolyte disorders, or drug toxicity.
- Reentry and abnormal automaticity are the pathophysiologic mechanisms that lead to tachydysrhythmias. Conduction disorders lead to bradydysrhythmias.
- Disorders arising in the atrium:
  - (1) **Sinus Tachycardia** — rapid, regular rhythm at a rate of 100-180 beats per minute with normal P wave and QRS complex
    - Causes:
      - fever
      - emotional/physical stress
      - heart failure
      - hyperthyroidism
      - medications — caffeine, atropine, epinephrine, and isoproterenol
    - Clinical Manifestations:
      - occasional palpitations
      - decreased activity tolerance
      - hypotension
      - angina pectoris
    - Medical Management
      - correct the underlying cause

223

— antidysrhythmic therapy:
- digitalis
- beta-adrenergic inhibiting agents (e.g., propranolol)
- calcium channel blockers—diltiazem, nifedipine

— bedrest to decrease metabolic demand
— supplemental oxygen

(2) **Sinus Bradycardia** — SA node fires at a rate less than 60 beats per minute with normal P wave and QRS complex

— Causes:
— Valsalva's maneuver (increase vagal tone)
— medications — digitalis, quinidine, procainamide
— myocardial infarction
— hyperkalemia
— hypothyroidism

— Clinical Manifestations:
— may be asymptomatic
— fatigue
— lightheadedness or syncope
— ectopic beats

— Medical Management:
— correct the underlying cause
— antidysrhythmic therapy:
- beta-adrenergic agonists (isoproterenol)
- vagolytics (atropine)

— temporary/permanent pacemaker placement

(3) **Sinus Dysrhythmia** — changes in the automaticity of the SA node which cause it to fire at varying speeds. ECG has normal P wave, PR interval, and QRS complex.

— Causes:
— alteration in vagal tone — speeds up with inhalation and slows down during exhalation

— Clinical Manifestations:
— usually asymptomatic

— Medical Management
Intervention usually not required.

(4) **Premature Atrial Contractions (PACs)** — most often result from enhanced automaticity of the atrial muscle. ECG shows P waves that occur

early and differ from normal sinus P waves in direction, size, and/or shape.
— Causes:
  — stress
  — fatigue
  — alcohol
  — smoking
  — coronary artery disease
  — heart failure
  — medications — digitalis, quinidine, and procainamide
— Clinical Manifestations:
  — palpitations or "missed beats"
— Medical Management:
  — correct the underlying cause
  — antidysrhythmic therapy:
    • quinidine
    • procainamide

(5) **SA Conduction Defects** — the impulse from the SA node is either (a) not generated in the SA node (sinus arrest) or (b) not conducted from the SA node (sinus exit block). During SA arrest neither the atria nor the ventricles are stimulated which produces a pause in the rhythm. In sinus exit block, there is a conduction delay between the SA node and the atrial muscle, but the rhythm of SA node discharge remains constant and uninterrupted.
— Causes:
  — coronary artery disease
  — myocardial infarction
  — hypertensive disease
  — medications — digitalis and quinidine
— Clinical Manifestations:
  — may be asymptomatic
  — lightheadedness or syncope
— Medical Management:
Intervention usually not necessary
  — correct the underlying cause
  — antidysrhythmic therapy:
    • vagolytics (atropine)
    • sympathomimetics (isoproterenol)
— Surgical Management:
  — pacemaker insertion — see "Pacemakers", p. 474.

(6) **Paroxysmal Atrial Tachycardia (PAT)** — is the sudden onset of rapid firing from an ectopic atrial pacemaker. The rate is 160-230 beats per minute, alternating with normal sinus rhythm. PAT is due to the reentry phenomenon. The P waves are upright in Lead II, narrow and peaked. At faster rates, the P waves may become lost in the preceding T wave.

— Causes:
  — digitalis toxicity
  — myocardial infarction
  — cardiomyopathy
  — caffeine, smoking, alcohol
— Clinical Manifestations:
  — palpitations
  — lightheadedness
  — syncope
— Medical Management:
  — vagotonic maneuvers (stimulating the vagus nerve to slow the heart) — carotid sinus massage, Valsalva's maneuver (bearing down as with a bowel movement)
  — antidysrhythmic therapy:
    • propranolol
    • verapamil
  — synchronized cardioversion — the use of electricity to convert a dysrhythmia to normal sinus rhythm. The electrical discharge is synchronized with the client's QRS complex to avoid discharge during the repolarization phase when the ventricles are most vulnerable to develop ventricular fibrillation (VF).

(7) **Atrial Flutter** — rapid firing of an ectopic atrial focus. Atrial rate is 250-350 beats per minute. P waves are bidirectional, producing a "saw-toothed" pattern. The AV node cannot conduct all the atrial impulses that bombard it; therefore, the ventricular rate is always slower than the atrial rate.

— Causes:
  — coronary artery disease
  — mitral valve disease
  — pulmonary embolism
  — post cardiac surgery

- — Clinical Manifestations:
  - — palpitations
  - — chest pain
- — Medical Management:
  - — synchronized cardioversion
  - — antidysrhythmic therapy:
    - digitalis
    - quinidine
    - verapamil
    - propranolol
    - procainamide
- ⑧ **Atrial Fibrillation** — rapid, chaotic atrial depolarization. ECG reveals erratic or no P waves and a baseline that appears to be irregular and undulating. The ventricular rhythm is irregular with rates ranging from 50 to 200 beats per minute.
  - — Causes:
    - — congestive heart failure
    - — pericarditis
    - — cor pulmonale
    - — organic heart disease
    - — post cardiac surgery
  - — Clinical Manifestations:
    - — may be asymptomatic
    - — irregular pulse
    - — pulse deficit between apical and radial pulses
    - — palpitations
    - — angina
    - — heart failure
    - — exercise intolerance
  - — Medical Management:
    - — synchronized cardioversion
    - — antidysrhythmic therapy:
      - digoxin
      - diltiazem, nifedipine
      - quinidine
      - procainamide
    - —anticoagulant therapy to decrease the risk of thrombi formation from blood that pools in the atria because of inadequate contraction of the atrial muscle
- Disorders arising within the atrioventricular (AV) junction

(1) **Junctional Rhythms** — upward spread of an impulse from the atrioventricular (AV) junction to the atria rather than the normal downward transmission of impulses from SA node to the AV junction. ECG shows P wave inversion in Lead II and PR interval less than 0.12 second. The major junctional dysrhythmias are (a) premature junctional contractions — single, early firing of a junctional ectopic focus, (b) junctional escape rhythm — if the SA node experiences decreased automaticity, a junctional escape rhythm at a rate of 40 to 60 beats per minute will take over, and (c) junctional tachycardia — a junctional rate that exceeds 60 beats per minute.

— Causes:
  — ischemia
  — myocardial infarction
  — digitalis toxicity
  — hyperkalemia
— Clinical Manifestations:
  — activity intolerance
  — lightheadedness
— Medical Management:
  — synchronized cardioversion
  — antidysrhythmic therapy:
    • vagolytics (atropine)
    • quinidine
  — pacemaker insertion - see "Pacemakers", p. 474

(2) **First-Degree Atrioventricular Block** — conduction in atrioventricular node slows so that the PR interval is greater than 0.20 second.

— Causes:
  — coronary artery disease
  — increased vagal tone
  — congenital anomalies
  — digitalis toxicity
— Clinical Manifestations:
  — none
— Medical Management:
    Usually requires no intervention
  — discontinuation of digitalis if due to toxicity

(3) **Second-degree Atrioventricular (AV) Block**
    This dysrhythmia indicates increased conduction disruption at the AV junction. An intermittent

228

block prevents the depolarization wave through the bundle of His. This results in intermittently dropped QRS complexes. Atrial depolarization continues without disturbance, and normal-appearing P waves occur at regular intervals. The degree of AV block and the number of dropped QRS complexes vary. This results in a discrepancy between the atrial and ventricular rates. QRS complexes appear normal.

(a) Mobitz Type I (Wenckebach's Phenomenon) — recurrent cycles in which the PR interval becomes progressively prolonged until eventually a QRS complex is dropped.

- Causes:
    - coronary artery disease
    - digitalis toxicity
    - myocardial infarction
- Clinical Manifestations:
    - usually asymptomatic
    - irregular pulse
    - vertigo
    - weakness

(b) Mobitz Type II — PR intervals remain constant; P waves are normal and are followed by normal QRS complexes until suddenly a ventricular beat is dropped.

- Causes:
    - ischemia
    - digitalis or quinidine toxicity
    - myocardial infarction
- Clinical Manifestations:
    - irregular pulse
    - weakness
    - syncope
- Medical Management:

    Intervention not required as long as the ventricular rate remains adequate for perfusion

    - correct underlying cause
    - assessment for progression to a higher degree of block
    - antidysrhythmic therapy:
        - atropine
        - isoproterenol

- temporary or permanent pacemaker placement —see "Pacemakers", p. 474
- withholding of cardiac depressant drugs (digitalis)

(4) **Third-Degree AV Block (complete heart block)**
— all impulses from the atria are blocked, and the action of the atria and ventricles becomes completed disassociated; that is, the atria and the ventricles each have their own pacemaker and beat independently of each other. ECG shows regular P to P intervals, regular R to R intervals, and no consistent PR intervals.

— Causes:
— fibrotic or degenerative changes in the conduction system
— myocardial infarction
— myocarditis
— congenital anomalies
— drug toxicities (digitalis, procainamide, quinidine, verapamil)
— post cardiac surgery

— Clinical Manifestations:
— angina
— hypotension
— heart failure
— signs/symptoms of decreased cardiac output

— Medical Management:
— pacemaker insertion — see "Pacemakers", p. 474
— antidysrhythmic therapy:
- isoproterenol (accelerates ventricular rate)

- Disorders arising in the ventricles

Ventricular dysrhythmias arise below the level of the AV junction. Ventricular dysrhythmias are generally more serious and life-threatening than are atrial or junctional dysrhythmias because they develop in association with intrinsic heart disease. Conversely, atrial dysrhythmias frequently arise in normal hearts affected by emotions, fatigue, etc. Also, ventricular dysrhythmias usually cause greater hemodynamic compromise (e.g., hypotension, heart failure, and shock). The independent contraction of the ventricles results in reduced stroke volume and, therefore, reduced cardiac output.

(1) **Premature Ventricular Contractions (PVCs)** —
are caused by the firing of an irritable focus in the
ventricle. On the ECG, a wide and bizarre QRS
appears, interrupting the underlying rhythm.
  — Causes:
    — hypoxia
    — hypokalemia
    — hypocalcemia
    — coronary artery disease
    — acidosis
    — heart failure
    — medications — digitalis, tricyclic antide-
      pressants
    — myocardial infarction
  — Clinical Manifestations:
    — present only if develops into ventricular
      tachycardia or ventricular fibrillation
  — Medical Management:
    PVCs are innocuous as long as they remain
    infrequent or isolated. They require interven-
    tion when they are: (1) frequent (more than 6
    per minute), (2) coupled with normal beats
    (bigeminy), (3) multiform, (4) occurring in
    pairs, (5) occurring as a result of acute myocar-
    dial infarction, or (6) falling on the T wave
    (vulnerable period).
    — Type I and Type II antidysrhythmics (quini-
      dine, lidocaine, Tambocor, propranolol)
(2) **Ventricular Tachycardia (VT)** — occurs when an
irritable ectopic focus in the ventricles takes over
the role of the pacemaker. It is characterized by a
rapidly occurring series of PVCs (three or more)
with no normal beats between. P waves are
absent; QRS complex is wide and bizarre. The
ventricular rate ranges between 130 to 170 beats
per minute.
  — Causes:
    — all factors that cause PVCs can ini-
      tiate ventricular tachycardia
    — most frequently develops after myocardial
      infarction
  — Clinical Manifestations:
    VT, an extremely dangerous dysrhyth-
    mia, produces a very low cardiac output that
    can quickly lead to cerebral and myocardial
    ischemia.

- may be asymptomatic
- hypotension
- non-palpable peripheral pulse
- change in level of consciousness
- at any time, ventricular tachycardia can deteriorate into ventricular fibrillation
- Medical Management:
  - defibrillation if client loses consciousness
  - antidysrhythmic therapy:
    - lidocaine

(4) Ventricular Fibrillation (VF) — characterized by an extremely rapid, erratic impulse formation and conduction. ECG tracing displays bizarre fibrillatory wave patterns, and it is impossible to identify P waves, QRS complexes, and T waves. Ventricular fibrillation causes abrupt cessation of effective blood flow and death results within minutes without immediate intervention.

- Causes:
  - severe myocardial damage
  - hypothermia
  - R-on-T phenomenon—the downward slope of the T wave is the most vulnerable period. If the heart is stimulated at this time, it often cannot respond in an organized fashion and VT or VF may be precipitated.
  - hypoxia
  - electrocution
  - electrolyte imbalance
  - drug toxicity (quinidine, procainamide, digitalis)
- Clinical Manifestations:
  - unresponsiveness
  - no palpable pulse
- Medical Management:
  - CPR and defibrillation
  - epinephrine in order to increase myocardial responsiveness to defibrillation

(5) Bundle Branch Block (BBB) — impaired conduction in one of the bundle branches (distal to the bundle of His), and thus the ventricles do not depolarize simultaneously. The ECG tracing shows a wide and notched QRS complex. These disturbances in conduction result in either a right bundle branch block (RBBB) or a left bundle branch block

(LBBB). Because of its association with left ventricular disease, LBBB has a worse prognosis.

— Causes:
  — myocardial fibrosis
  — coronary artery disease
  — myocardial infarction
  — pulmonary embolism
  — congenital anomalies
— Clinical Manifestations:
  — asymptomatic
— Medical Management:

  No specific intervention, however, if RBBB exists along with block in one of the fascicles of the left bundle, the one remaining fascicle represents the only conduction pathway; therefore, a pacemaker may be inserted.

(6) Pre-excitation Syndrome — occurs when part or all of the ventricle is re-entered by a depolarization wave traveling down a congenital or acquired conducting pathway between the atrium and ventricle. Wolff-Parkinson-White (WPW) syndrome is an example.

— Clinical Manifestations:
  — may be asymptomatic
  — sudden chest pain
  — shortness of breath
  — palpitations
  — syncope
— Medical Management:
  — vagotonic maneuvers
  — cardioversion
  — propranolol administration

SURGICAL MANAGEMENT OF DYSRHYTHMIAS

Surgery can be used to treat dysrhythmias when medications or cardioversion fail. Surgical methods include:

- pacemaker placement — see "Pacemakers", p.474
- chemical ablation — alcohol or phenol is injected into involved areas of the myocardium through an angioplasty catheter. Postoperative care is the same as that for angioplasty. See "Coronary Artery Disease", p. 189.
- mechanical ablation - abnormal pathway is surgically dissected or treated with a cryoprobe. Prior to

surgery, the myocardium is mapped to isolate the area to be treated. Postoperative care is the same as for other forms of heart surgery. See "Cardiac Surgery", p. 119.

- automatic implantable cardioverter defibrillator (AICD) — placement of a system that consists of a pulse generator and sensor that continuously monitors the heart's rhythm and delivers a countershock when it detects a dysrhythmia. This implanted system does not require as much energy as external defibrillation because less energy is lost when the impulse is directly applied to the heart. The AICD is implanted surgically into a pouch in the abdominal wall through a thoracotomy incision. Two conditions for AICD placement are (1) survival of one or more episodes of sudden death resulting from ventricular tachycardia or ventricular fibrillation, and (2) recurrent refractory, life-threatening ventricular dysrhythmias that can develop into ventricular tachycardia or ventricular fibrillation despite antidysrhythmic therapy. See "Cardiac Surgery", p. 119.

NURSING MANAGEMENT

MEDICAL

- Monitor heart rhythm continuously.
- Assess skin temperature, lung sounds, heart sounds, and peripheral pulses.
- Monitor laboratory values — drug levels, enzyme levels, electrolyte levels.
- Administer antidysrhythmics as prescribed.
- Administer supplemental oxygen therapy as prescribed.
- Maintain a quiet, restful environment.

SURGICAL

- See "Pacemakers", p. 474.
- See "Cardiac Surgery", p. 119.

FOCUSED DISCHARGE CARE

- Instruct the client regarding:

- — importance of taking antidysrhythmic agents as prescribed
- — importance of household member(s) to be trained in CPR
- — how to obtain emergency medical attention
- — importance of follow-up laboratory/clinic visits
- See "Pacemakers", p.474.
- See "Cardiac Surgery", p. 119.
- Additional instructions for AICD clients:
  - — AICD follow-up testing (every 2 months)
  - — need to wear medical alert identification and to carry a cardioverter defibrillator identification card
  - — avoidance of contact sports
  - — avoidance of strong magnetic fields
  - — need to inform doctors/dentists of the device
  - — procedure to follow if shock occurs
  - — need to report audible beeping tones coming from the pulse generator in the abdomen

(For more information, see pp. 706-716 of Polaski and Tatro, *Luckmann's Core Principles and Practice of Medical-Surgical Nursing.*)

E

Encephalitis (Viral)

- Encephalitis is inflammation of the brain parenchyma.
- The two most common causes of encephalitis are arbovirus and herpes simplex Type I virus.

  (1) Arbovirus encephalitis is transmitted via a mosquito or tick bite. It commonly occurs in late summer and early fall. Clinical manifestations are gradual: headache, nausea, vomiting, listlessness and fever. After a few days, seizures, stiff neck and coma develop. Fever and neurological signs subside within two weeks unless the client develops irreversible central nervous system changes or dies.

  (2) Herpes simplex virus encephalitis occurs at any time of the year and particularly in middle-aged adults. Clinical manifestations are acute with headache, fever, vomiting, visual field deficits and seizures. Temporal lobe swelling can lead to herniation, coma and brain death. The prognosis is grave with a mortality rate above 30 per cent. The client may die within two weeks and of those who survive, many are left with severe neurologic and mental disabilities. Nursing management includes protection from injury due to combative, restless or confused behavior and support to the client's family.

(For more information, see pp. 362-363 of Polaski and Tatro, *Luckmann's Core Principles and Practice of Medical-Surgical Nursing.*)

Endometrial (Uterine) Cancer

OVERVIEW

- Endometrial cancer is cancer of the uterus. It is the second most common genital malignancy. One in 100 women in the United States will develop uterine cancer.
- Endometrial cancer is related to the hormone estrogen because estrogen is the primary stimulant of endometrial proliferation.
- Risk factors include:
  — exogenous estrogen replacement therapy for long periods without concomitant progesterone therapy
  — obesity (increased estrogen production and storage)
  — history of pelvic irradiation
  — hyperestrogenism (early menarche, late menopause, dysfunctional uterine bleeding, delayed onset of ovulation)
  — old age
  — history of other reproductive cancer
  — family history
  — history of infertility or habitual abortion
  — history of diabetes or hypertension
  — white race
  — postmenopausal bleeding
- Primary prevention includes weight loss and proper use of estrogen.
- Early detection is important. Women at menopause and older should have a yearly pelvic examination and Pap smear. Women at high risk should have periodic endometrial tissue sample biopsies.

CLINICAL MANIFESTATIONS

- abnormal uterine bleeding

MEDICAL MANAGEMENT

- progesterone
- chemotherapy and hormonal therapy with estrogen and tamoxifen is used to treat late stages

237

- irradiation

SURGICAL MANAGEMENT

- total abdominal hysterectomy and bilateral salpingo-oophorectomy (TAH-BSO) alone or in combination with radiation therapy

NURSING MANAGEMENT

See "Uterine Tumors, Benign", p. 646, for care following a TAH-BSO; "Radiation Therapy", p. 543; and "Chemotherapy", p. 145.

(For more information, see pp. 1484-1485 of Polaski and Tatro, *Luckmann's Core Principles and Practice of Medical-Surgical Nursing.*)

Endometriosis

OVERVIEW

- Endometriosis is an abnormal condition in which endometrial tissue (which normally lies in the uterine cavity) is located in other sites.
- The abnormally located tissue usually is confined to the pelvic cavity, typically the ovary or dependent portion of the pelvic peritoneum. Tissue also may be found outside the pelvis, although rarely.
- The misplaced tissue responds to hormonal stimulation and bleeds, leading to scarring, inflammation and adhesions.
- This disorder most commonly is found in premenopausal women aged 30 to 40 years. It appears to be a hereditary disorder, although the cause is unknown.

CLINICAL MANIFESTATIONS

- pain, beginning before the menstrual period and lasting until several days after the period ends

- dyspareunia (pain during vaginal intercourse)
- menstrual irregularities
- infertility in the absence of tubal obstruction

MEDICAL MANAGEMENT

- analgesics
- oral contraceptives, progesterone or both to induce a pseudopregnancy (symptoms subside during pregnancy)
- Danazol (Danocrine) to induce ovarian suppression or pseudomenopause

SURGICAL MANAGEMENT

- carbon dioxide laser treatment to vaporize adhesions and endometrial implants
- removal of the uterus, as many implants as possible and some ovarian tissue if the client does not wish to have any more children
- radical surgery involving removal of the uterus, ovaries, tubes and as many implants as possible. Although this procedure is almost completely effective, it does cause surgically induced menopause and sterility

NURSING MANAGEMENT

- Nursing care of the woman with endometriosis is individualized and depends on the severity of her symptoms, age, and child-bearing status. Nursing care includes helping the woman through the diagnostic process as she considers the various treatment options.

(For more information, see pp. 1479-1481 of Polaski and Tatro, *Luckmann's Core Principles and Practice of Medical-Surgical Nursing.*)

Endotracheal Tubes

OVERVIEW

- An endotracheal tube is a long, slender, hollow tube inserted into the trachea via the nose or mouth. It passes through the vocal cords and the distal tip is positioned just above the bifurcation of the main stem of the bronchus. For short term management, oral intubation may be used due to the risk of sinusitis with nasal intubation. A tracheostomy may be performed for prolonged intubation.
- Indications for endotracheal intubation include:
  — relief of airway obstruction
  — prevention of aspiration
  — facilitation of tracheal suctioning
  — facilitation of artificial ventilation
- After placement of an endotracheal tube, tube placement can be verified by bilateral auscultation and chest x-ray examination to ensure aeration of both sides of the chest. The point at which the tube meets the lips or nostrils is recorded in the nurse's notes, using the numbers listed on the side of the tube. The tube is secured with adhesive tape or specially designed endotracheal tube holders.
- Endotracheal tubes have soft plastic cuffs designed to inflate with a high enough volume of air to seal the trachea while exerting the lowest possible pressure on the tracheal wall. Low cuff pressure is necessary to prevent impeded circulation to the tracheal mucosa, which may lead to stenosis and necrosis of the trachea.
- Extubation is the removal of the endotracheal tube. This is done when the client demonstrates adequate arterial oxygen levels, tidal volume, vital capacity and negative inspiratory force, as well as a level of consciousness to sustain spontaneous respiration. If the client has been on mechanical ventilation, the client will need to be weaned from the ventilator prior to extubation (see "Mechanical Ventilation", p. 437). Only health team members qualified to reintubate can extubate a client. Extubation requires a physician order.

- To extubate, the endotracheal tube is suctioned, the cuff deflated and the tube removed.
- After extubation, the client is placed on oxygen and assessed for signs of respiratory distress, hypoxia (restlessness, irritability, tachycardia, tachypnea) and decreased PaO_2 or increased $PaCO_2$.
- Possible complications due to endotracheal intubation are tracheal necrosis, tracheal trauma from self-extubation and aspiration from inability to seal the airway.

NURSING MANAGEMENT

- Discuss the purpose of the tube.
- Discuss that suctioning will last about 15 seconds at most.
- Provide reassurance.
- Use a suction catheter that does not exceed one-third to one-half the diameter of the airway being suctioned.
- Suction PRN. Provide oxygen and hyperinflate the client's lungs by delivering 5 or 6 breaths with a manual resuscitation bag before and after suctioning.
- Limit suctioning to fifteen seconds.
- Keep the suction level below 120 mm Hg.
- During suctioning, monitor for cardiac dysrhythmias.
- Assess for clinical manifestations of airway obstruction requiring suctioning: noisy, wet respirations; visible mucous bubbling into the artificial airway; rhonchi identified by auscultation; restlessness; increased pulse and respirations; and an increase in peak inspiratory pressures, if client is on continuous mechanical ventilation.
- Provide adequate hydration and humidification to thin secretions.
- Do not instill normal saline via the endotracheal tube before suctioning to loosen secretions, as research has shown this practice to be unsafe. (1995)
- Monitor color, odor, and amount of sputum.
- Provide a means of communication for the client — pen and pad of paper or a picture board.
- Perform frequent oral hygiene.
- Perform oral suctioning above the cuff frequently.
- Monitor the cuff pressure (should be below 20 cm H_2O).

- Use the minimal leak technique to inflate the cuff (see p.526 (Table 20-4), Polaski and Tatro, *Luckmann's Core Principles and Practice of Medical-Surgical Nursing.*)

- Monitor for cuff leaks:
    — pilot balloon is not filling when air is injected
    — client is able to talk when cuff is inflated
    — air is heard leaking during positive-pressure breathing
    — food is able to be suctioned up through the tube
      Anticipate possible reintubation since the client is at risk for aspiration.
- Monitor the point at which the tube meets the lip or nostrils (should match number documented when placed).
- Retape if necessary.
- Assess for nasal or oral breakdown or necrosis, depending upon site of the tube.
  See also, "Mechanical Ventilation", p. 437.

(For more information, see pp. 521-523 of Polaski and Tatro, *Luckmann's Core Principles and Practice of Medical-Surgical Nursing.*)

Enteral Nutrition

OVERVIEW

- Enteral nutrition is nutrition the client takes in via the gastrointestinal tract. It may be administered through a nasogastric, gastric, duodenal, or jejunal tube if the client is unable to take the nutrition orally.
- Major advantages of gastrointestinal feedings over parenteral nutrition are that they help maintain gastrointestinal structure, gastrointestinal motility and the mucosal barrier.
- Problems associated with tube feedings include a variety of fluid and electrolyte disturbances and diarrhea.
- Tube feedings may be administered continuously,

intermittently (given amount is administered over set intervals several times daily) or by bolus (a specified volume of formula is poured through an Asepto syringe or funnel attached to the gastrointestinal tube and allowed to drip in by gravity).

NURSING MANAGEMENT

- Initiate tube feeding at a low rate and gradually increase as prescribed until client is receiving the desired amount of formula.
- Keep head of bed elevated 45 degrees for continuous feedings.
- Keep the head of the bed elevated 30 degrees and turn the client on the right side for at least 30 minutes after bolus feedings.
- Check the placement of the tube by aspirating for gastric contents or injecting air with a syringe while listening over the stomach for the movement of air. For bolus feedings, check prior to each feeding. For continuous feedings, every 4 hours. Always check prior to medication administration.
- Check gastric residuals before each feeding (for bolus feedings) or every four to eight hours. Stop the tube feeding and notify physician of high residuals according to agency policy. Reinstill the feeding to prevent excessive fluid and electrolyte loss.
- Monitor for signs of intolerance, such as cramping, diarrhea, nausea, vomiting and aspiration.
- The feeding tube should be flushed with water followed by cola after intermittent feedings, every four hours during continuous feedings, and after any medications are administered through the tube.
- If an obstruction occurs, try flushing the tube with water or cola.
- Monitor for diarrhea and report to physician (decreasing the rate or concentration of the feeding may alleviate the problem).
- Monitor for possible complications:
  — nausea, vomiting
  — plugging of the tube
  — dislocation of the tube into the trachea or lungs
  — aspiration
- Provide instructions to the client/significant other on home enteral feedings.
- Refer to a home health care agency as appropriate.

(For more information, see pp. 1032-1033 of Polaski and Tatro, *Luckmann's Core Principles and Practice of Medical-Surgical Nursing.*)

Epilepsy

OVERVIEW

- Epilepsy is a paroxysmal neurologic disorder causing recurrent episodes of (1) loss of consciousness, (2) convulsive movements or other motor activity, (3) sensory phenomena, or (4) behavioral abnormalities.
- Epilepsy is always recurrent. An isolated single seizure does not mean the client has epilepsy. Seizures may be caused by brain tumors, head trauma or metabolic disturbances. A tendency to cerebral dysrhythmia is inherited, not the actual seizure disorder itself.
- The following are important terms which may be used when discussing epilepsy:
  - (1) prodromal phase — a vague change that occurs in emotional reactivity or affective responses (e.g., depression or anxiety) that may precede the seizure by minutes or hours
  - (2) aura — a brief, sensory experience that occurs a few seconds before the seizure. It may be an odor or a feeling of weakness or dizziness.
  - (3) ictus — seizure phase
  - (4) "epileptic cry" — a cry occurring with some seizures; caused by a thoracic and abdominal spasm, which expels air through the glottis
  - (5) seizure — a paroxysmal, uncontrolled, abnormal discharge of electrical activity in the brain's gray matter; causes events that interfere with normal function
  - (6) post-ictal - the postseizure phase during which the client experiences some change in consciousness, behavior or activity
  - (7) status epilepticus — the state in which a client has continuous seizures or seizures in rapid succession lasting at least thirty minutes. This

is a medical emergency and may result in permanent damage to the brain. Status epilepticus may be precipitated by the sudden withdrawal of anticonvulsant medication.
- Approximately 0.5 to 1.0 per cent of people in the United States have epileptic seizures.

CLINICAL MANIFESTATIONS

Generalized Seizures

- Generalized Tonic Clonic (grand mal)
  — sudden loss of consciousness
  — tonic phase - entire body stiffens in rigid contraction
    — respirations may be interrupted temporarily and cyanosis may be present
    — jaws are fixed and the hands clenched
    — eyes open wide, pupils are fixed and dilated
    — lasts 30 to 60 seconds
  — clonic phase
    — rhythmic, jerky contraction and relaxation of all body muscles, especially the extremities
    — incontinence of urine or feces
    — saliva blown from the mouth (creates a froth at the lips)
    — biting of lips, tongue and inside of the mouth

This entire episode may last two to five minutes, after which the client may go into a post-ictal sleep lasting thirty minutes to several hours. This may be followed by depression, confusion or headache pain.
- Petit Mal (Absence) Seizures
  — brief periods of altered consciousness (periods of "absence") lasting five to thirty minutes
  — usually begin during childhood and diminish or disappear after puberty
- Minor Motor Seizures
  — myoclonic — involuntary jerking contractions of major muscles
  — akinetic — momentary loss of muscle movement
  — atonic — total loss of muscle tone

- Partial Motor Seizures
  - begin with convulsive twitching in an upper extremity
  - involuntary movements of an area may spread centrally and involve the entire limb, that side of the face and the lower extremity. This progression or "spread" is known as the Jacksonian march.
- Partial Sensory Seizures — experiencing sensory phenomena from a focus in a specific area; clients may see flashing lights, or experience numbness or tingling
- Partial Seizures with Complex Symptoms — "psychomotor seizures" or "partial complex seizures"
  - automatism (such as purposeless repetitive activities, e.g., lip smacking, chewing, patting a part of the body, picking at clothes) while in a dreamy state
  - usually last two to three minutes, but may last up to fifteen minutes

MEDICAL MANAGEMENT

- antiepileptic drugs — usually single drug therapy is used, e.g., phenytoin (Dilantin), carbamazepine (Tegretol)
- investigational drugs — lamotrigine and vigabatrin

SURGICAL INTERVENTION

- cortical resection of the anterior temporal lobe for complex partial seizures

NURSING MANAGEMENT

- Initiate seizure precautions.
- Monitor for seizure activity.
- Administer anticonvulsants.

During a seizure
- If possible, move to a place of safety.
  - If in bed, raise padded side-rails.
  - If sitting or standing, lower to floor.
  - Move objects out of the way.
- Turn client to one side to maintain patent airway and prevent aspiration.

- Document when seizure started and describe it (presence of aura, tonic clonic movements, area where seizure began, eye deviation, generalized or unilateral activity, labored or frothy respirations, incontinence, and client's behavior during post-ictal period).

During status epilepticus
- Be aware that this is a medical emergency and will result in permanent brain damage or death if not treated rapidly.
- Maintain a patent airway and prevent aspiration (Position on side, suction and provide oxygenation. Endotracheal intubation may be needed.)
- Assess client continuously.
- Protect client from injury.
- Anticipate laboratory studies for blood chemistries, liver function tests and toxicology.
- Administer IV lorazepam (first line of treatment) and then loading dose of phenytoin. Other medications, such as valium or phenobarbital may be prescribed.
- Anticipate general anesthesia or a barbiturate coma, if unable to control with medications.
- Provide emotional support to significant others.

FOCUSED DISCHARGE CARE

- Instruct client/significant other regarding:
  — medication — importance of taking daily even if no seizures occur, method of action and possible side effects. (Gingival hyperplasia [excessive gum tissue growth] may occur with phenytoin. Instruct client to brush teeth two to three times daily. Discuss possible need to have gingival tissues excised every six to twelve months. Diplopia and ataxia are other possible side effects.)
  — avoidance of factors that may trigger seizures (flickering lights, stress, lack of sleep, emotional upset, alcohol use)
  — using safety measures for certain activities (e.g., swimming or horseback riding) and avoidance of dangerous activities
  — avoidance of overprotecting the client
  — local laws on driving motor vehicles
  — what to do if seizure occurs:
    — lie on ground (when aura occurs, if client has aura)

247

- — loosen clothing
- — protect head (place something under it)
- — remove sharp objects from environment
- — do not insert anything into mouth (clients do not swallow their tongues)
- — position on side
- — stay with client until consciousness returns
- — call ambulance, if: seizure lasts over ten minutes, respiratory difficulty occurs, injury occurs, another seizure occurs or the client is pregnant
- — importance of wearing identification stating client has epilepsy and name of physician
- Provide emotional support for possible feelings of anger, poor self image, self consciousness, guilt or depression.
- Refer to National Epilepsy League, National Association to Control Epilepsy or local support groups.

(For more information, see pp. 354-360 of Polaski and Tatro, *Luckmann's Core Principles and Practice of Medical-Surgical Nursing*.)

Epistaxis

OVERVIEW

- Epistaxis (nosebleed) may result from irritation, trauma, infection or tumors. It also may result from systemic disease (hypertension, atherosclerosis or blood dyscrasias) or systemic treatment (chemotherapy or anticoagulants).

MEDICAL MANAGEMENT

- Application of pressure by pinching the anterior portion of the nose for 5-10 minutes and application of ice compresses.
- Cauterization of the bleeding vessel with silver nitrate.
- Nasal packing is most effective for anterior nasal bleeding. A water soluble ointment is applied to one-

half inch gauze and inserted into the anterior nasal cavities and left in place for 48-72 hours.
- For posterior nasal bleeding, a posterior plug may be needed in addition to nasal packing. A small red rubber catheter is passed through the nose into the oropharynx and mouth. A gauze pack is tied to the catheter, and the catheter is withdrawn, moving the pack into the nasopharynx and posterior nose. Strings from the pack are tied around a rolled gauze. Strings from the oral cavity are taped to the client's face to prevent dislodgement of the plug. Posterior plugs are left in for 5 days.

SURGICAL MANAGEMENT

- internal maxillary or ethmoid artery ligations, if the above interventions fail

NURSING MANAGEMENT

MEDICAL

- Monitor for changes in vital signs.
- Monitor for bleeding from the anterior nares.
- Monitor for posterior bleeding manifested by increased swallowing or presence of blood in the throat.
- Change nasal drip pad PRN.
- Encourage use of humidification, adequate fluids, and frequent mouth care to prevent dryness and crusting of secretions.
- If nasal packing or posterior plugs are present, monitor for hypoxia. Ensure intactness of the packing or plug. Assess the oral cavity for proper placement of the plug. If the plug is visible, notify the physician for repositioning.

FOCUSED DISCHARGE CARE

Instruct client regarding:
- minimal activity for 10 days — avoidance of strenuous exercise
- no blowing of the nose
- sneezing only with the mouth open
- no lifting, stooping, or straining

- use of water soluble lubricant at the entrance of the nose and around the nares for comfort

(For more information, see pp. 562-563 of Polaski and Tatro, *Luckmann's Core Principles and Practice of Medical-Surgical Nursing.*)

Esophageal Neoplasms

OVERVIEW

- Cancer of the esophagus may be manifest as either squamous cell carcinoma or adenocarcinoma of the esophageal mucosa. Adenocarcinoma occurs less often than squamous cell carcinoma.
- The incidence of esophageal cancer is twice as high in men as in women. The incidence of squamous cell cancer of the esophagus in the United States is 4 per 100,000 males.
- Risk factors include long-term use of alcohol and tobacco combined with poor nutrition. The presence of achalasia, hiatal hernia, reflux, stricture or poor oral hygiene also increases the risk.

CLINICAL MANIFESTATIONS

- dysphagia, odynophagia (pain upon swallowing)

MEDICAL MANAGEMENT

Treatment depends upon the location of the tumor, size of the tumor, metastases and the condition of the client.
- radiation therapy, used alone or in conjunction with surgery (radiation therapy reduces tumor size and slows tumor growth)

SURGICAL MANAGEMENT

- esophageal dilation to treat strictures and tumor obstruction

- esophagectomy — removal of all or part of the esophagus (the resected esophagus is replaced with a dacron graft)
- esophagogastrostomy — resection of the lower portion of the esophagus and anastomosis of the remainder to the stomach
- esophagoenterostomy — resecting the esophagus and replacing it with a segment of the descending colon
- gastrostomy or jejunostomy tube placement as needed for nutrition

NURSING MANAGEMENT

MEDICAL

- Monitor nutritional status and caloric intake.
- Obtain daily weights.
- Monitor intake and output.
- Provide tube feedings or total parenteral nutrition..
- Maintain skin integrity around the gastrostomy feeding tube:
  - wash area with gentle soap and water and dry thoroughly twice a day
  - apply protective ointments, such as zinc oxide or Karaya
- Keep in upright position to prevent aspiration of secretions.
- Provide receptacle for saliva and mucous secretions when client unable to swallow.
- Assist with frequent oral care.
- Provide emotional support to assist with coping with poor prognosis and change in body image.
- See "Chemotherapy", p. 145.

SURGICAL

PREOPERATIVE CARE

In addition to routine preoperative care:
- Provide hyperalimentation or tube feedings for nutritional support for 2 to 3 weeks preoperatively.
- Perform oral care four times per day.
- Perform bowel preparation as prescribed if esophagoenterostomy will be performed.

In addition to routine postoperative care:

- See "Mechanical Ventilation," p. 437, if client on mechanical ventilation.
- Administer analgesics as prescribed to assist with effective turning, coughing and deep breathing.
- Place in semi-Fowler's to prevent reflux.
- Maintain chest tube patency; assess for amount and color of drainage.
- Monitor intake and output (client will be NPO for 4 to 5 days).
- Monitor nasogastric drainage (bloody for the first 24 hours, then a greenish-yellow color).
- Monitor anastomosis site (leakage is common for 5-7 days after surgery).
- Assess all wounds for signs of bleeding, drainage or separation of the suture lines.
- Reinitiate oral intake with sips of water as prescribed. Position upright and monitor for signs of leakage at the anastomosis site. If client tolerates sips, slowly advance to pureed and semi-solid foods.
- Instruct on importance of small, frequent feedings, sitting upright for meals and for 1 hour after meals.

FOCUSED DISCHARGE CARE

- Instruct client/significant other regarding:
  — nutritional support
  — wound care and healing
  — respiratory care
  — wound and respiratory complications and when to contact physician
  — recurrence of symptoms may mean development of an esophageal stricture or tumor regrowth.
- Refer to home health agency as needed.
- Refer to support groups (American Cancer Society, Hospice) as appropriate.

(For more information, see pp. 1025-1027 of Polaski and Tatro, *Luckmann's Core Principles and Practice of Medical-Surgical Nursing.*)

Extracellular Fluid Volume Deficit

OVERVIEW

- An extracellular fluid volume deficit (ECFVD) is a decrease in intravascular and interstitial fluids. Extracellular fluid volume deficit is a serious fluid imbalance. ECFVD can lead to cellular fluid loss owing to fluid shifting from the cells to the vascular fluid to restore fluid balance.
- The pathophysiologic changes related to ECFVD are usually related to changes in sodium levels. Serum sodium concentration is increased with ECFVD due to insufficient water intake or water loss. The increased serum sodium concentration causes a shifting of water from the cells to the vascular space to decrease the hyperosmolality that occurs with water loss. This shift causes cells to shrink and cellular dehydration to occur.
- There are two major types of ECFVD: (1) hyperosmolar fluid volume deficit — fluid loss is greater than the solute (sodium) loss, and (2) iso-osmolar fluid volume deficit — equal proportions of fluid and solute loss.
- ECFVD commonly occurs with severe vomiting or diarrhea, traumatic injuries with excessive blood loss, third space fluid shifts and insufficient water or fluid intake.

CLINICAL MANIFESTATIONS

- thirst (thirst mechanism may be depressed in elderly or debilitated client)
- decreased skin turgor
- dry mucous membranes
- dry, cracked lips or tongue
- soft and sunken eyeballs
- apprehension and restlessness; coma with severe deficit
- elevated temperature
- tachycardia
- hypotension
- narrowed pulse pressure (difference between systolic and diastolic pressure readings)
- flattened neck veins in supine position

- weight loss
- oliguria (less than 30 ml/hr)
- laboratory findings:
  — increased osmolality
  — increased or normal serum sodium
  — hyperglycemia (due to hemoconcentration)
  — elevated hematocrit
  — increased urine specific gravity

MEDICAL MANAGEMENT

If the deficit has existed for more than 24 hours, it is dangerous to correct it too rapidly.
- fluid and electrolyte replacement
- blood replacement
- measures to control fluid/electrolyte loss as indicated:
  — antidiarrheal agents
  — antiemetics
  — nasogastric tube placement

SURGICAL MANAGEMENT

To correct the source of fluid deficit, e.g.,control hemorrhage, relieve intestinal obstruction (causes vomiting), relieve esophageal obstruction (causes difficulty swallowing), etc.

NURSING MANAGEMENT

- Administer fluid/electrolyte replacement.
- Monitor vital signs including orthostatic blood pressure.
- Assess for signs of fluid overload — cerebral edema, congestive heart failure (may occur if replacement fluids are given too rapidly).
- Assess intake and output.
- Daily weights.
- Administer antiemetics or antidiarrheals as prescribed.
- Monitor for signs of increasing fluid loss (increased drainage from NG tube, chest tube or wound site, etc.).
- Provide frequent oral care.
- Implement measures to maintain skin integrity.
- Monitor laboratory findings — BUN, hematocrit, serum sodium, serum osmolality, specific gravity.

FOCUSED DISCHARGE CARE

Discharge care is based on the etiologic factor(s) causing extracellular fluid volume deficit.

(For more information, see pp. 39-41 of Polaski and Tatro, *Luckmann's Core Principles and Practice of Medical-Surgical Nursing.*)

Extracellular Fluid Volume Excess

OVERVIEW

- Extracellular fluid volume excess (ECFVE) is increased fluid retention in the intravascular and interstitial spaces (fluid overload).
- With a fluid volume excess, the fluid pressure is greater than usual at the arterial end of the capillary. Fluid is pushed into the tissue spaces. Peripheral and pulmonary edema may result.
- Causes of ECFVE include:
  — heart failure — impaired pumping action
  — renal disorders — decreased sodium and water excretion
  — cirrhosis of the liver — decreased serum protein and albumin levels, therefore, oncotic pressure is decreased, resulting in less fluid reabsorption from the tissue spaces
  — lymphatic obstruction — blocked lymph channels, increasing tissue oncotic pressure
  — tissue injury — increased movement of plasma protein into tissue, increasing oncotic pressure
  — increased ingestion of foods containing high amounts of sodium — increase water retention
  — excessive amounts of IV fluids containing sodium — increase water retention
  — Cushing's syndrome (hyperaldosteronism) — increased sodium and water retention

CLINICAL MANIFESTATIONS

- dyspnea
- crackles in the lungs
- cyanosis
- constant irritating cough (due to fluid accumulation in the alveolar sacs)
- neck vein engorgement in semi-Fowler's position
- hand vein engorgement
- bounding pulse
- elevated blood pressure
- S_3 gallop
- pitting edema of the lower extremities
- sacral edema
- weight gain
- malaise, confusion, headache and lethargy (secondary to cerebral edema)
- laboratory findings:
  - decreased serum osmolality (indicates there are fewer solutes in proportion to the fluid volume)
  - serum sodium may be normal, decreased or elevated (depending upon the amount of sodium retention or water retention)
  - decreased hematocrit (hemodilution)
  - decreased urine specific gravity

MEDICAL MANAGEMENT

- diuretic therapy
- fluid restriction
- low-sodium diet
- management of underlying disorder — heart failure, cirrhosis, renal disease, etc.

NURSING MANAGEMENT

- Administer diuretics as prescribed and monitor effectiveness.
- Assess for signs/symptoms of congestive heart failure — neck vein distention, S_3 gallop, shortness of breath, rales, etc.
- Assess for signs/symptoms of cerebral edema — malaise, confusion, lethargy, etc.
- Monitor vital signs.

- Monitor laboratory values — electrolytes, osmolality, specific gravity, arterial blood gases, renal profile, liver enzymes.
- Monitor intake and output.
- Daily weights.
- Maintain fluid restriction.
- Maintain low sodium diet.
- Frequent skin care to edematous areas.

FOCUSED DISCHARGE CARE

Instruct client regarding:
- dietary modifications — low sodium
- importance of medication regime
- signs of fluid overload and need to report to physician:
  — weight gain
  — increased edema
  — increased shortness of breath
- importance of follow-up appointments

(For more information, see pp. 41-44 of Polaski and Tatro, *Luckmann's Core Principles and Practice of Medical-Surgical Nursing*.)

Extracellular Fluid Volume Shift

OVERVIEW

- A fluid volume shift is a change in the location of extracellular fluid between the intravascular and the interstitial spaces.
- There are two types of fluid shift: (1) vascular fluid to interstitial space leading to a fluid volume deficit (hypovolemia), and (2) interstitial fluid to vascular fluid space leading to fluid volume excess (hypervolemia).
- Fluid that shifts into the interstitial space due to increased capillary permeability or increased vascu-

lar fluid volume and remains there, is referred to as third space fluid. Third space fluid is physiologically useless because it does not circulate to provide nutrients.

- Clinical causes of fluid shift include: crushing injuries, extensive burns, perforated ulcer, intestinal obstruction, lymphatic obstruction and large venous thrombosis.

CLINICAL MANIFESTATIONS

Fluid shift from vascular to interstitial (resembles shock)
- skin pallor
- cold extremities
- weak, rapid pulse
- hypotension
- oliguria
- decreased level of consciousness

Fluid shift from interstitial to vascular (resembles fluid overload)
- bounding pulse
- crackles
- neck vein engorgement
- elevated blood pressure

MEDICAL MANAGEMENT

- determination/treatment of the cause of the fluid shift
- management of hypovolemia:
  — fluid replacement
  — vasoactive agents
- management of overload:
  — diuretics
  — fluid restriction

NURSING MANAGEMENT

- Monitor vital signs.
- Administer prescribed treatments for hypovolemia or hypervolemia.
- Measure abdominal girth daily, if ascites is present.
- Daily weights.
- Monitor intake and output.
- Assess neurological status.

- Provide frequent skin care to edematous areas.
- Monitor laboratory findings — electrolytes, renal profile, serum ammonia levels.
- Provide frequent oral care

FOCUSED DISCHARGE CARE

Discharge care is based on the etiologic factor(s) causing fluid shift.

(For more information, see pp. 44-45 of Polaski and Tatro, *Luckmann's Core Principles and Practice of Medical-Surgical Nursing.*)

F

Flail Chest

- A flail chest consists of fractures of two or more adjacent ribs on the same side, and possibly the sternum, with each bone fractured into two or more segments.
- The flail segment no longer has bony or cartilaginous connections with the rest of the rib cage. Lacking attachment to the thoracic skeleton, the flail section "floats", moving independently of the chest wall during ventilation, and causes a paradoxical motion.
- During paradoxical motion, the flail portion of the chest and its underlying lung tissue are "sucked in" with inspiration and ballooned out with expiration. This diminishes the ability to achieve an adequate tidal volume and to cough adequately. Hypoventilation and hypoxemia may result without prompt intervention.
- Paradoxical motion also causes mediastinal flutter [movement of the mediastinal structures (heart, trachea, esophagus) in a swinging, back and forth motion] which may affect circulatory dynamics, causing elevated venous pressure, impaired filling of the right side of the heart and decreased arterial pressure.
- Signs and symptoms of flail chest are excruciating pain; cyanosis; severe dyspnea; anxiety; rapid, shallow grunting respirations, and obvious paradoxical movement of the chest wall.
- Treatment is usually intubation and mechanical ventilation.

(For more information, see pp. 1578-1579 of Polaski and Tatro, *Luckmann's Core Principles and Practice of Medical-Surgical Nursing.*)

Fracture, Hip

OVERVIEW

- Hip fractures are divided into three types: (1) femoral neck, (2) inter-trochanteric, and (3) subtrochanteric.
- Hip fractures are the leading traumatic injury in the elderly. Two contributing factors seen in the elderly are loss of postural stability with increased incidence of falls and decreased bone mass.

CLINICAL MANIFESTATIONS

- shortened, externally rotated hip
- ecchymosis
- pain, tenderness

MEDICAL MANAGEMENT

- Buck's traction (skin traction) — realigns fracture and reduces muscle spasms until surgery can be performed
- analgesia

SURGICAL MANAGEMENT

- placement of internal fixation device (screw, pin, nail)
- total hip arthroplasty — joint replacement

NURSING MANAGEMENT

MEDICAL

- Apply Buck's traction.
- Administer PRN analgesics.
- Monitor skin for signs of breakdown.

SURGICAL

Internal Fixation — See "Rheumatoid Arthritis", p. 561, for care of client with hip joint replacement.

261

In addition to routine postoperative care:

- Maintain repaired limb so it is internally rotated and in a neutral or abducted position.
  — Place a pillow or an A-frame between the client's legs to maintain abduction.
  — Place a trochanter roll beside the external aspect of the thigh to prevent external rotation.
  — Never adduct the operated leg past the body's midline.
- Encourage client to perform in-bed exercises for upper and lower extremities.
  — Place trapeze to facilitate upper arm and shoulder strength.
- Implement passive and active range of motion exercises.
- Consult physical therapy for assisted ambulation, exercises, transfer techniques and adaptive devices as prescribed.
- Monitor for signs/symptoms of hip dislocation.
- Turn the client only with a physician's order.
  — When helping the client turn:
    — avoid adduction and excessive movement of the operated limb
    — prevent strain on the hip
    — keep the leg and hip in proper alignment
- Avoid acute flexion of the operated hip by not elevating the head of the bed greater than 40 degrees.
- Keep operated limb extended, well supported and elevated when client is allowed to sit in a chair. Follow prescribed amount of weight bearing.
- Remind client not to cross legs.
- Administer PRN analgesics.
- Monitor for signs/symptoms of deep vein thrombosis (redness, warmth, pain in calf, positive Homan's sign).
- Provide meticulous skin care and monitor for signs of skin breakdown.
- Monitor for clinical manifestations of compartment syndrome (caused by bleeding or edema into a compartment which consists of muscle, bone, nerves and blood vessels wrapped by a fibrous membrane); pallor, pulselessness, paresthesias, pain and paralysis.

FOCUSED DISCHARGE CARE

- Instruct client regarding:
  — avoidance of crossing legs
  — avoidance of putting excess weight on operated leg
  — use of supportive devices (canes, crutches, or walkers)
  — safe home environment
  — need to stop at least once every hour when traveling long distances
  — daily exercises as ordered by physician
  — nutritious diet low in fat, high in fiber with plenty of fluids
  — avoidance of weight gain that may cause stress on the femoral repair

(For more information, see pp. 1312-1316 of Polaski and Tatro, *Luckmann's Core Principles and Practice of Medical-Surgical Nursing.*)

Fracture of the Femur

OVERVIEW

- Femoral shaft fractures occur most often in young or middle-aged people. Fractures of the proximal femur are more common in the elderly.

CLINICAL MANIFESTATIONS

- marked displacement and deformity
- extensive soft tissue damage
- swelling
- pain

MEDICAL MANAGEMENT

- splint application
- traction

- cast

SURGICAL MANAGEMENT

- placement of internal fixation devices (rods, nails, plates or screws)

NURSING MANAGEMENT

- See "Casts", p. 128.
- See "Traction", p. 622.

FOCUSED DISCHARGE CARE

- See "Casts", p. 128.

(For more information, see p. 1316 of Polaski and Tatro, *Luckmann's Core Principles and Practice of Medical-Surgical Nursing.*)

Fracture of the Pelvis

OVERVIEW

- Pelvic fractures occur in nearly 30 per cent of all multiple trauma injuries.

CLINICAL MANIFESTATIONS

- hypotension - resulting from hemorrhage
- pain

MEDICAL MANAGEMENT

- bedrest and traction (less severe fracture)
- analgesia

SURGICAL MANAGEMENT

- open reduction with internal fixation

NURSING MANAGEMENT

* See "Traction", p.622.

FOCUSED DISCHARGE CARE

* See "Traction", p. 622.

(For more information, see p. 1316 of Polaski and Tatro, *Luckmann's Core Principles and Practice of Medical-Surgical Nursing.*)

Fractured Ribs

* Rib fractures usually are associated with a blunt injury, such as a fall, blow to the chest or the impact of a steering wheel during an automobile accident.
* Clinical manifestations include:
  — localized pain and tenderness over the fracture area on inspiration and palpation
  — shallow respirations
  — guarding of the chest
* Fractured ribs predispose the client to atelectasis and pneumonia due to shallow breathing and ineffective coughing.
* Bone splinters from fractured ribs may cause a pneumothorax or hemothorax.
* Treatment involves rest, local heat and analgesics. (Strapping the ribs is not recommended because it increases the incidence of atelectasis and pneumonia.)
* Intercostal nerve blocks may be used if ventilation is significantly impaired due to pain.
* The pain from fractured ribs lasts five to seven days. Healing is complete in approximately six weeks.

(For more information, see p. 1578 of Polaski and Tatro, *Luckmann's Core Principles and Practice of Medical-Surgical Nursing.*)

Fractured Sternum

- Sternal fractures usually result from blunt deceleration injuries, such as the impact from the steering wheel in a motor vehicle accident.
- Other injuries typically accompany sternal fractures, such as flail chest; hemothorax; pneumothorax; ruptured aorta, trachea, bronchus or esophagus; and pulmonary or myocardial contusions.
- Clinical manifestations include sharp, stabbing pain; crepitus; and tenderness, swelling and discoloration over the fracture site.
- Treatment is aimed at the associated injuries. Analgesics and possibly nerve blocks are given for pain. Surgical fixation may be performed for severe sternal fractures.

(For more information, see p. 1578 of Polaski and Tatro, *Luckmann's Core Principles and Practice of Medical-Surgical Nursing.*)

Fractures, General Information

OVERVIEW

- A fracture is a disruption of normal bone continuity that occurs when more stress is placed on a bone than it is able to absorb. Surrounding soft tissue injury often also occurs.
- Classification of fractures:
  — Closed (simple) — uncomplicated with intact skin over the fracture site
  — Open (compound) — a break in the skin is present over the fracture site
  — Complete — fracture line extends through the entire bone substance
  — Incomplete (partial) — fracture line extends part way through the bone (also called willow, green-stick or hickory-stick fracture)

— Displaced - bone fragments are separated at the fracture line
— Comminuted — more than one fracture line and bone fragments are crushed or broken into several pieces
— Impacted or compression — one bone fragment is forcibly driven into another adjacent bone fragment
— Complicated — associated with injury to surrounding structures, such as nerves, blood vessels, joints
— Pathologic — fracture occurs due to underlying bone disorders, such as osteoporosis or tumor; usually occurs with minimal trauma

CLINICAL MANIFESTATIONS

- deformity
- swelling
- bruising (from subcutaneous bleeding)
- muscle spasm (involuntary muscle contraction near the fracture)
- tenderness
- pain
- impaired sensation (numbness)
- loss of normal function
- crepitus
- hypovolemic shock (from blood loss or other injuries)
- abnormal mobility of the affected part

MEDICAL MANAGEMENT

- traction — to align bone fragments
- closed reduction — manual application of traction to restore bone alignment
- cast application
- management of shock

SURGICAL MANAGEMENT

- open reduction — an incision is made and the fracture is aligned under direct vision
- internal fixation device placement (insertion of screws, plates, pins, wires, nails or rods)

NURSING MANAGEMENT

- Apply traction as prescribed.
- Administer PRN analgesics.
- Assess for signs/symptoms of arterial damage:
  — variable or absent pulse
  — swelling
  — pallor or patch cyanosis distal to the fracture
  — pain
  — poor capillary return
  — coolness of the extremity
  — paralysis or sensory loss distal to fracture
- Assess for signs/symptoms of compartment syndrome (caused by bleeding or edema within a compartment which consists of muscles, bones, nerves and blood vessels wrapped by fibrous membrane):
  — ischemic pain
  — pain with elevation (due to increased arterial inflow)
  — paresthesias
  — diminished or absent pulses
  — coolness or pallor
- Assess for signs/symptoms of fat embolism (may occur 24 to 48 hours after injury):
  — altered mental status
  — tachypnea
  — tachycardia
  — hypoxemia
  — petechiae
  — fever
- Assess for signs/symptoms of infection:
  — increased temperature
  — rapid pulse
  — pain
  — drainage
- Monitor for signs/symptoms of shock and administer prescribed therapy.
- Consult with physical/occupational therapy for prescribed exercises, ambulation techniques and adaptive devices.

See "Casts", p. 128. See "Traction", p. 622.

FOCUSED DISCHARGE CARE

Discharge instruction will be determined by type/location of fracture and selected treatment regime.

See "Casts", p. 128.

(For more information, see pp. 1306-1312 of Polaski and Tatro, *Luckmann's Core Principles and Practice of Medical-Surgical Nursing*.)

Fractures, Specific Sites

Also see, "Fractures, General Information", p. 266.

FRACTURE OF THE TIBIA AND FIBULA

- Most commonly casted after reduction.
- Complex fractures may require traction or internal fixation.

FRACTURE OF THE FOOT

- Minimally displaced fractures are treated with open walking shoes, casts or braces.
- Open reduction and casting may be necessary.

FRACTURE OF THE HUMERUS

- Common fracture in the elderly.
- Impacted fractures of the proximal humerus are treated with a sling.
- Displaced fractures of the proximal humerus are treated with surgical open reduction and fixation with pins.
- Fractures of the shaft of the humerus are usually managed with traction via a hanging arm cast or splint. Sometimes the fracture is surgically reduced and repaired with rods, plates or screws.
- Nonunion is common and bone grafting may be required.
- Fractures of the condyles of the humerus are usually treated with open reduction and internal fixation devices.

FRACTURE OF THE RADIUS AND ULNA

- Colles' fracture is a fracture of the distal radius from a fall on an outstretched hand. It is treated with open reduction and internal fixation, splints, casts or external fixation, depending upon severity.
- The radius and ulna usually fracture together. Closed reduction with casting is the most common form of treatment.

FRACTURE OF THE OLECRANON

- Usually results from a fall onto the elbow.
- Treatment includes closed reduction and long arm casting for six to eight weeks.

FRACTURE OF THE WRIST AND HAND

- Closed reduction and casting are the most common treatment for six to twelve weeks.
- Fractures of the metacarpals and phalanges are seldom displaced. They are immobilized with splints.

See "Casts", p. 128.
See "Traction", p. 622, for care of the client in traction.
See "Fractures, General Information", p. 266, for information on closed reduction.

(For more information, see pp. 1316-1317 of Polaski and Tatro, *Luckmann's Core Principles and Practice of Medical-Surgical Nursing.*)

Frostbite

- Frostbite is damage to tissues and blood vessels as a result of prolonged exposure to cold. The fingers, toes, nose and ears are most often affected.
- There may be initial numbness, paresthesia and pallor of the affected part. Severe pain, swelling, erythema and blistering may occur once the client is

in a warm environment. Necrosis and gangrene may develop in severe cases.
- Treatment is rewarming of the affected part with tepid water (about 105° F.). Massage never is used as it may result in further tissue damage. Bulky dressings are applied and a bed cradle may be needed.

(For more information, see p. 1588 of Polaski and Tatro, *Luckmann's Core Principles and Practice of Medical-Surgical Nursing.*)

Ganglion

OVERVIEW

- A ganglion is the most common benign soft tissue mass in the hand, consisting of a round cyst-like lesion overlying or adjacent to the wrist joint or tendon.
- The synovium surrounding the tendon degenerates, allowing the tendon sheath to buckle and weaken.
- Onset may be sudden or gradual and may be post-traumatic.
- Ganglion most frequently is seen in the second to sixth decade of life.
- There is a female predominance.

CLINICAL MANIFESTATIONS

- localized pain exacerbated by dorsiflexion of the wrist
- freely moveable mass

MEDICAL MANAGEMENT

- aspiration of the ganglion followed by injection of corticosteroid into the joint
- nonsteroidal anti-inflammatory agents

SURGICAL MANAGEMENT

- ganglion excision

NURSING MANAGEMENT

Treatment is generally done on an outpatient basis.

(For more information, see pp. 1300-1301 of Polaski and Tatro, *Luckmann's Core Principles and Practice of Medical-Surgical Nursing.*)

Gastric Cancer

OVERVIEW

- Gastric cancer refers to malignant neoplasms in the stomach, usually adenocarcinoma.
- Stomach cancer is twice as common in men as in women, more common in whites, and frequent in clients with pernicious anemia.
- The incidence in the United States has been declining, but it is still the sixth most common cause of death from cancer.
- Risk factors include Helicobacter pylori (H. pylori) infection, wood or tobacco smoke, chronic gastritis, nitrite food preservatives and carcinogens in the diet, such as pickled foods and salted fish.

CLINICAL MANIFESTATIONS

Early symptoms are vague and indefinite. Other symptoms occur late, so diagnosis is usually at a late stage.
- weight loss, vague indigestion, anorexia
- blood in stool, anemia
- palpable mass, ascites, bone pain from metastasis

MEDICAL MANAGEMENT

- chemotherapy
- radiation

SURGICAL MANAGEMENT

- partial or complete gastrectomy (removal of the stomach) and removal of associated lymph nodes
- palliative gastroenterostomy — surgical creation of a passage between the stomach and small intestine

NURSING MANAGEMENT

- See "Chemotherapy", p. 145, and "Radiation Therapy", p. 543.
- Administer analgesics and assess effectiveness.
- Administer total parenteral nutrition (TPN) or jejunostomy tube feedings.

- See "Peptic Ulcer Disease", p. 493, for information on surgical procedures.

FOCUSED DISCHARGE CARE

- Instruct client/significant other regarding:
  — pain management
  — TPN therapy
  — jejunostomy feedings
  — wound care
  — signs/symptoms of infection
  — signs/symptoms of complications and to report to physician
- Make home health care referral for TPN therapy/jejunostomy feedings.
- Refer to support groups, e.g., I Can Cope, Hospice.

(For more information, see pp. 1048-1049 of Polaski and Tatro, *Luckmann's Core Principles and Practice of Medical-Surgical Nursing.*)

Gastritis, Acute

OVERVIEW

- Acute gastritis is inflammation of the gastric mucosa caused by ingestion of a corrosive, erosive or infectious substance.
- Aspirin, non-steroidal anti-inflammatories, digitalis, steroids, acute alcoholism and food poisoning may also cause this disorder.
- Risk factors include ingestion of gastric irritants such as aspirin, alcohol, and caffeine. There is also greater incidence in clients who are heavy smokers.
- Gastritis may also occur secondary to a variety of diseases or it may follow treatments such as chemotherapy and radiation therapy.

CLINICAL MANIFESTATIONS

- epigastric discomfort, abdominal tenderness, cramping, eructation, severe nausea and vomiting, hematemesis, and gastrointestinal bleeding
- diarrhea, if due to food poisoning

MEDICAL MANAGEMENT

- phenothiazines to treat vomiting
- antacids or H_2 antagonists
- NPO status, then slow introduction of simple bland substances

NURSING MANAGEMENT

- Assist to assess factors that increase symptoms (e.g., stress, fatigue) and ways to reduce these.
- Administer antacids as prescribed.
- Maintain NPO status if nausea and vomiting present; slowly initiate a bland diet.

FOCUSED DISCHARGE CARE

- Instruct client regarding:
  — signs/symptoms of gastrointestinal bleeding and to report these to physician
  — foods and beverages to avoid
  — stress reduction
  — use of antacids
- Refer to smoking cessation program.

(For more information, see pp. 1037-1038 of Polaski and Tatro, *Luckmann's Core Principles and Practice of Medical-Surgical Nursing*.)

Gastritis, Chronic

OVERVIEW

- Chronic gastritis is inflammation of the gastric mucosa in one of three forms:

(1) Superficial gastritis — causes a reddened, edematous mucosa with hemorrhages and small erosions.

(2) Atrophic gastritis — occurs in all layers of the stomach.

(3) Hypertrophic gastritis — causes a dull and nodular mucosa with irregular, thickened or nodular rugae.

- Aspirin, non-steroidal anti-inflammatories, digitalis, steroids, cigarette smoking and acute alcoholism may cause this disorder. Infection with the Helicobacter pylori organism and advanced age are also risk factors.
- Peptic ulcer disease or gastric surgery may lead to chronic gastritis.

CLINICAL MANIFESTATIONS

Symptoms are vague and may be absent.
- anorexia, dyspepsia, belching, nausea and vomiting
- a feeling of fullness, vague epigastric pain and intolerance of spicy or fatty foods

MEDICAL MANAGEMENT

- bland diet, small frequent meals
- antacids, anticholinergics, sedatives
- avoidance of foods that cause symptoms
- corticosteroids
- Vitamin B_{12} if pernicious anemia is present

SURGICAL MANAGEMENT

- If conservative measures have not controlled bleeding, surgery may be necessary.

NURSING MANAGEMENT

- Maintain NPO status if nausea and vomiting are severe.
- Administer antacids (Gaviscon is antacid of choice).
- Assist to assess factors that increase symptoms (e.g., stress, fatigue) and explore ways to reduce these.

FOCUSED DISCHARGE CARE

- Instruct client regarding:
  — signs/symptoms of recurrence
  — avoidance of aggravating foods and beverages
  — use of medications/antacids
  — signs/symptoms of gastrointestinal bleeding
  — methods to reduce stress
  — need for follow-up and periodic testing for development of gastric cancer (clients are at increased risk for cancer following Helicobacter pylori [H. pylori] infection or atrophic gastritis)
- Refer to smoking cessation program.

(For more information, see pp. 1038-1039 of Polaski and Tatro, *Luckmann's Core Principles and Practice of Medical-Surgical Nursing*.)

Gastroesophageal Reflux Disease

OVERVIEW

- Gastroesophageal reflux disease (GERD) is a term used to describe a syndrome resulting from esophageal reflux. Esophageal reflux is the backward flow of gastric contents into the esophagus.
- Reflux exposes the esophageal mucosa to the gastric contents and gradually breaks down the esophageal mucosa (this is referred to as reflux esophagitis).
- The exact cause of GERD seems to be an inappropriate relaxation of the lower esophageal sphincter (LES).
- Risk factors include: nicotine; high-fat foods; xanthine derivatives (including theophylline and caffeine drinks); ganglionic stimulants; beta-adrenergic agents; and high levels of estrogen and progesterone.

CLINICAL MANIFESTATIONS

- heartburn, dysphagia, acid regurgitation, water brash (the release of salty secretions in the mouth) and eructation

- burning sensation in the epigastric region that moves up and down
- pain that may radiate to the back, neck, or jaw
- pain after meals relieved by antacids or fluids
- pain worsened with supine position or when stomach is distended

MEDICAL MANAGEMENT

- antacid therapy — 1 hour before and 2-3 hours after a meal
- histamine receptor antagonists, e.g., ranitidine (Zantac) or famotidine (Pepcid)
- bethanecol (Urecholine) to increase lower esophageal sphincter pressure and prevent reflux
- metoclopramide (Reglan) to increase the rate of gastric emptying
- dietary changes (see Nursing Management below)

SURGICAL MANAGEMENT

- Nissen fundoplication — the gastric fundus is wrapped around the distal esophagus and sutured to itself.
- Hill's operation — involves narrowing the esophageal opening and anchoring the stomach and distal esophagus to the median arcuate ligament.
- Belsey's repair — plicating the anterior and lateral aspects of the stomach onto the distal esophagus.

NURSING MANAGEMENT

MEDICAL

- Instruct on use of medications/antacids.
- Provide pain medications; monitor effectiveness.
- Instruct on dietary management:
  — Eat four to six small meals/day.
  — Drink adequate fluids at meals to promote food passage.
  — Eat slowly and chew food thoroughly.
  — Avoid extremely hot or cold foods, spices, coffee, alcohol, fats, citrus juices and chocolate.
  — Avoid eating and drinking for 3 hours before retiring to prevent nocturnal reflux.

— Elevate the head of bed 6 to 8 inches to prevent nocturnal reflux.
— Lose weight (if overweight).
— Avoid tobacco, salicylates or phenylbutazone.

SURGICAL

In addition to routine postoperative care:
- Maintain patent chest tube (if the thoracic approach was used).
- Assess for signs/symptoms of wound infection.
- Assist the client with coughing and deep breathing, even though postoperative breathing can be painful.
- Maintain NG tube patency to prevent distention.
- Slowly advance diet as prescribed (fluids are resumed in 24 hours).

AFTER FUNDOPLICATION:

- Monitor for gas-bloat syndrome (occurs if the fundus wrap is too tight, causing bloating and the inability to eructate).
- Avoid carbonated beverages and drinking with a straw.
- Instruct to report to physician dysphagia, epigastric fullness, bloating or excessive rumbling.

FOCUSED DISCHARGE CARE

Instruct client regarding:
- substances to avoid (alcohol, aspirin, chocolate and caffeine)
- diet (see Nursing Management above)
- keeping head of bed elevated for sleeping
- signs/symptoms of recurrence and to report to physician (nausea, vomiting, hematemesis or symptoms of obstruction)
- ambulating after meals
- the availability of support groups for weight loss and smoking cessation

SURGICAL

- avoidance of straining the incision for at least 6 weeks after surgery

- avoidance of lifting heavy objects
- signs/symptoms of infection to report to physician

See also "Hiatal Hernia", p. 330.

(For more information, see pp. 1020-1022 of Polaski and Tatro, *Luckmann's Core Principles and Practice of Medical-Surgical Nursing*.)

Genital Herpes

OVERVIEW

- Genital herpes is one of the most common sexually transmitted diseases (STD).
- Peak incidence is in the adolescent and young adult.
- It is caused by herpes simplex virus type II.
- The herpes simplex virus organism is in the exudate of the lesion. The disease can be transmitted while a lesion is present and for 10 days after it has healed.
- Genital herpes usually is transmitted by direct contact during sexual activity, but transmission is possible by fomites, such as towels used by an infected client.
- Potential complications include aseptic meningitis, transverse myelitis, and spontaneous abortion.
- The major problem of herpes simplex virus (HSV) infections is recurrence. About one half to three quarters of infected clients have recurrence within one year of the first episode.

CLINICAL MANIFESTATIONS

Symptoms generally occur 3 to 7 days after contact.
- Acute Phase:
  - paresthesia/burning at site of exposure
  - painful genital vesicles that ulcerate, crust and heal with a scar in 2-4 weeks
  - fever, chills, muscle aches
- Latent Phase — herpes virus lies dormant, probably in the sacral ganglion until triggered by stress, infection, trauma, etc.

— asymptomatic
- Recurrent Phase:
  — symptoms similar to acute phase, although usually less severe

MEDICAL MANAGEMENT

All contacts of clients with active lesions should be evaluated and if symptomatic, treated. Genital herpes is a chronic disease; there is no cure.
- acyclovir (Zovirax) orally for 5 to 10 days

NURSING MANAGEMENT

- Administer acyclovir as prescribed.
- Maintain isolation precautions.
- Provide palliative measures — sitz baths, cool applications and analgesics.

FOCUSED DISCHARGE CARE

Instruct client regarding:
- importance of completing acyclovir regime
- information about the disease, transmission, treatment and follow-up
- measures to avoid autoinoculation from the genital area to other body sites.
- the need to evaluate all sexual contacts and, if symptomatic, the need to be treated
- the need to avoid sexual contact during initial and recurrent infections
- the use of condoms in latent phases as there is a risk of transmission even though symptoms are not present

(For more information, see pp. 1510-1511 of Polaski and Tatro, *Luckmann's Core Principles and Practice of Medical-Surgical Nursing.*)

Genital Warts

OVERVIEW

- Genital warts are caused by the human papillomavirus (HPV).
- Genital warts are the fourth most common sexually transmitted disease (STD).
- Warts occur 1-2 months after exposure.
- HPV can cause laryngeal papillomatosis in infants born to mothers with vaginal warts.
- Clients with genital warts are at increased risk for genital malignancy, such as cancer of the vulva, cervix or penis.

CLINICAL MANIFESTATIONS

- Warts occur in multiple, painless clusters on the vulva, vagina, cervix, perineum, anorectal area, urethral meatus, or glans penis.
- Oral and pharyngeal lesions can also occur.

MEDICAL MANAGEMENT

All contacts should be evaluated and, if symptomatic, treated. Recurrence is high. There is no cure; treatment only ameliorates the symptoms.

- topical application of podophyllin in compound with tincture of benzoin.

SURGICAL MANAGEMENT

- cryotherapy with liquid nitrogen or a cryoprobe
- carbon dioxide laser, electrocautery, or surgical excision for extensive warts

NURSING MANAGEMENT

- Apply topical treatment as prescribed.

FOCUSED DISCHARGE CARE

Instruct the client regarding:

- information about the disease, transmission, and treatment
- need to treat all sexual partners if symptomatic
- if pregnant, the possibility of infecting the baby
- importance of annual Pap smear and follow-up due to increased risk of genital malignancy

(For more information, see pp. 1511-1512 of Polaski and Tatro, *Luckmann's Core Principles and Practice of Medical-Surgical Nursing.*)

Giantism

OVERVIEW

- Giantism is a disturbance of growth that arises from an over-secretion of growth hormone (GH).
- Giantism, an overgrowth of the long bones, develops in children before the age when the epiphyses of the bones close. Clients may grow to nine feet tall.
- Giantism results from growth hormone secreting adenomas of the anterior pituitary glands.

CLINICAL MANIFESTATIONS

- Extreme height

MEDICAL MANAGEMENT

- irradiation of the pituitary gland to destroy tumor

- bromocriptine (Parlodel) to reduce the levels of growth hormone and decrease tumor size

SURGICAL MANAGEMENT

- The treatment of choice is a surgical hypophysectomy to remove the tumor (approach through inner aspect of upper lip). Partial or complete removal of the pituitary gland occurs during resection of pituitary tumors.

NURSING MANAGEMENT

SURGICAL

Postoperative Care

In addition to routine postoperative care:
- Assess for signs of cerebral edema and rising intracranial pressure:
  — elevated blood pressure
  — widened pulse pressure
  — decreased pulse rate
  — pupil changes
  — altered respiratory pattern
- Assess for signs of target gland deficiencies (the pituitary no longer produces tropic hormones):
  — adrenal insufficiency
  — hypothyroidism
  — diabetes insipidus (ADH deficiency)
- Assess for signs of meningitis (elevated temperature, headache, irritability, and nuchal rigidity).
- Provide frequent oral hygiene.
- Observe the client for rhinorrhea after nasal packing is removed (can indicate a cerebrospinal fluid leak).
- Encourage client to avoid coughing, sneezing, or blowing his nose.

FOCUSED DISCHARGE CARE

Instruct client regarding:
- importance of taking daily replacement hormones

- need for client/significant other to demonstrate medication injection technique if client not able to tolerate oral medications
- signs of under and over-dosage
- need to call for dosage adjustment if experiencing physical or emotional stress
- dietary modifications
- need to report persistent post-nasal drainage
- need to avoid sneezing, coughing, and bending from the waist for specified period of time
- need for Medic Alert bracelet and card.

Glaucoma

OVERVIEW

- Glaucoma includes a group of ocular disorders characterized by increased intraocular pressure, optic nerve atrophy and visual field loss.
- Intraocular pressure is determined by the rate of aqueous production in the ciliary body and the resistance of outflow of aqueous from the eye. Increased intraocular pressure (usually greater than 23 mm Hg) may result from hyperproduction of aqueous or obstruction of the outflow. As aqueous fluid builds up in the eye, the increased pressure inhibits blood supply to the optic nerve and retina. These tissues become ischemic and gradually lose function.
- The terms open (wide) and closed (narrow) describe the width of the angle between the cornea and iris. Narrow anterior chamber angles predispose clients to an acute onset of angle-closure glaucoma.

- It is estimated that over 50,000 people in the United States are blind as a result of glaucoma. The incidence is about 1.5 per cent and in blacks between the ages of 45 and 65, the prevalence is five times that of whites.
- Types of glaucoma:
  — primary open-angle glaucoma
    — bilateral
    — insidious in onset
    — slow to progress
    — symptoms appear late when vision is impaired by damage to the optic nerve
    — cause — degenerative changes resulting in decreased outflow of aqueous
  — angle-closure glaucoma
    — acute onset
    — develops only in an eye in which the anterior chamber is anatomically narrowed
    — cause — sudden blockage of the anterior angle by the base of the iris
  — secondary glaucoma
    — etiologic factors
      - postoperative edema
      - trauma
      - lens displacement
      - hemorrhage into the anterior chamber
      - inflammation of aqueous filtering mechanism
      - tumor encroachment

CLINICAL MANIFESTATIONS

- visual changes — blind spots in periphery, decreased visual acuity, loss of contrast sensitivity
- angle-closure glaucoma — pain, blurred vision or vision loss, rainbow halos around lights, nausea and vomiting
- increased intraocular pressure
- cupping or indentation of optic nerve disc

MEDICAL MANAGEMENT

- topical miotics — constrict pupils and increase outflow (pilocarpine hydrochloride)
- topical epinephrine — increases outflow
- topical beta-blockers — suppress secretion of aqueous (timolol maleate)

- oral carbonic anhydrase inhibitors — reduce production of aqueous (acetazolamide [Diamox])
- oral osmotic agents — glycerin (Glyrol), isosorbide (Ismotic)
- IV osmotic agents — mannitol (glaucoma crisis)

SURGICAL MANAGEMENT

- laser trabeculoplasty — creation of an opening in the trabecular meshwork to facilitate outflow
- filtering procedures (trephination, trabeculectomy, thermal sclerostomy, sclerectomy) — creation of an outflow channel from the anterior chamber into the subconjunctival space where the aqueous is absorbed through the conjunctival vessels
- cyclocryotherapy - (application of a freezing tip) - damages the ciliary body, thus decreasing the production of aqueous

NURSING MANAGEMENT

MEDICAL

- Administer eye drops and oral medications as prescribed.
- Implement appropriate safety measures.

SURGICAL

POSTOPERATIVE CARE

In addition to routine postoperative care:
- Maintain eye pad and shield in place.
- Instruct client not to lie on operative side.
- Observe for signs of increased intraocular pressure (pain, nausea).
- Assist with ambulation and activities of daily living.

FOCUSED DISCHARGE CARE

Instruct client regarding:
- disease process and importance of medications in preventing loss of vision
- technique for instilling eye drops

- signs/symptoms of increased intraocular pressure (pain, nausea, decreased vision) and to report to physician
- rationale for eye protection (shield or glasses at all times). Not all physicians order eye protection.
- measures to prevent intraocular pressure increase:
  — no bending at the waist
  — no lifting of heavy objects
  — no straining during bowel movements
  — avoidance of coughing and vomiting
- Postoperative
  — signs/symptoms of infection (redness, swelling, drainage, blurred vision or pain)
  — how to cleanse the eye with warm water
  — instruct not to rub or apply pressure over closed eye (could damage healing tissue)
- safety in the home environment
- importance of follow-up visits

(For more information, see pp. 437-450 of Polaski and Tatro, *Luckmann's Core Principles and Practice of Medical-Surgical Nursing.*)

Glomerulonephritis, Acute

OVERVIEW

- Glomerulonephritis is a term that encompasses a wide variety of diseases, most of which are caused by changes in the immune system which results in changes in the glomerular portion of the kidney.
- Damage occurs due to trapping of circulating antigen-antibody complexes within the glomerulus or by the fixing of antibodies to the glomerular basement membrane.
- There are 2 forms of acute glomerulonephritis:
  (1) Postinfectious glomerulonephritis—usually caused by a beta-hemolytic streptococcal infection elsewhere in the body. It occurs about 21 days after a respiratory or skin infection.

(2) Infectious glomerulonephritis — caused by a beta-hemolytic streptococcal infection or another bacterial, viral or parasitic infection in the body. It occurs during or within a few days of the original infectious process.

CLINICAL MANIFESTATIONS

- sudden onset of hematuria and proteinuria
- fever, chills, weakness, pallor, nausea and vomiting
- generalized edema, ascites, pleural effusion, congestive heart failure
- headache, hypertension
- oliguria or anuria for several days
- signs/symptoms also may be insidious or mild with reports of anorexia, vague weakness, lethargy

MEDICAL MANAGEMENT

Interventions aim to eliminate antigens, alter the immune balance and inhibit or alleviate inflammation to prevent further renal damage.
- antibiotic therapy
- diuretics, antihypertensives and restriction of dietary sodium and water to treat volume overload and hypertension
- corticosteroids and immunosuppressive agents

NURSING MANAGEMENT

- Monitor for complications: congestive heart failure with pulmonary edema, increased intracranial pressure or renal failure.
- Obtain daily weights.
- Monitor intake and output.
- Maintain fluid restriction and provide hard candies or ice chips for thirst.
- Measure edematous areas daily.
  Monitor laboratory results: BUN, creatinine.
- Monitor vital signs.
- Maintain bedrest or activity restrictions.
- Provide good skin care and change position frequently.
- Protect the client from infection since the client has increased susceptibility due to an altered immune response.

FOCUSED DISCHARGE CARE

- Instruct client regarding:
  — high calorie, controlled protein, low sodium diet to avoid protein catabolism and to rest the kidney
  — avoidance of infection
  — avoidance of stressors on the kidneys
  — need for follow-up testing of renal function.
- If client develops renal failure and requires dialysis, see "Renal Failure, Chronic", p. 554, and "Dialysis", p. 215.
- Also see "Glomerulonephritis, Chronic", p. 290.

(For more information, see pp. 952-955 of Polaski and Tatro, *Luckmann's Core Principles and Practice of Medical-Surgical Nursing.*)

Glomerulonephritis, Chronic

OVERVIEW

- Chronic glomerulonephritis is characterized by an often slow and silent onset with signs and symptoms not occurring until years later.
- All forms of acute glomerulonephritis can progress to a chronic state.
- Hypertension is a cardinal sign of chronic glomerulonephritis. Associated manifestations may include epistaxis, signs of arteriosclerosis, cardiomegaly, edema, hemorrhage into the kidneys, lungs, retina, or cerebrum.

CLINICAL MANIFESTATIONS

- hypertension, malaise, weight loss, mental cloudiness, metallic taste in the mouth, polyuria, and nocturia

MEDICAL MANAGEMENT

- dialysis, transplant and control of symptoms, such as edema and hypertension

- anti-inflammatory agents and anticoagulants

NURSING MANAGEMENT

- Monitor for signs/symptoms of complications.
- Assess for relief of symptoms.
- Instruct on disease and management.
- Provide support; discuss coping strategies to deal with long-term illness.

Also see "Glomerulonephritis, Acute", p. 288; "Dialysis", p. 215; "Renal Failure, Chronic", p. 554; and "Renal Transplantation", p. 557.

(For more information, see p. 955 of Polaski and Tatro, *Luckmann's Core Principles and Practice of Medical-Surgical Nursing.*)

Gonorrhea

OVERVIEW

- Gonorrhea is caused by the gram-negative diplococcus Neisseria gonorrhoeae.
- This disease continues to be one of the most common sexually transmitted diseases (STD). It is easily transmitted by sexual contact, and there is a large carrier population (i.e., people who have no symptoms but carry the organism and can transmit the disease).
- Teenagers and young adults are at highest risk; the highest rates occur in the 20 to 24 year old age group.
- Gonorrhea may be divided into two groups:
  — local - involves the mucosal surfaces of the urethra, cervix, rectum, pharynx, and conjunctiva
  — systemic - includes polyarthritis, dermatitis, endocarditis, or meningitis, secondary to bacteremia.
- There is no lasting immunity that prevents reinfection.

CLINICAL MANIFESTATIONS

- Female:
  - — may be asymptomatic
  - — thick, purulent vaginal discharge
  - — genital irritation
  - — dysuria and frequency
  - — red, swollen vulva
  - — pharyngeal infection
- Male:
  - — may be asymptomatic
  - — urethral discharge
  - — dysuria, frequency
  - — pharyngeal infection
- Disseminated (systemic), either sex:
  - — bacteremia
  - — arthritis
  - — dermatitis

MEDICAL MANAGEMENT

All contacts within the preceding 30 days should be examined, cultured, and treated presumptively.

- ceftriaxone sodium (Rocephin) one intramuscular dose, followed by doxycycline hyclate (Vibramycin Hyclate)
- repeat culture after therapy completed

NURSING MANAGEMENT

- Administer antibiotics as prescribed.
- Monitor temperature.

FOCUSED DISCHARGE CARE

Instruct client regarding:

- importance of taking the complete course of antibiotics and follow-up culture
- information about the disease, how it spreads, and treatment regime
- importance of identifying and treating sex partners
- importance of abstinence or use of a male or female condom until infection is cured
- the possibility of reinfection and infection of sexual partners
- the increased risk of infection with multiple sexual partners

- medication administration:
  — take 1 to 2 hours after meals
  — avoid iron, dairy products and antacids

(For more information, see pp. 1505-1507 of Polaski and Tatro, *Luckmann's Core Principles and Practice of Medical-Surgical Nursing.*)

Gout/Gouty Arthritis

OVERVIEW

- Gout is a metabolic disorder by which purine (protein) metabolism is altered and the by-product, uric acid, accumulates. In the body, uric acid is made by the enzymatic breakdown of tissue and dietary purines. Hyperuricemia develops because of under-secretion or oversecretion of uric acid. In addition to accumulating in the blood, uric acid accumulates in the synovial fluid, myocardium, kidneys, and ears. When uric acid levels reach a certain level, they crystallize and the crystals, called tophi, are deposited in connective tissue. Because the crystals are deposited in connective tissue, gout is classified as a form of arthritis.
- Gout is classified as primary or secondary
  — *Primary*—caused by an inherited defect of purine metabolism leading to increased or decreased renal excretion.
  — *Secondary* — an acquired condition, following hematopoietic or renal disorders. Also may develop from the rapid induction of chemotherapy, radiation therapy or from the use of aspirin, thiazide, mercurial diuretics, and some antituberculosis medications. Alcohol ingestion and starvation increase serum urate levels.
- Primary gout accounts for 80 per cent of all cases, of which 95 per cent occur in males. The initial attack of gout occurs in the fourth or fifth decade of life.

CLINICAL MANIFESTATIONS

Clinical manifestations of gout develop in three stages:

- Stage I — asymptomatic hyperuricemia (> 7.0 mg/dL).
- Stage II — hyperuricemia persists through all the stages
  — rapid development of acute attack; often develops overnight with symptoms subsiding within one week. Following initial attack, client may be asymptomatic for years. Eventually other attacks occur.
  — redness, swelling, tenderness in one joint
  — fever, tachycardia, malaise, anorexia
  — pruritis and local desquamation may be noted as the edema subsides
- Stage III — permanent changes in multiple joints with restrictions in movement
  — tophi on the ears, hands, elbows, feet, and knees
  — possible renal and cardiac disorders, uric acid renal stones, renal colic, hypertension and atherosclerosis.

MEDICAL MANAGEMENT

ACUTE ATTACK

- colchicine and nonsteroidal anti-inflammatory agents to reduce pain and inflammation
- adrenocorticotropic hormone or steroids for resistant cases of gout
- allopurinol to block formation of uric acid
- probenecid to promote resorption of uric acid deoposits and excretion of uric acid
- low purine diet

LONG TERM MANAGEMENT

- allopurinol
- probenecid
- low purine diet

NURSING MANAGEMENT

Instruct client regarding:
- pain management
- ice to inflamed joints
- bedrest until pain subsides
- avoidance of foods high in purine (liver, kidneys, sweetbreads, mussels, anchovies, consomme)

- increasing fluid intake
- avoidance of beer, ale, and wine (moderate amounts of distilled alcohol do not seem to precipitate gouty attacks)
- need for gradual weight loss
- medications and long term side effects
- signs of colchicine toxicity (nausea, vomiting, diarrhea)
- no aspirin products when taking uricosuric agents (antagonistic effect)
- need for follow-up laboratory tests

(For more information, see pp. 231-232 of Polaski and Tatro, *Luckmann's Core Principles and Practice of Medical-Surgical Nursing.*)

Guillain-Barre´ Syndrome

OVERVIEW

- Guillain-Barre´ syndrome (GBS) is an inflammatory disease of unknown etiology that involves degeneration of the myelin sheath of peripheral nerves.
- GBS affects people of all ages and races.
- In one-half to two-thirds of cases, an upper respiratory or gastrointestinal infection precedes the onset of the syndrome by 1 to 4 weeks.
- The characteristic feature of GBS is ascending weakness, usually beginning in the lower extremities and spreading, sometimes rapidly to the trunk, upper extremities, and face with maximal deficit by 4 weeks in 90 per cent of cases.
- Improvement and recovery occur with remyelination. If nerve axons are damaged, some residual deficits may remain. Recovery is usually maximal at 6 months with 85 to 90 per cent of clients recovering completely.

CLINICAL MANIFESTATIONS

- weakness

- paresthesia (tingling sensation) of the limbs
- loss of deep tendon reflexes
- deep, aching muscle pain in shoulder girdle and thighs
- respiratory compromise or failure — dyspnea, decreased breath sounds, decreased tidal volume
- autonomic dysfunction — orthostatic hypotension, hypertension, pupillary disturbances, sweating dysfunction, cardiac dysrhythmias, paralytic ileus, and urinary retention
- facial weakness, dysphagia, diplopia

MEDICAL MANAGEMENT

- supportive therapy
- plasmapheresis - to remove circulating antibodies

NURSING MANAGEMENT

- Monitor cardiac and respiratory status.
- Monitor laboratory arterial blood gas results.
- Monitor results of daily pulmonary function studies.
- Assure respiratory support equipment is maintained at bedside (oxygen, ambu bag).
- Assess ability to perform self care and provide assistance based on level of client's ability.
- Collaborate with physical and occupational therapy for adaptive devices and exercises.
- Monitor for signs of deep vein thrombosis or pulmonary embolism while on bedrest.
- Initiate appropriate safety measures.
- Provide measures to prevent skin breakdown.

FOCUSED DISCHARGE CARE

- Instruct the client/family regarding:
  — disease process and prognosis
  — use of adaptive devices
  — prevention of skin breakdown
  — exercise regime
  — need for clinic follow-up visit
- Refer to available community resources (e.g., home health care agency).

(For more information, see p. 385 of Polaski and Tatro, *Luckmann's Core Principles and Practice of Medical-Surgical Nursing.*)

H

Hallux Valgus

OVERVIEW

- The hallux valgus (bunion) deformity is the most common disorder of the foot. It is defined as a painful swelling of the bursa mucosa when the great toe deviates laterally at the metatarsophalangeal joint.
- Hallux valgus may be congenital or caused by wearing ill-fitting shoes.
- There is a female predominance.

CLINICAL MANIFESTATIONS

- pain
- deformity of great toe
- callous formation on bottom of the feet

MEDICAL MANAGEMENT

- metatarsal pads
- corticosteroid injections
- analgesics

SURGICAL MANAGEMENT

- bunionectomy (bone resection of first metatarsal) and insertion of Kirschner wires vertically through the toe that remain in place three weeks

NURSING MANAGEMENT

Treatment is generally done on an outpatient basis.

(For more information, see p. 1301 of Polaski and Tatro, *Luckmann's Core Principles and Practice of Medical-Surgical Nursing*.)

Hammer Toe

OVERVIEW

- Hammer toe deformity is a flexion contracture of the proximal interphalangeal joint with extension or slight hyperextension of the distal interphalangeal joint.
- Hammer toe often accompanies hallux valgus deformity (bunion).
- There is a female predominance, occurring in adolescents and young adults.

CLINICAL MANIFESTATIONS

- pain on ambulation with alterations in stride length
- presence of corns on dorsum of toe

MEDICAL MANAGEMENT

- use of toe cushions
- removal of corns
- passive stretching exercises

SURGICAL MANAGEMENT

- resection of proximal phalanx

NURSING MANAGEMENT

Treatment is generally done on an outpatient basis.

(For more information, see p. 1301 of Polaski and Tatro, *Luckmann's Core Principles and Practice of Medical-Surgical Nursing.*)

Headaches, Cluster (Histamine Headaches)

- Cluster headaches sometimes are classified as a

form of migraine. They are excruciatingly painful, unilateral and tend to occur in clusters.

- Numerous episodes may occur over a few days or weeks, followed by a remission with no symptoms for months or years.
- Cluster headaches begin suddenly and may last only a few minutes or as long as two to three hours. There may be excruciating, throbbing or steady pain arising high in the nostril and spreading to one side of the forehead, around and behind the affected eye. The nose and affected eye may water.
- Indomethacin (the medication of choice) and tricyclic antidepressants may be used to prevent the occurrence of cluster headaches. Once the headache occurs, applying cold may help, but most interventions are ineffective because of the shortness of the episodes.
- Supportive care is important because clients may feel depressed over their condition and fearful of another episode.

(For more information, see p. 366 of Polaski and Tatro, *Luckmann's Core Principles and Practice of Medical-Surgical Nursing.*)

Headaches, Migraine

OVERVIEW

- Migraine headaches are paroxysmal disorders characterized by recurrent throbbing headaches.
- The early neurologic symptoms are due to constriction of intracranial vessels. The later, throbbing headache is due to dilation of branches of the external carotid artery. The underlying mechanism causing this spasm and dilation is unknown.
- There are many factors that can precipitate migraines:
  — perfectionist tendencies
  — fatigue
  — excess sleep
  — hunger

— stress
— bright lights
— emotional excitement
— excessive smoking
— drinking alcoholic beverages
— menstruation and ovulation
— chocolate, cheese, citrus fruits, coffee, dairy products and pork products

CLINICAL MANIFESTATIONS

CLASSIC OR TYPICAL MIGRAINE

- an aura or prodromal phase precedes the headache with depression, irritability, restlessness or transient neurological disturbances. It may last several minutes or several hours.
- headache pain, which may be vise-like, dull, pressing, boring, throbbing or hammering — it is usually unilateral and may be localized to the front, back or side of the head
- hypersensitivity of all sensory organs
- photophobia
- vertigo, tremor
- nausea, vomiting, diarrhea
- arteries of the head become prominent, and the amplitude of their pulsation increases

ATYPICAL OR COMMON MIGRAINE

- sudden headache with or without prodromal phase — may be unilateral or generalized
- nausea and vomiting may or may not be present

MEDICAL MANAGEMENT

- ergot preparations, only effective if taken 30 to 60 minutes after headache onset
- codeine sulfate, diphenhydramine hydrochloride or meperidine for pain
- prophylactic beta-adrenergic blockers to reduce frequent episodes
- medication adjustment during menstrual cycles (menstruation and ovulation can trigger migraines)
- elimination of tyramine in diet

NURSING MANAGEMENT

- Instruct client/significant other regarding:
  - factors that trigger migraines
  - use of pressure on the common carotid artery and the affected superficial artery to reduce pain
  - identifying and avoiding dietary triggers
  - stress reduction
  - use of ice on the back of the neck and lying in a dark, quiet room to reduce the pain
- Refer to appropriate resources for relaxation training and biofeedback, if desired.

(For more information, see pp. 364-366 of Polaski and Tatro, *Luckmann's Core Principles and Practice of Medical-Surgical Nursing.*)

Head Trauma

OVERVIEW

- Head trauma is any injury to the scalp, skull or brain.
- Head trauma results in more deaths than all other causes combined for Americans under the age of 34 years.
- Motor vehicle accidents are the main cause of head injuries. Other causes are assaults, falls and accidents.
- Head trauma may be categorized by describing the injury:
  - blunt trauma — complex injuries involving several cranial structures, including brain parenchyma and vessels. Because the brain is able to move within the skull, movement of the brain can result in injuries at different locations.
  - penetrating injuries — those made by foreign bodies such as a knife or bullet
  - coup injury - injury at the point of impact — because of movement within the skull, the same blow may cause injury on the opposite side of the brain, that is, a contrecoup injury

- Scalp injuries can cause lacerations, hematomas and contusions or abrasions to the skin. They may bleed profusely.
- There are three types of skull fractures:
  (1) linear skull fractures — appear as thin lines radiographically
     — do not require treatment
  (2) depressed skull fractures — palpable, can be seen radiographically
     — may require surgery
  (3) basilar skull fractures — occur in bones over the base of the frontal and temporal lobes
     — rarely seen radiographically
- Types of brain injuries include:
  — open head injuries — those that penetrate the skull
  — closed head injuries — those from blunt trauma
  — concussions — head trauma that may result in retrograde amnesia and loss of consciousness for five minutes or less
     — there is no break in the skull or dura and no damage is seen on CT or MRI
     — the client may have headache, nausea and vomiting
  — contusions — cause more damage than concussions
     — contusions damage the brain substance itself, causing multiple areas of petechial and punctate hemorrhage and bruised areas

CLINICAL MANIFESTATIONS

SKULL FRACTURES

- cerebrospinal fluid or other drainage from the ear or nose
- blood behind the eardrum
- periorbital ecchymosis (bruising around the eyes)
- bruise over the mastoid (Battle's sign)
- signs of cranial nerve damage

CEREBRAL CONTUSIONS

- findings vary depending upon the area of injury

Brain Stem Contusions

- unresponsive or comatose
- respiratory, pupillary, eye movement and motor abnormalities may occur

Scalp Injuries

- lacerations, hematomas, contusions, abrasions

MEDICAL MANAGEMENT

Severe head injury

There is a high association of cervical fracture with head injury; therefore, lateral cervical spine radiographs are obtained before the client's head is moved.

- prompt recognition and treatment of hypoxia and acid-base imbalances which, if left untreated, contribute to further cerebral edema
- airway management and adequate oxygenation
- management of shock
- osmotic diuretics to reduce intracranial pressure (ICP)
- management of nutrition and gastrointestinal function
- management of fluid and electrolyte balance
- antiseizure medications
- histamine antagonists to prevent stress ulcers

SURGICAL MANAGEMENT

Simple Skull Depressions

- elevation of the depressed bone fragment and repair of the dura

Compound Depressed Skull Fractures

- debridement of the scalp, skull and devitalized brain and cleansing of the wound

NURSING MANAGEMENT

Immediately following injury:
- Immobilize head and neck until cervical injury ruled out.

- Avoid flexion, hyperextension and rotation of the neck.
- If respiratory resuscitation is needed, use the jaw thrust maneuver.
- Maintain patent airway and support ventilatory function.
- Document baseline neurological assessment.

After initial stabilization:
- Monitor neurological status every hour until stable:
  — Assess level of consciousness, responsiveness.
  — Assess pupillary size, position, direct and consensual responses.
  — Assess extraocular movements.
  — Note verbalization and response to verbal commands by checking hand grip and release, leg movement, dorsiflexion and plantar flexion.
- Monitor for complications:
  — hematoma formation — assess for signs/symptoms of increasing intracranial pressure.
  — infection — assess for signs/symptoms of meningitis.
  — acute hydrocephalus — assess for signs/symptoms of increasing intracranial pressure.
  — adult respiratory distress syndrome — assess for signs/symptoms of hypoxemia, pulmonary congestion, atelectasis and ventricular failure.
- Monitor temperature and maintain normothermia with antipyretic agents or hypothermia blanket.
- Elevate head of bed 30 degrees or as prescribed; keep head in neutral position (use sandbags).
- Monitor vital signs every one to four hours.
- Report high urine output (over 200 ml/hr for two consecutive hours).
- Monitor electrolytes and serum osmolality.
- Monitor urine osmolality and specific gravity.
- Avoid extreme hip flexion (increases intracranial pressure)
- Monitor hemoglobin and hematocrit (loss of blood will result in decreased cerebral perfusion).
- Assess for signs of bleeding: abdomen, chest, pelvis, urinary tract, long bones and extremities.
- Begin early range of motion as prescribed.
- Reposition every two hours.
- Use splints to maintain functional position of hands, arms, legs and feet.
- Facilitate referral to physical/occupational therapy.

- Assess and maintain skin integrity.
- Assess corneal reflex; apply artificial tears or lubricant and tape eyes closed or use patches as necessary.
- Observe for otorrhea or rhinorrhea.
- Test clear, watery fluid for glucose using a test strip.
- Observe blood-tinged fluid for halo sign.
- Do not suction nasally if anterior fossa fracture is present or if basilar fractures are suspected.
- Instruct not to blow nose, cough or inhibit sneeze; sneeze through an open mouth.
- Provide mouth care every four hours; assess for thrush.
- Monitor daily caloric and protein intake.
- Monitor daily weights.
- If tube feeding present, assess for dehydration and provide free water.
- Assess client for pain if restless.
- Reduce environmental stimuli.
- Perform intermittent urinary catheterization as prescribed.
- Begin bladder training as soon as possible.
- Administer stool softeners, laxatives, suppositories as needed.
- Check daily for impaction.
- Orient to person, time and place.
- Devise alternative methods of communicating as needed.
- Assist with gradual progression of activity.
- Encourage to discuss concerns/fears.

FOCUSED DISCHARGE CARE

If the client has mild head injury or is not hospitalized, instruct client/significant other to monitor client for 24 hours and take client to hospital if any of the following occur:
- increased drowsiness or confusion
- inability to be awakened
- vomiting, convulsions
- bleeding or drainage from the nose or ears
- weakness in either arm or either leg
- blurring of vision, slurred speech
- enlargement or shrinkage of one pupil

If the client is hospitalized longer than 48 hours and requires rehabilitation:

- Facilitate referral to rehabilitation program.
- Communicate with rehabilitation facility to ensure continuity of care.

(For more information, see pp. 341-359 of Polaski and Tatro, *Luckmann's Core Principles and Practice of Medical-Surgical Nursing.*)

Hearing Impairment

OVERVIEW

- Hearing impairment ranges from difficulty in understanding words or hearing certain sounds to total deafness.
- Hearing impairment affects one of every fifteen Americans.
- Factors that may cause hearing loss are: scarring or perforation of the tympanic membrane, toxic substances, noise exposure, trauma to the head or ear, age, and infectious diseases (measles, mumps and meningitis).
- Preventive measures include:
  — early, adequate treatment of diseases
  — prevention of trauma to the ear
  — early detection of hearing loss
  — monitoring effects of ototoxic drugs
  — monitoring and prevention of noise pollution
  — periodic ear examinations.

CLINICAL MANIFESTATIONS

- loss of discrimination (the ability to understand what is spoken)
- tinnitus (hearing a roaring, cricket-like or musical sound)
- hearing distorted or abnormal sounds
- excessively loud speech
- constant need for clarification of conversation
- constant requests to repeat information
- tilted head when listening

- failure to respond or inappropriate response to communication.

MEDICAL MANAGEMENT

- aural rehabilitation to teach the client more effective use of vision, touch and vibration, plus maximizing the use of any remaining hearing ability
- hearing aids
- implantable hearing devices
- assistive listening devices (for use with a television, radio or telephone)
- hearing education for speech (lip) reading and sign language

SURGICAL MANAGEMENT

- rare, but may be used to alleviate a conductive hearing loss component or to stop progressive hearing loss

NURSING MANAGEMENT

- Be aware that hearing aids usually amplify all sounds including background noise.
- Facilitate communication with client:
  — minimize background noise
  — gain the client's attention by raising an arm or hand
  — stand so that your face is in light to assist client to speech read
  — speak facing the client
  — speak clearly in a normal tone
  — do not smile, chew gum or cover the mouth when talking
  — use phrases to convey meaning rather than one word answers. State the major topic of discussion first and then give details.
  — encourage use of the hearing aid
  — in a group, repeat important statements and avoid asides to other members in the group
  — do not avoid conversation with a client who has a hearing loss.
- Encourage client to remain socially active.

307

FOCUSED DISCHARGE CARE

Instruct client regarding:
- closed-caption services for the television
- a telephone device for the deaf (TDD)
- sign language classes
- electrical devices for the doorbell
- light-activated special devices such as alarms
- amplification of all sounds and background noise when using a hearing aid; avoid noisy, crowded environments

(For more information, see pp. 465–471 of Polaski and Tatro, *Luckmann's Core Principles and Practice of Medical-Surgical Nursing.*)

Heat Exhaustion

OVERVIEW

- Heat exhaustion occurs after sustained exposure to heat. It is caused by lack of water or salt or both.
- Heat exhaustion from loss of water occurs most often in the elderly, the ill, or the unconscious client, because they are unable to verbalize their thirst. Heat exhaustion from lack of salt occurs mainly in clients who have moved to hot climates but have not acclimated to the weather.

CLINICAL MANIFESTATIONS

Heat exhaustion from lack of water:
- intense thirst with dehydration
- fatigue
- muscle incoordination
- agitation
- impaired judgment
- body temperature exceeds 104° F. (40.6° C.)
- hot, dry and flushed skin
- hypotension (blood shunted into peripheral circulation for cooling)
- seizures

- muscle rigidity, tremors
- dysrhythmias

Heat exhaustion from lack of salt
- weakness and fatigue
- severe headache
- muscle cramps

MEDICAL MANAGEMENT

- replacement of water and salt
- antipyretics

NURSING MANAGEMENT

- Administer fluid and salt replacement therapy.
- Monitor body temperature.
- Monitor intake and output.
- Ensure adequate rest.
- Administer antipyretics.
- Implement safety measures.

FOCUSED DISCHARGE CARE

Instruct client regarding:
- measures to prevent recurrence

(For more information, see p. 307 of Polaski and Tatro, *Luckmann's Core Principles and Practice of Medical-Surgical Nursing.*)

Heatstroke

- Heatstroke is an emergency and requires immediate treatment for survival.
- There are two forms of heatstroke: classic heatstroke and exertional heatstroke.
  — Classic heatstroke usually is seen in the poor, the elderly, the chronically ill, clients with heart disease, the obese and alcoholics. Hot humid weather lasting three or more days increases the risk of heatstroke in these clients. The mechanism for classic heatstroke is not known but involves the

failure of the heat regulating mechanism with cessation of sweating. Signs and symptoms include rectal temperature greater than 106° F.; hot dry skin; absence of sweating (in most cases); tachycardia; rapid, weak respirations; hypotension; lethargy; stupor; coma; and muscle flaccidity.

— Exertional heatstroke is more common in laborers, farmers, athletes and clients who work in boiler rooms or foundries. Symptoms are similar to classic heatstroke except sweating occurs, and the temperature is lower (about 102 to 104° F.) than in classic heatstroke. Piloerection (gooseflesh), nausea, vomiting, unsteady gait and incoherent speech also occur. Clients with exertional heatstroke tend to develop more lactic acidosis and severe bleeding problems than clients with classic heatstroke.

NURSING MANAGEMENT

Immediate nursing management involves rapidly reducing body temperature via immersion in ice water, if possible, for classic heatstroke. Placement of wet, cold sheets; sponging with cold water; or a hypothermia blanket may be used for exertional heatstroke or as a secondary treatment for classic heatstroke if an ice water bath is not available.

- The client should be placed in a cool place with adequate circulation of cool air and with most of the clothing removed.
- Monitor rectal temperature continuously.
- Insert an intravenous line.
- Monitor cardiac rhythm continuously.
- Obtain frequent vital signs.
- Administer chlorpromazine or diazepam as prescribed to reduce shivering.
- Insert urinary catheter.
- Provide supplemental oxygen as prescribed.

(For more information, see p. 307, 1588 of Polaski and Tatro, *Luckmann's Core Principles and Practice of Medical-Surgical Nursing.*)

Hemophilia

OVERVIEW

- Hemophilia is a genetically transmitted coagulation disorder.
- There are three major types of hemophilia: Hemophilia A (classic hemophilia), Hemophilia B (Christmas disease) and von Willebrand's disease.
  — Hemophilia A — factor VIII deficiency
  — Hemophilia B — factor IX deficiency
  — von Willebrand's disease — factor VIII deficiency and defective platelet function.
- Classic hemophilia makes up 80 per cent of the hemophilias.

CLINICAL MANIFESTATIONS (HEMOPHILIA A)

- slow, prolonged, persistent bleeding from cuts or scratches
- delayed bleeding that follows minor injuries
- bleeding into deep subcutaneous and intramuscular tissue
- easy bruising
- joint pain — secondary to hemorrhage into joints
- platelet function, platelet count, bleeding time and prothrombin time are normal
- factor VIII is missing from the plasma

MEDICAL MANAGEMENT (HEMOPHILIA A)

- factor VIII or IX concentration transfusion
- packed red blood cell replacement if severe blood loss
- topical bleeding control — applying pressure, packing area with fibrin foam, topical hemostatics, such as thrombin
- joint immobilization
- analgesics and corticosteroids for joint pain
- desmopressin — increases plasma factor VIII activity

NURSING MANAGEMENT (HEMOPHILIA A)

- Administer factor VIII replacement.

- Institute ordered measures to control topical bleeding.
- Assess the factor VIII level prior to even a minor invasive procedure.
- Assess all body systems for signs of bleeding.
- Administer analgesics.
- Immobilize affected joints until swelling subsides, then begin range of motion exercises.
- Monitor daily laboratory findings — CBC, factor VIII level.
- Institute bleeding precautions:
  - no intramuscular or subcutaneous injections
  - soft toothbrush
  - electric razor
  - hold venipuncture sites
  - safety measures for ambulation
- Provide emotional support.

FOCUSED DISCHARGE CARE

- Instruct client regarding:
  - disease process and treatment regime
  - factor VIII administration (life-long therapy)
  - precautions to prevent bleeding:
    - no contact sports
    - soft toothbrush
    - electric razor
    - care when preparing food
    - care when doing yard work
    - safety precautions
  - emergency administration of factor VIII and methods to control bleeding if injury occurs
  - signs/symptoms of complications and when to call physician
  - importance of laboratory and clinic follow-up visits
  - need to wear a Medic-Alert bracelet
- Refer to available community resources.

(For more information, see pp. 874-876 of Polaski and Tatro, *Luckmann's Core Principles and Practice of Medical-Surgical Nursing.*)

Hemorrhoids

OVERVIEW

- Hemorrhoids are perianal varicose veins. They may be internal or external.
- Hemorrhoids may result from the many anastomoses between the plexuses or from the lack of valves in the veins of the superior hemorrhoidal plexus, which leads into the portal vein.
- Enlargement of hemorrhoids is caused by increased intra-abdominal pressure.
- Pregnancy, congestive heart failure, prolonged sitting or standing, cirrhosis with portal hypertension, constipation, diarrhea and prolonged straining with defecation contribute to hemorrhoid development and enlargement.

CLINICAL MANIFESTATIONS

- enlarged mass at the anus (external hemorrhoids)
- bright red bleeding, prolapse, rectal itching and constipation (internal hemorrhoids)

MEDICAL MANAGEMENT

- treatment of constipation (fiber, increased fluids, stool softeners, hydrophilic psyllium preparations)
- heat application and astringent lotions to relieve pain
- topical anesthetic or steroid preparations

SURGICAL MANAGEMENT

- ligation — placement of a rubber band around the neck of the hemorrhoid through an anoscope (for internal hemorrhoids only)
- cryosurgery — freezing of the hemorrhoids, performed infrequently
- laser removal — burning off the hemorrhoid with a laser
- hemorrhoidectomy — excision of the vein with the area left open to heal by granulation (high success rate) or sutured closed

NURSING MANAGEMENT

Postoperative Care

In addition to routine postoperative care:

- Monitor for urinary retention.
- Monitor for hemorrhage.
- Provide warm sitz baths 3 to 4 times daily after a hemorrhoidectomy.
- Apply zinc oxide ointment for perianal irritations.
- Instruct to wipe area very gently.
- Warn that fainting can occur due to pain and vagal stimulation during the first postoperative bowel movement.

FOCUSED DISCHARGE CARE

Instruct client regarding:

- measures to avoid constipation
- monitoring stool for blood
- high fiber diet
- adequate fluid intake
- use of bulk laxatives or mineral oil
- use of cold packs followed by warm sitz baths 3 to 4 times per day
- good cleansing of the peri-anal area

(For more information, see pp. 1084-1085 of Polaski and Tatro, *Luckmann's Core Principles and Practice of Medical-Surgical Nursing.*)

Hemothorax

- Hemothorax is the presence of blood in the pleural space. Hemothorax may be present in clients with chest injuries.
- A small amount of blood (less than 300 ml) may cause no symptoms and require no treatment (the blood will be reabsorbed spontaneously).
- A large amount (1400 to 2500 ml) may be life-threatening because of resultant hypovolemia and compression of the lung. Clinical manifestations may

include dullness to percussion on the affected side, tachycardia, hypotension and shock.

- For severe distress, the physician may insert a 16-gauge needle into the fifth or sixth intercostal space at the mid-axillary line to aspirate the blood.
- A chest tube catheter may be inserted and connected to a closed drainage system.
- An initial drainage of 500 to 1000 ml is considered moderate. Continued large amounts of drainage (200 ml or more per hour) may indicate a need for emergency thoracotomy.

(For more information, see pp. 1577-1578 of Polaski and Tatro, *Luckmann's Core Principles and Practice of Medical-Surgical Nursing.*)

Hepatic Encephalopathy

OVERVIEW

- Hepatic encephalopathy encompasses a spectrum of central nervous system (CNS) disturbances. These may appear in conjunction with severe liver injury, liver failure or a portal shunt.
- Hepatic encephalopathy is characterized by elevation of ammonia levels in the blood and cerebrospinal fluid. Normally, the liver converts ammonia into glutamine, which is stored in the liver and later converted to urea and excreted through the kidneys. Blood ammonia rises when the liver cells are unable to perform this function due to liver cell damage or necrosis. With a portal shunt, serum ammonia levels may rise since the blood bypasses the liver and is directly shunted into the systemic venous circulation.
- Mental status changes occur with high ammonia levels because ammonia is a central nervous system (CNS) toxin, causing altered CNS metabolism and function.
- Ammonia is produced when protein is broken down in the gastrointestinal tract by bacteria. In clients with impaired liver function, any process that in-

315

creases protein in the intestine, such as increased dietary protein or gastrointestinal bleeding, causes elevated blood ammonia levels.

CLINICAL MANIFESTATIONS

- fatigue, restlessness, irritability
- impaired memory, decreased attention span, impaired concentration, decreased rate of response
- personality changes, sleep pattern reversal
- deterioration in handwriting
- asterixis (rapid extension and flexion of the fingers and wrists when the arms are extended and the hands dorsiflexed — also called liver flap)
- drowsiness, confusion
- lethargy
- hyperventilation with respiratory alkalosis
- severe confusion, inability to follow commands
- coma, unresponsiveness to painful stimuli
- absence of reflexes
- decerebrate or decorticate posturing

MEDICAL MANAGEMENT

- dietary protein restriction
- neomycin to reduce bacteria in the intestinal tract
- lactulose to bind ammonium ions in the bowel, which are then eliminated
- prevention of gastrointestinal bleeding
- fluid and electrolyte replacement
- respiratory support for hypoxia

NURSING MANAGEMENT

- Discuss need for low protein diet.
- Monitor for signs/symptoms of gastrointestinal bleeding: bright red blood in stools or dark tarry stools (bleeding increases protein in the gastrointestinal tract, which will produce ammonia when it is broken down).
- Monitor for therapeutic effect of lactulose (usual goal is 2 to 3 soft stools daily).
- Maintain adequate fluid volume (hypovolemia may precipitate hepatic encephalopathy).
  — Monitor intake and output.
  — Monitor vital signs.

- — Measure central venous pressure hourly.
- — Administer IV fluids as ordered.
- Monitor electrolyte and pH levels (electrolyte or acid-base disturbances may precipitate encephalopathy).
- Monitor neurological status and perform neurological checks frequently.
- Assess for possible side effects of diarrhea and vitamin K deficiency with neomycin therapy, due to depletion of intestinal flora.
- Assess for possible side effects of ototoxicity and nephrotoxicity with neomycin use.
- Maintain safety precautions (especially if confused/agitated).
- Prevent and treat hypoxia which may precipitate encephalopathy.
- Protect from infection.
- Avoid use of depressants which may precipitate coma.
- Review medications and avoid use of medications solely metabolized by the liver (metabolism by the kidney preferred). Discuss with physician.
- Provide good skin care and good pulmonary hygiene for the client with decreased level of consciousness.

FOCUSED DISCHARGE CARE

- Instruct client/significant other regarding:
  - — signs/symptoms of encephalopathy/worsening encephalopathy and to call physician
  - — medications — action and side effects
  - — need for low protein diet
  - — signs/symptoms of gastrointestinal bleeding and other complications of cirrhosis
  - — safety precautions
- Refer to chemical dependency group or support group such as Alcoholics Anonymous.

See also, "Cirrhosis", p. 164.

(For more information, see pp. 1130-1133 of Polaski and Tatro, *Luckmann's Core Principles and Practice of Medical-Surgical Nursing*.)

Hepatitis, Alcoholic

- Alcoholic hepatitis is an acute or chronic inflammation of the liver caused by parenchymal necrosis from heavy alcohol ingestion.
- This condition is the most frequent cause of cirrhosis.
- Clinical manifestations usually follow a recent bout of heavy drinking: anorexia, nausea, abdominal pain, splenomegaly, hepatomegaly, jaundice, ascites, fever and encephalopathy.
- Nursing intervention includes a high-vitamin, high-carbohydrate diet; folic acid supplements and parenteral fluids.
- The prognosis is poor, particularly if the client continues to use alcohol.

(For more information, see pp. 1119-1120 of Polaski and Tatro, *Luckmann's Core Principles and Practice of Medical-Surgical Nursing.*)

Hepatitis, Chronic

- Chronic hepatitis exists when liver inflammation continues beyond a period of 3 to 6 months. It may be manifest as chronic persistent hepatitis (CPH) or chronic active hepatitis (CAH).
- CPH is benign and seldom progressive. CAH is more serious.
- Untreated CAH has a high mortality rate. Death results from hepatic failure, bleeding varicies, hepatic encephalopathy, or primary hepatocellular carcinoma.
- Clinical manifestations of CAH are: jaundice, fever, bleeding tendencies, liver necrosis, abdominal pain, severe weakness, arthralgias and extrahepatic abnormalities (such as thyroiditis, hemolytic anemia, amenorrhea, arthritis, urticaria and glomerulonephritis).
- Treatment of symptomatic CAH may include steroids for 3 to 5 years or azathioprine with smaller

steroid doses. Bedrest is encouraged during the active phase of disease.
- Nursing management includes:
  — supportive care
  — instructing client on steroid therapy, possible side effects and not to abruptly stop medication
  — instructing client/significant other on signs/symptoms to report to physician
  — discussing importance of compliance with follow-up
- See also, "Hepatitis, Viral", p. 319.

(For more information, see p. 1119 of Polaski and Tatro, *Luckmann's Core Principles and Practice of Medical-Surgical Nursing.*)

Hepatitis, Viral

OVERVIEW

- Hepatitis is inflammation of the liver. There are 5 types of viral hepatitis:
  (1) Hepatitis A (also called short incubation hepatitis, infectious hepatitis and MS_1 hepatitis) — caused by an enterovirus, it is transmitted primarily by the fecal-oral route, although parenteral transmission can occur, though rarely. It also may be transmitted through contaminated shellfish or via the airborne route if there are copious secretions. Causes of epidemics include infected water, milk, food and raw shellfish from contaminated waters. The incubation period is 15 to 45 days.
  (2) Hepatitis B — transmitted via the blood of an infected client, but also may be spread through semen, saliva, sexual contact or the fecal-oral route. It may be spread by carriers. The hepatitis B virus (HBV) can survive on surfaces up to one week. The incubation period is 28 to 180 days. Up to 10 per cent of persons infected with HBV

become chronic carriers and may be at risk for cirrhosis, liver cancer, and death.

(3) Hepatitis C— transmitted parenterally through the blood, by personal contact and possibly by the fecal-oral route. It may be spread by carriers. The incubation period is 7 to 8 weeks.

(4) Delta Hepatitis— transmitted only through blood contact. It is a defective RNA virus that must coexist with HBV. The incubation period is 28 to 180 days.

(5) Hepatitis E — transmitted by the fecal-to-oral route, contaminated water, and poor sanitation. It is seen in Asia, Africa, and Mexico, but is not common in the United States. The incubation period is 15 to 64 days. May be similar to Hepatitis A in infectiousness. Full recovery is likely with no chronic carrier state.

- Risk factors for each type of hepatitis are:
  (1) Hepatitis A —
    — handling feces or contaminated articles
    — working with animals imported from areas where hepatitis A is endemic
  (2) Hepatitis B -
    — health care workers
    — multiple blood transfusions or dialysis
    — homosexually active males
    — morticians
    — persons who undergo tattooing
    — intravenous drug abusers
    — infected heterosexuals via body fluids
  (3) Hepatitis C —
    — similar risk factors as for hepatitis B
  (4) Delta Hepatitis —
    — same risk factors as for hepatitis B
  (5) Hepatitis E —
    — similar to those associated with Hepatitis A
- Preventive measures include:
  (1) Hepatitis A
    — good personal hygiene and handwashing
    — avoidance of shellfish or polluted fishing waters
    — monitoring of eating establishments by local health authorities
    — isolating newly imported animals for 2 months
    — prophylactic immune globulin (IG) (protects for 2 months)

(2) Hepatitis B
  — using body substance isolation when handling blood or body fluids
  — screening donors' blood for hepatitis B virus surface antigen (HB$_s$Ag)
  — use of volunteers rather than paid donors for blood products
  — encouraging clients who are having elective surgery to donate their own blood
  — good personal hygiene by clients with hepatitis B or carriers
  — vaccination with hepatitis B immune globulin (HBIG) after exposure (passive immunization)
  — use of hepatitis B vaccine (active immunization) before exposure. It may be used in conjunction with HBIG after documented exposure to hepatitis B.
(3) Hepatitis C
  — similar measures as for hepatitis B
(4) Delta Hepatitis
  — similar measures as for hepatitis B
(5) Hepatitis E
  — vaccine not available in United States

CLINICAL MANIFESTATIONS

Symptoms vary from client to client. Hepatitis B and delta hepatitis usually produce the most severe symptoms, although some clients may be asymptomatic.
- jaundice, lethargy, irritability, fatigue, weakness
- myalgia, arthralgia, anorexia
- nausea, vomiting, abdominal pain in right upper quadrant, diarrhea, constipation
- flu-like symptoms, fever
- pruritus
- dark urine, clay-colored stools
- bleeding tendencies
- anemia
- drowsiness
- hepatic encephalopathy
- asterixis (rapid extension and flexion of the fingers and wrists when the arms are extended and the hands are dorsiflexed, also called "liver flap")

MEDICAL MANAGEMENT

- rest
- proper diet high in protein (if not encephalopathic), carbohydrates and calories
- Hepatitis A— immune globulin (IG) for prophylaxis or post exposure
- Hepatitis B— for prophylaxis, hepatitis B immune globulin (HBIG) is usually given in 3 doses—the second and third doses are given 1 month and 6 months after initial dose. For post exposure, HBIG or the standard form (IG) may be administered.
- antiemetics for nausea and vomiting
- cholestyramine or ursodiol for pruritus (binds with bile salts in the intestine)

NURSING MANAGEMENT

- Monitor mental status and assess for early signs of hepatic encephalopathy (ask patient to write name every shift — deterioration of handwriting is an early sign of encephalopathy).
- Consider possible effects of medications on liver function before administering.
- Assess for asterixis.
- Monitor hemoglobin and hematocrit.
- Monitor for signs/symptoms of bleeding.
- Encourage a reasonable activity level and frequent rest periods (excess activity can possibly lead to liver failure).
- Assist with activities of daily living as needed.
- Implement measures to prevent complications of immobility.
- Encourage adequate nutrition.
  — Avoid heavy, greasy foods.
  — Provide good breakfast (usually best tolerated meal).
  — Devise dietary plan high in protein (unless encephalopathic), high in carbohydrates and moderate in fat.
  — Suggest multiple small meals.
  — Instruct to avoid alcohol (hepatotoxic agent).
- Discuss disease and its treatment, and how to prevent recurrence and spread.

- Provide opportunities for discussion of feelings/concerns regarding duration and cost of illness and effects of illness on future health.
- Administer oral cholestyramine as prescribed for pruritus.
- Administer oral antihistamines for itching as prescribed.

FOCUSED DISCHARGE CARE

Instruct client regarding:
- slowly returning to former activity levels to avoid a relapse
- obtaining adequate rest
- diet
- how to avoid reinfection or infecting other family members
- avoidance of alcohol and medications such as aspirin or sedatives which are hepatotoxic
- avoidance of sexual activity until physician permits
- need for follow-up visits to ensure liver is healing and no damage has occurred

See also "Hepatitis, Chronic", p. 318.

(For more information, see pp. 1113-1119 of Polaski and Tatro, *Luckmann's Core Principles and Practice of Medical-Surgical Nursing*.)

Herniated Intervertebral Disc

OVERVIEW

- Displacement of intervertebral disc material may be referred to as prolapse, herniation, rupture or extrusion of the disc. These interchangeable terms indicate loss of integrity of the disc between two vertebrae. Ruptured intervertebral discs may occur at any level of the spine; however, lumbar discs are the most likely to rupture.
- Compression of spinal nerve roots may result from herniation of the disc. If compression remains un-

treated, weakness or paralysis of the innervated muscle group may result.

- Risk factors include:
  — heavy physical labor
  — strenuous exercise
  — weak abdominal and back muscles
  — use of poor body mechanics.

CLINICAL MANIFESTATIONS

RUPTURED LUMBAR DISC

- lower back pain that radiates down the posterior thigh
- muscle spasm
- aggravation of pain by straining (coughing, defecation, bending, lifting and straight-leg raising)
- depression of deep tendon reflexes
- hyperesthesia in the area of distribution of affected nerve roots

RUPTURED CERVICAL DISC

- stiff neck
- shoulder pain that radiates down the arm into the hand
- paresthesias and sensory disturbances in the hand

MEDICAL MANAGEMENT

- anti-inflammatory agents
- muscle relaxants
- analgesics
- ultrasonic heat treatment
- localized moist heat application
- localized ice application
- progressive muscle strengthening exercises
- bedrest — initially with progressive activity schedule
- brace, corset or cervical collar

SURGICAL MANAGEMENT

- laminectomy — surgical removal of the posterior arch of a vertebra, exposing the spinal cord for removal of the portion of the nucleus pulposus that

is protruding or ruptured from a herniated intervertebral disc
- spinal fusion — placement of a bone graft in the disc
interspace that grows and fuses the two vertebrae
together thus immobilizing them. Bone chips may be
placed between vertebral bodies where a disc was
removed. The bone graft may be obtained from a
bone bank or a region of the client's iliac crest. An
anterior or posterior surgical approach may be taken.
- microsurgical techniques to remove ruptured discs
cause less trauma and preserve tissue integrity.

NURSING MANAGEMENT

MEDICAL

- Administer anti-inflammatory and analgesic agents
and muscle relaxants as prescribed.
- Apply heat/cold applications as prescribed.
- Collaborate with physical therapy for a progressive
exercise/activity schedule.

SURGICAL

POSTOPERATIVE CARE

In addition to routine postoperative care:
Cervical Laminectomy or Fusion
- Assess for possible complications:
  (1) posterior approach
    — soft tissue hematoma
    — air embolism
    — migration of the bone graft (spinal fusion) —
      radicular pain suddenly recurs
    — wound dehiscence
    — spinal cord compression
  (2) anterior approach
    — laryngeal nerve damage
    — injury to neck structures, such as carotid ar-
      teries, trachea, or esophagus
    — spinal cord compression
    — migration of the bone graft (spinal fusion)
- Assess neurological status:
  — movement of shoulders and extremities
  — presence of numbness or tingling
  — changes in sensation

325

(Progressive worsening of motor and sensory function may indicate spinal cord edema or hemorrhage compressing the spinal cord.)
- Maintain soft cervical collar.
- Keep head flat (except for small folded blanket).
- Assist with repositioning, avoid any jarring movements.
- Initiate out-of-bed activities as prescribed with collar in place.
- Implement measures to relieve sore throat (anterior approach) — throat lozenges, viscous lidocaine, humidified air, minimal talking.
- Assure that emergency respiratory equipment is readily available.
- Prevent flexion of the neck.
- Administer PRN analgesics and assess effectiveness.

Lumbar Laminectomy or Fusion
- Assess for possible complications:
  - epidural hematoma (a surgical emergency)
  - injury to nerve roots
  - migration of bone graft (spinal fusion)
  - injury to nearby structures
  - urinary retention
  - paralytic ileus
- Assess neurological status:
  - movement of extremities
  - presence of numbness or tingling
  - changes in sensation
    (Progressive worsening of motor and sensory function may indicate spinal cord edema or hemorrhage compressing the spinal cord.)
- Position as ordered (in immediate postoperative period)
  - laminectomy — client is not turned for 1 to 2 hours and is left flat
  - spinal fusion — bed is generally kept flat
  - microdiscectomy — head of bed elevated to position of comfort
- Reposition side-to-side using log-rolling technique.
- Initiate out-of-bed activities as ordered.
  - laminectomy — usually first or second postoperative day
  - spinal fusion — bedrest maintained longer
- Administer PRN analgesics and muscle relaxants as prescribed. Assess effectiveness.

- Collaborate with physical therapy regarding progressive activity/exercise program and adaptive devices (braces, corsets, etc.).
- Assess for distended bladder.
- Assess for paralytic ileus.

FOCUSED DISCHARGE CARE

Instruct client regarding:
- walking restrictions
- driving restrictions
- lifting restrictions
- work restrictions
- use of adaptive devices
- wound care

(For more information, see pp. 406–412 of Polaski and Tatro, *Luckmann's Core Principles and Practice of Medical-Surgical Nursing.*)

Herniations

OVERVIEW

- A hernia is the abnormal protrusion of an organ, tissue or part of an organ through the structure that normally contains it.
- Hernias occur due to defects in the integrity of the muscular wall and increased intra-abdominal pressure.
- The most common hernias are:
  — inguinal
    — indirect — occurs through inguinal ring and follows the inguinal canal
    — direct - occurs through the abdominal wall in an area of muscular weakness
  — femoral — occurs through the femoral ring and gradually pulls the peritoneum and urinary bladder into the sac

— umbilical — due to increased abdominal pressure, as with obese or multiparous women
— incisional (ventral) — occurs at a site of previous surgical incision that healed inadequately.

MEDICAL MANAGEMENT

- mechanical reduction, if the hernia is not strangulated or incarcerated
- truss - a firm pad held in place by a belt; worn daily and applied before arising

SURGICAL MANAGEMENT

- hernia repair — excision of the hernia sac, returning the herniated contents (usually intestine) back to their normal position and closing the muscle tightly over the area

NURSING MANAGEMENT

Surgical

Postoperative Care
In addition to routine postoperative care:
- Instruct the client to splint incision when coughing or sneezing to provide incisional support.
- Ensure the client voids after surgery.
- Assure the client that the hernia will not recur in the immediate postoperative period.
- Inguinal Hernia Repair:
  — Apply an ice pack to the incisional area.
  — Assess scrotal area for swelling in male clients:
    — elevate scrotum and instruct to wear a scrotal support when the client is out of bed.

FOCUSED DISCHARGE CARE

Medical

- Ensure client knows how to wear truss or binder.
- Instruct client on signs/symptoms of hernia strangulation and to report immediately to physician.
- Encourage weight reduction program for obese clients.
- Instruct client to assess for any skin irritation under binder.

- Instruct client regarding:
  — no heavy lifting for 4 to 6 weeks after surgery
  — signs/symptoms of infection
  — wound care
- If binder will be worn at home, instruct how to assess skin for irritation and to evaluate the effectiveness of the system.

(For more information, see pp. 1087-1088 of Polaski and Tatro, *Luckmann's Core Principles and Practice of Medical-Surgical Nursing.*)

Herpes Zoster

- Herpes zoster (or shingles) is an infection caused by the same virus that causes varicella (or chicken pox).
- After one to two days of pain, itching and hyperesthesia, clusters of grouped vesicles appear unilaterally along cranial or spinal nerve dermatomes. Because they follow nerve pathways, the lesions do not cross the body's midline; however, the nerves of both sides may be involved.
- The eruption clears in about two weeks unless the period between the pain and the eruption is longer than two days. In the latter case, a prolonged convalescence may be expected.
- Residual pain, post-herpetic neuralgia and itching are the major problems with herpes zoster. The pain may last weeks or months to years.
- Medical management:
  — use of the antiviral agent, acyclovir (Zovirax)
  — systemic corticosteroids in clients over age 50
  — analgesics and sedatives
- Nursing management:
  — Administer and assess effectiveness of prescribed analgesics.
  — Provide other measures for pain relief: application of cool compresses, use of cooling antipruritic preparations.

- Instruct client and significant other on mode of transmission and ways to prevent.
- Instruct client and significant other on measures to prevent secondary infection.
- Provide emotional support and discuss with client and significant others that continued intervention and long-term support will be needed.

(For more information, see pp. 1354-1355 of Polaski and Tatro, *Luckmann's Core Principles and Practice of Medical-Surgical Nursing*.)

Hiatal Hernia

OVERVIEW

- A hiatal hernia (diaphragmatic hernia) is a condition in which the cardiac sphincter becomes enlarged allowing the stomach to pass into the thoracic cavity.
- There are 2 types:
  (1) sliding hernias —the upper stomach and the gastroesophageal junction are displaced upward into the thorax (most common)
  (2) rolling or paraesophageal hernias — the gastroesophageal junction stays below the diaphragm, but all or part of the stomach pushes through to the thorax.
- Risk factors include obesity, pregnancy or ascites.

CLINICAL MANIFESTATIONS

Sliding
- heartburn 30 to 60 minutes after meals
- substernal pain

Rolling
- no symptoms of reflux
- fullness after a meal
- chest pain, worse when recumbent

MEDICAL MANAGEMENT

See "Gastroesophageal Reflux Disease", p. 277.

SURGICAL MANAGEMENT

If the client does not respond to medical treatment, the client may be treated surgically, the same as for "Gastroesophageal Reflux Disease", see p. 277.

NURSING MANAGEMENT

See "Gastroesophageal Reflux Disease", p. 277.

FOCUSED DISCHARGE CARE

MEDICAL

See "Gastroesophageal Reflux Disease", p. 277.

SURGICAL

Following hiatal hernia repair
- Instruct client regarding:
  — appropriate diet modifications
  — drug therapy
  — positioning
  — avoid straining the incision for at least 6 weeks after surgery
  — avoidance of lifting heavy objects
  — avoidance of stair climbing for several days
  — signs/symptoms of incisional infection and to report to physician
  — eating several small meals daily rather than three large meals
  — available weight loss and smoking cessation support groups as appropriate

(For more information, see pp. 1022-1023 of Polaski and Tatro, *Luckmann's Core Principles and Practice of Medical-Surgical Nursing*.)

Hodgkin's Disease

OVERVIEW

- Hodgkin's disease is a lymphoma that results in uncontrolled proliferation of lymphocytes.
- Hodgkin's arises in the lymphoid tissues, that is, lymph nodes, thymus, spleen and lymphoid tissues of the gastrointestinal tract. It is characterized by painless enlargement of lymph nodes with progression to extralymphatic sites, such as the spleen and liver.
- Lymphomas are classified as either (1) Hodgkin's — containing the Reed-Stenberg cell, or (2) non-Hodgkin's —without Reed-Stenberg cell.
- Hodgkin's staging classifications are:
  - Stage I — involves a single lymph node region
  - Stage II — involves two or more lymph node regions on the same side of the diaphragm
  - Stage III — involves lymph node regions on both sides of the diaphragm
  - Stage IV — diffuse or disseminated involvement of one or more extralymphatic tissues
- Hodgkin's is a disease of young adults, primarily occurring between the ages of 20 and 40 years. It affects men more than women.
- The complete remission rate for Hodgkin's is 75 to 90 per cent. There is a 10 to 20 per cent recurrence rate that varies with the stage of the disease.

CLINICAL MANIFESTATIONS

- painless, enlarged lymph nodes
- fevers and night sweats
- weight loss
- pruritus
- hepatosplenomegaly
- pain over enlarged lymph nodes after ingesting alcohol
- nonproductive cough, dyspnea (mediastinal involvement)
- edema of the face, neck, right arm (superior vena cava syndrome secondary to lymph node enlargement and compression)

- jaundice (bile duct obstruction)
- renal failure (ureteral obstruction by enlarged lymph nodes)
- progressive anemia with fatigue and malaise
- bone pain (vertebral compression)
- paraplegia (spinal cord compression)

MEDICAL MANAGEMENT

- chemotherapy — nitrogen mustard, oncovin, procarbazine, prednisone
- radiation therapy

NURSING MANAGEMENT

- Administer prescribed chemotherapy.
- See "Chemotherapy", p. 145.
- See "Radiation Therapy", p. 543.
- Monitor laboratory findings - CBC, BUN, creatinine, platelet count.
- Encourage balanced diet.
- Encourage rest.

FOCUSED DISCHARGE CARE

- Instruct client regarding:
  — disease process and treatment regime
  — see "Chemotherapy", p. 145
  — see "Radiation Therapy", p. 543
  — signs/symptoms to report to physician
  — importance of follow-up visits
- Refer to available community resources.

(For more information, see pp. 863-864 of Polaski and Tatro, *Luckmann's Core Principles and Practice of Medical-Surgical Nursing.*)

Human Immunodeficiency Virus (HIV) Infection

OVERVIEW

- Human immunodeficiency virus is the causative agent in the development of acquired immunodeficiency syndrome (AIDS), an advanced stage of disease along a continuum that ranges from asymptomatic HIV infection to the development of this most serious and debilitating condition.
- Once the initial HIV infection takes place, the virus may remain latent inside the cell for an undetermined amount of time. The main target of HIV infection is the T_4 cell. Once these cells are infected, either they are changed and rendered nonfunctional or their actual number is depleted. The normal number of T_4 cells is between 700 and 1300 T_4 cells/mm^3. Opportunistic infections most commonly occur when the T_4 cell count drops below 200. HIV-related malignancies and neurologies can occur at a higher count.
- The disease has grown to epidemic proportions since 1981.
- HIV infection has an extremely high mortality rate; over 90 per cent of clients who develop the most severe form of the disease will die within 4 years of an AIDS diagnosis. Most clients affected are between the ages of 20 and 49 years.
- Transmission of HIV occurs through horizontal transmission (from either sexual contact or parenteral exposure to blood and blood products) or through vertical transmission (from HIV-infected mother to infant). HIV is not transmitted by casual contact. Transmission always involves exposure to some body fluid of an infected client. The greatest concentrations of the virus have been found in blood, semen, cerebrospinal fluid, and cervical/vaginal secretions. Risk factors include:
  — homosexual activity
  — heterosexual activity associated with multiple sexual partners, receptive anal intercourse, presence of open lesions in the genital area, and sexual exposure without protection
  — direct blood to blood contact

- sharing contaminated needles
- transfusion of blood or blood products
- accidental needlestick
- blood exposure to non-intact skin or mucous membrane
- babies born to mothers who are HIV positive
- babies breastfed by HIV-positive mothers

CLINICAL MANIFESTATIONS

The first stage of HIV infection is the process of being exposed to HIV and becoming antibody-positive (sero-conversion). Some clients experience a mononucleosis-like illness consisting of fever, malaise, lymphadenopathy, rash, and at times, aseptic meningitis; others remain asymptomatic throughout this phase. Once the client is HIV positive, the continuum begins with a period of remaining asymptomatic. Although the length of this phase varies, it commonly ranges from 7 to 10 years. HIV disease begins to develop as the immune system becomes depleted or ineffective as a result of the virus' effect on the T-helper cell.

- lymphadenopathy
- skin rashes
- fevers
- fatigue
- drenching night sweats
- persistent diarrhea, weight loss
- oral thrush
- vaginal yeast infection
- pain related to peripheral neuropathies, myalgias, or malignancies
- evidence of opportunistic infections:
  — Pneumocystis carinii pneumonia (PCP)
    — number one killer of clients with AIDS
    — clinical manifestations:
      - fever
      - fatigue
      - weight loss
      - cough and dyspnea
      - clear lung sounds
  — Cytomegalovirus infection (CMV)
    — almost 90% of AIDS clients develop CMV during the course of their illness
      - CMV chorioretinitis
      - CMV colitis
      - CMV pneumonitis

- Herpes simplex virus (HSV)
  - clinical manifestations:
    - tingling and burning at the site of the vesicle (mouth, esophagus, genital or perirectal areas)
    - severe pain at the site of the lesion
    - dysphagia
- Toxoplasmosis
  - major opportunistic infection of the central nervous system
  - clinical manifestations:
    - headaches
    - seizures
    - hemiparesis
    - lethargy
    - personality changes
    - change in cognitive ability
- Cryptosporidium infection (intestinal protozoan infection)
  - clinical manifestations:
    - watery diarrhea
    - malaise
    - nausea and abdominal cramps
- Mycobacterium tuberculosis (MTB)
  - is often extrapulmonary involving the kidneys, liver, spleen, lymph nodes, and bone marrow
  - clinical manifestations:
    - fever
    - weight loss
    - night sweats
    - fatigue
    - lymphadenitis
- Candida albicans infection
  - fungus that causes infection of the mouth, esophagus, and vagina
  - clinical manifestations:
    - white, thick, cottage cheese-like exudate on the affected mucosa
    - atrophic form — smooth red patch on affected mucosa
    - difficulty and pain with swallowing
    - retrosternal burning
- Cryptococcus neoformans infection
  - clinical manifestations:
    - fever
    - headache

- subtle mental changes
- focal neurologic signs
- seizures
- coma
— Histoplasmosis
— clinical manifestations:
- fever
- weight loss
- HIV associated malignancies:
— Kaposi's sarcoma
— most common neoplasm affecting AIDS clients
— is often aggressive and disfiguring
— clinical manifestations:
- purplish-red, non-painful lesion appearing anywhere on the skin and may include lymph nodes, mucous membranes, and viscera
- lesion is flat or indurated and frequently progresses to a nodule
— Non-Hodgkin's lymphoma
— clinical manifestations:
- painless, enlarged lymph nodes
- fever
- malaise
- night sweats
- HIV neurologic disease (AIDS dementia complex)
— characterized by cognitive, motor, and behavioral dysfunction
— can involve the central and peripheral nervous systems
- HIV wasting syndrome
— greater than 10% loss of body weight
— clinical manifestations:
— cachexia
— persistent fever
— diarrhea

MEDICAL MANAGEMENT

- antiretroviral therapy - zidovudine (also known as Retrovir, ZDV, and formerly AZT)
- blood and blood product replacement therapy
- Dideoxyinosine (ddI) and Dideoxycytidine (ddC) — antiretroviral agents for clients with intolerance to zidovudine or significant disease progression despite treatment with these drugs

- opportunistic infection/ treatment:
  — Pneumocystis carinii pneumonia (PCP)
    — trimethoprim-sulfamethoxazole (Bactrim or Septra)
    — pentamidine
    — dapsone-trimethoprim
  — Cytomegalovirus infection
  — Herpes simplex
    — acyclovir
  — Toxoplasmosis
    — combination of sulfadiazine and pyrimethamine
  — Cryptosporidium infection
    — alleviation of symptoms associated with dehydration, fluid and electrolyte imbalance, and weight loss
  — Mycobacterium tuberculosis
    — ethambutol
    — isoniazid
    — rifampin
  — Candida albicans
    — topical and/or systemic antifungal therapy
  — Cryptococcus neoformans infection
    — topical and/or systemic antifungal therapy
  — Histoplasmosis
    — topical and/or systemic antifungal therapy
- HIV-associated malignancies treatment
  — radiation therapy
  — chemotherapy
  — interferon alpha
- HIV neurologic disease treatment
  — zidovudine
- complete blood counts at frequent intervals
- oral and enteral nutritional supplements

NURSING MANAGEMENT

- Administer antiretroviral and opportunistic infection therapy as prescribed.
- Monitor for side effects and effectiveness of medication therapy.
- Monitor laboratory findings—complete blood count, platelet count, culture reports, arterial blood gases.
- Assess respiratory status — rate, rhythm, use of accessory muscles.
- Administer supplemental oxygen.

- Monitor oxygen saturation levels at rest and with activity.
- Initiate a progressive activity program and monitor client's response.
- Provide frequent rest periods and a restful environment.
- Administer anti-inflammatory, anti-anxiety, or analgesics for pain control.
- Monitor intake and output.
- Daily weights.
- Provide dietary supplements.
- Institute appropriate safety measures for client with neurologic involvement.
- Inspect skin and oral, vaginal and rectal areas closely and provide meticulous hygiene.
- Facilitate/provide counseling and support regarding the issues of social stigma, potential losses to body image and child-bearing potential, changes in sexuality, and premature loss of life.

FOCUSED DISCHARGE CARE

- Instruct the client regarding:
  — importance of medication regime
  — strategies aimed at reducing the risk of transmission:
    — safe sex counseling
    — avoidance of sharing needles
    — care of household items
    — proper disposal of items soiled with body fluids
  — health maintenance:
    — maintaining adequate nutrition
    — weight management
    — exercise
    — smoking cessation
    — stress reduction
  — basics of routine skin care and inspection
  — proper oral, vaginal, and rectal hygiene
  — importance of drug and/or alcohol abuse counseling
  — importance of follow-up appointments
- Refer to available community resources.

(For more information, see pp. 182-192 of Polaski and Tatro, *Luckmann's Core Principles and Practice of Medical-Surgical Nursing.*)

Huntington's Disease

OVERVIEW

- Huntington's disease (HD) is a genetically transmitted degenerative neurologic disease.
- The disease is autosomal dominant, meaning that offspring of an affected person have a 50 per cent chance of inheriting the disease.
- The pathology of Huntington's disease involves degeneration of the striatum (caudate and putamen) in the basal ganglia. This leads to a reduction of some neurotransmitters and relatively higher concentrations of other neurotransmitters (dopamine and norepinephrine).
- The disease is characterized by abnormal movements (chorea), intellectual decline, and emotional disturbance.
- Signs and symptoms usually begin in the fourth and fifth decades. Women and men are equally affected.
- The disease is relentlessly progressive, leading to disability and death within 15 to 20 years, usually from respiratory complications.

CLINICAL MANIFESTATIONS

- restless and fidgety appearance
- rapid, jerky choreiform movements involving all muscles
- dysphagia
- poor balance
- hesitant, explosive speech
- bowel and bladder incontinence
- emotional disturbance — becomes negative, suspicious, and irritable
- depression
- psychosis
- temper outbursts, sexual promiscuity
- dementia

MEDICAL MANAGEMENT

There is no known treatment to cure or alter the course.

- dopamine blocker — Haloperidol (Haldol) — to control abnormal movements and some behavioral manifestations
- anti-anxiety medications — diazepam (Valium)
- antidepressants

NURSING MANAGEMENT

- Assess client's ability to do self-care activities and provide care as indicated.
- Collaborate with physical and occupational therapy for exercises and adaptive devices for ambulation and self care.
- Determine strategies to optimize communication.
- Initiate aspiration precautions.
- Maintain high caloric intake (required because of excessive movement).
- Initiate appropriate safety measures.
- Provide quiet, restful environment.
- Conserve client energy by spacing activities and allowing rest periods.

FOCUSED DISCHARGE CARE

- Instruct the client regarding:
    — disease process and prognosis
    — need to use good posture and swallowing techniques while eating and drinking to prevent aspiration
    — use of adaptive devices
    — home environment safety measures
- Refer to available community resources (e.g., Home Health Care).

(For more information, see pp. 383-385 of Polaski and Tatro, *Luckmann's Core Principles and Practice of Medical-Surgical Nursing.*)

Hydronephrosis

OVERVIEW

- Hydronephrosis is distention of the renal pelvis and calices by an obstruction of normal urine flow.
- The obstruction may be due to a calculus, tumor, scar tissue or a kink in the ureter.
- Treatment involves relieving the obstruction and preventing pyelonephritis from urinary stasis.
- After removal of the obstruction, diuresis occurs.

NURSING MANAGEMENT

The nurse performs the following interventions after relief of the obstruction:
- Monitor for potential fluid volume deficit due to increased urine output.
  — Obtain hourly outputs.
  — Monitor vital signs.
  — Obtain urine specific gravities, glucose, and albumin.
  — Monitor serum electrolytes and glucose.

(For more information, see p. 957 of Polaski and Tatro, *Luckmann's Core Principles and Practice of Medical-Surgical Nursing.*)

Hypercalcemia

OVERVIEW

- Hypercalcemia is a serum calcium level over 5.5 mEq/L.
- In hypercalcemia, cardiac and smooth muscle activity is decreased. Calcium in the blood stream impairs renal function and precipitates as a salt, forming renal stones.

- Causes of hypercalcemia include:
  — metastatic malignancy — causes bone destruction or increased secretion of ectopic parathyroid hormone (PTH)
  — hyperparathyroidism
  — thiazide diuretic therapy — causes calcium retention
  — prolonged immobilization
  — excessive intake of calcium and Vitamin D
  — hypophosphatemia
  — metabolic acidosis — decreases calcium elimination

CLINICAL MANIFESTATIONS

- anorexia, nausea, vomiting, decreased peristalsis, abdominal distention
- weakness, fatigue
- difficulty concentrating
- lethargy, confusion, coma
- ECG changes — shortened ST segment, lengthened QT interval
- dysrhythmias, heart block
- signs of digitalis toxicity
- cardiac arrest
- polyuria, kidney stones, renal failure
- bone pain and fracture
- serum calcium greater than 5.5 mEq/L

MEDICAL MANAGEMENT

- determination/treatment of underlying cause
- intravenous normal saline with furosemide (Lasix) — promotes urinary calcium excretion
- cardiac monitoring
- antitumor antibiotic therapy — mithramycin C – inhibits action of PTH on osteoclasts in bone tissue reducing decalcification
- calcitonin therapy — inhibits effect of PTH and increases urinary calcium excretion
- corticosteroid therapy — decreases serum calcium by competing with vitamin D, resulting in decreased intestinal absorption of calcium
- phosphate therapy
- etidronate disodium therapy — reduces bone reabsorption of calcium

- aggressive hydration—to flush calcium through the kidneys
- dietary modification — low calcium

NURSING MANAGEMENT

- Administer prescribed therapy.
- Assess ECG for rhythm changes.
- Assess bowel sounds every 8 hours.
- Assess neurological status.
- Encourage fluid intake (particularly fluids with acid, such as prune and cranberry juices), unless contraindicated.
- Monitor laboratory findings — serum calcium.
- Monitor for signs of digitalis toxicity if on digoxin (calcium enhances the action of digitalis) — bradycardia, nausea, vomiting, blurred vision.
- Strain urine for renal calculi.
- Institute appropriate safety measures.
- Reposition cautiously to prevent pathologic fractures.
- Encourage high fiber foods to prevent constipation.

FOCUSED DISCHARGE CARE

Discharge care is based on the etiologic factor(s) causing hypercalcemia.

(For more information, see pp. 63-65 of Polaski and Tatro, *Luckmann's Core Principles and Practice of Medical-Surgical Nursing.*)

Hyperglycemia and Diabetic Ketoacidosis

OVERVIEW

- Hyperglycemia and diabetic ketoacidosis are acute complications of diabetes mellitus. Hyperglycemia is an elevated blood glucose over 120 mg/100 ml. Hyperglycemia results when glucose cannot be transported to the cells because of lack of insulin. Due to the lack of carbohydrates for cellular fuel, the liver converts its glycogen stores back to glucose (glycogenolysis) and increases biosynthesis of glucose (gluconeogenesis). This causes blood glucose levels to rise even higher. In insulin dependent diabetes mellitus (IDDM), the need for cellular fuel grows more critical and the body begins to draw on its fat and protein stores for energy. This results in the production of ketone bodies which accumulate in the blood (ketosis) and are excreted in the urine (ketonuria). Metabolic acidosis develops from the acidic effects of the ketones acetoacetate and betahydroxybutyrate. This condition is called diabetic ketoacidosis. It may cause the client to lose consciousness, a condition called diabetic coma.

- The process of catabolizing fats for fuel gives rise to four pathologic events:
  (1) incomplete lipid metabolism
  (2) dehydration
  (3) metabolic acidosis
  (4) electrolyte and acid-base imbalances
- Diabetic ketoacidosis is primarily a complication of insulin dependent diabetes mellitus, although it can occur in non-insulin dependent clients in periods of extreme stress.
- Diabetic ketoacidosis is an emergency.
- Causes of diabetic ketoacidosis and hyperglycemia include:
  — taking too little insulin
  — omitting doses of insulin
  — failing to meet increased need for insulin due to stress, infection, surgery, trauma, pregnancy or puberty
  — developing insulin resistance due to insulin antibodies.
- Prevention includes:
  — taking insulin as prescribed
  — monitoring blood glucose frequently
  — monitoring urine ketones when blood glucose rises
  — recognizing signs/symptoms of infection and other stressors that may precipitate diabetic ketoacidosis
  — calling physician for anorexia, nausea, vomiting, diarrhea, ketonuria for greater than eight hours,

febrile illness or infection, or any signs/symptoms of acidosis.

CLINICAL MANIFESTATIONS

- hot, dry skin
- nausea, vomiting
- flushed appearance
- dry mucous membranes
- sunken eyeballs
- Kussmaul's respirations (deep and rapid respirations) or tachypnea
- fruity or acetone odor of the breath
- abdominal pain and rigidity
- ECG changes due to potassium imbalance
- alteration in level of consciousness
- hypotension
- tachycardia
- polyuria (early sign)
- oliguria or anuria (late sign)
- stupor or coma (late sign)

MEDICAL MANAGEMENT

Goals are to (1) correct fluid and electrolyte imbalances, (2) restore normal circulating blood volume, (3) shift from a state of fat catabolism to carbohydrate catabolism, and (4) identify and correct the factors precipitating the ketoacidosis.

NURSING MANAGEMENT

- Monitor blood glucoses every one to two hours.
- Administer low dosage IV insulin as prescribed. Never administer subcutaneous insulin to someone in diabetic ketoacidosis. The subcutaneous tissue is dehydrated and poorly perfused.
- Administer fluid replacement (initially isotonic saline) as prescribed.
- Monitor hemodynamic readings, vital signs and level of consciousness every one to two hours.
- Maintain nasogastric tube to suction as ordered.
- Assess fluid status:
  — hematocrit
  — weight
  — lung sounds

- — skin turgor
- — intake and output.
- Monitor bowel sounds.
- Administer blood, albumin and plasma volume expanders as ordered for circulatory collapse.
- Monitor for signs/symptoms of hyperkalemia (usually present in first four hours of intervention) and hypokalemia (usually develops 4 to 24 hours after the initial intervention).
  - — signs/symptoms of hyperkalemia include: bradycardia, weakness, flaccid paralysis, oliguria, peaked T waves, loss of P wave, a widened QRS complex, and possible cardiac arrest.
  - — signs/symptoms of hypokalemia include: weakness, flaccid paralysis, paralytic ileus, flattening or inversion of the T wave, prolonged QT intervals and cardiac arrest
  - — do not administer potassium to a client with low urine output (hyperkalemia may result).
  - — encourage foods and liquids high in potassium when able to tolerate eating and drinking.
- Monitor sodium chloride and phosphate levels and replace as ordered.
- Administer sodium bicarbonate as prescribed to correct metabolic acidosis.
- Monitor level of consciousness and neurological status and notify physician promptly of any changes (may signal the onset of cerebral edema).

FOCUSED DISCHARGE CARE

Instruct client regarding:
- causes of diabetic ketoacidosis and how to prevent
- monitoring of blood glucose and when to take extra insulin
- monitoring of urine ketones when blood glucose is high
- when to contact physician

See also, "Diabetes Mellitus", p. 208, and "Hyperglycemic, Hyperosmolar, Nonketotic Coma", p. 348.

(For more information, see pp. 1188-1192 of Polaski and Tatro, *Luckmann's Core Principles and Practice of Medical-Surgical Nursing.*)

Hyperglycemic, Hyperosmolar, Nonketotic Coma (HHNK)

OVERVIEW

- Hyperglycemic, hyperosmolar, nonketotic coma (HHNK) is an acute complication of diabetes. It is a variant of diabetic ketoacidosis and is characterized by extreme hyperglycemia (800 to 2000 mg/100 ml), mild or undetectable ketonuria and the absence of acidosis.
- It is most often seen in older aged clients with noninsulin dependent diabetes mellitus (NIDDM). The major difference between HHNK and diabetic ketoacidosis is the lack of ketonuria with HHNK. This is because there is some insulin secretion in NIDDM, so the mobilization of fats for energy is avoided.
- In the absence of adequate insulin, blood glucose levels rise and water moves from the interstitial spaces and cells into the blood by osmosis. Fluid and glucose are lost through the urine. Eventually dehydration results and the client becomes obtunded.
- Precipitating factors for HHNK are stress, infection and certain medications (thiazide diuretics, steroids and phenytoin).

CLINICAL MANIFESTATIONS

- polyphagia — excessive hunger
- polydipsia — abnormal thirst
- polyuria — frequent urination
- glucosuria — glucose in the urine
- dehydration
- abdominal discomfort
- hyperpyrexia
- hyperventilation
- changes in sensorium, coma
- hypotension
- shock

MEDICAL MANAGEMENT

- fluid and electrolyte replacement
- insulin therapy

NURSING MANAGEMENT

- Replace fluids as prescribed (usually isotonic saline initially).
- Administer potassium, sodium, chloride and phosphates intravenously as prescribed.
- Administer IV insulin via an infusion pump.
- Monitor fluid volume and electrolyte levels.
- Monitor blood glucose levels.

FOCUSED DISCHARGE CARE

Instruct client regarding:
- causes of HHNK and how to prevent
- monitoring of blood glucose, and when to call physician or take extra insulin

See also, "Diabetes Mellitus", p. 208, and "Hyperglycemia/ Diabetic Ketoacidosis", p. 344.

(For more information, see p. 1192 of Polaski and Tatro, *Luckmann's Core Principles and Practice of Medical-Surgical Nursing.*)

Hyperkalemia

OVERVIEW

- Hyperkalemia is an elevated potassium level over 5.0 mEq/L.
- Hyperkalemia decreases the cell membrane's threshold causing the cell to become more excitable. This results in increased nerve and muscle irritability.
- There are three major causes of hyperkalemia:
  — retention of potassium
    — causes:
      • renal insufficiency
      • adrenal insufficiency
      • hypoaldosteronism
      • potassium-sparing diuretics
      • blood transfusion (contains potassium)
  — excessive release of cellular potassium

- — causes:
  - crushing injuries
  - severe burns
  - severe infection
  - metabolic acidosis
  - use of a perfusion pump during surgery
  — excessive intravenous or oral administration of potassium
- Clients at risk for hyperkalemia are those with insufficient renal function and decreased urinary output (80 to 90 per cent of potassium is excreted by the kidneys).

CLINICAL MANIFESTATIONS

- initially tachycardia then bradycardia
- ECG changes — peaked, narrow T wave; widened QRS complex; depressed ST segment; widened PR interval; wide flat P wave
- ectopic beats
- hypotension
- weakened cardiac contraction, cardiac arrest
- nausea
- explosive diarrhea, intestinal colic
- paresthesia
- muscle weakness, paralysis
- muscle cramps
- oliguria and later anuria
- elevated serum osmolality
- serum potassium greater than 5.0 mEq/L

MEDICAL MANAGEMENT

- determination/treatment of underlying cause
- cardiac monitoring
- sodium bicarbonate administration (promotes potassium uptake by the cell)
- potassium-wasting diuretic therapy
- calcium gluconate infusion — decreases antagonistic effect of excess potassium on the myocardium
- infusion of insulin and glucose — promotes potassium uptake into cells
- cation exchange resin — polystyrene sulfonate (Kayexalate) — induces diarrhea and potassium loss
- dietary modification — low potassium

- peritoneal dialysis or hemodialysis for marked renal failure

NURSING MANAGEMENT

- Administer prescribed therapy.
- Monitor cardiac rhythm and assess for changes.
- Assess neuromuscular status.
- Monitor laboratory findings — potassium level, renal profile.
- Monitor intake and output.
- Daily weights.
- Implement appropriate safety measures.
- Encourage diet low in potassium.

FOCUSED DISCHARGE CARE

Discharge care is based on the etiologic factor(s) causing hyperkalemia.

(For more information, see pp. 57-59 of Polaski and Tatro, *Luckmann's Core Principles and Practice of Medical-Surgical Nursing.*)

Hypernatremia

OVERVIEW

- Hypernatremia is a serum sodium level over 145 mEq/L. It occurs in approximately one per cent of hospitalized clients and carries a high mortality rate.
- Hyperosmolality of extracellular fluid (ECF) promotes a shift of water from the cells to the extracellular fluid by osmosis. More sodium is available to move across the excitable membrane which results in earlier membrane depolarization.
- There are three types of hypernatremia:
  — hypovolemic hypernatremia — total body water is greatly decreased relative to sodium
    — causes:

- severe hyperglycemia
- osmotic diuresis
- profuse diaphoresis
- decreased thirst
- diarrhea without fluid replacement
- fluid replacement with hyperosmolar solutions

— euvolemic hypernatremia — total body water is decreased relative to sodium
  — causes:
    - excess fluid loss from skin or lungs
    - diabetes insipidus
— hypervolemic hypernatremia — total body water is normal or near normal relative to the increased sodium
  — causes:
    - hypertonic tube feedings
    - administration of concentrated saline solutions
    - excessive salt intake

CLINICAL MANIFESTATIONS

- anorexia, nausea, vomiting
- dry, flushed skin due to decreased interstitial fluid
- dry, sticky mucous membranes
- dry, rough tongue
- elevated body temperature
- restlessness, agitation, irritability due to cerebral cellular dehydration
- lethargy, stupor, coma
- muscle twitching, hyperreflexia
- seizures
- elevated blood pressure (hypervolemic type)
- decreased blood pressure (hypovolemic type)
- erratic heart rate due to myocardial depression as sodium ions compete with calcium ions in the slow channels of the heart
- oliguria, urine dark and concentrated
- serum sodium greater than 145 mEq/L
- increased serum osmolality

MEDICAL MANAGEMENT

- determination/management of the underlying cause

- sodium reduction and fluid loss replacement therapy — 0.2 per cent or 0.45 per cent NaCl or 5 per cent dextrose in water
- diuretic therapy — furosemide (Lasix)
- dietary management — low sodium
- fluid restriction (hypervolemic)

NURSING MANAGEMENT

- Administer hypo-osmolar electrolyte solution.
- Administer diuretics as prescribed.
- Monitor vital signs.
- Assess neurologic status.
- Assess cardiac status.
- Monitor intake and output.
- Monitor laboratory findings — electrolytes, osmolality.
- Encourage oral intake (hypovolemic type).
- Maintain fluid restriction (hypervolemic type).
- Provide frequent oral and skin care.
- Maintain sodium restricted diet.

FOCUSED DISCHARGE CARE

Discharge care is based upon the etiologic factor(s) causing hypernatremia.

(For more information, see pp. 51-53 of Polaski and Tatro, *Luckmann's Core Principles and Practice of Medical-Surgical Nursing.*)

Hyperparathyroidism

OVERVIEW

- Hyperparathyroidism is a disorder caused by overactivity of one or more of the parathyroid glands.
- The normal function of parathyroid hormone (PTH) is to increase bone resorption, thereby maintaining the proper balance of calcium and phosphorus ions. Excess circulating PTH leads to bone damage,

hypercalcemia, renal failure, and decreased phosphate levels.
- Hyperparathyroidism is classified as:
  — Primary - normal regulatory relationship between serum calcium levels and PTH is interrupted secondary to adenoma or hyperplasia.
  — Secondary - glands are hyperplastic from malfunction of another organ system, i.e., renal failure, carcinoma with bone metastasis.
  — Tertiary - PTH production is irrepressible in clients with low or normal calcium levels.
- Hyperparathyroidism usually occurs in clients over 60 years of age and affects women more often than men (about 2 to 1).

CLINICAL MANIFESTATIONS

- backache, joint pain, pathologic fractures of the spine, ribs, and long bones
- polyuria, polydipsia, kidney stones
- thirst, nausea, anorexia, constipation, ileus, abdominal pain
- listlessness and depression

MEDICAL MANAGEMENT

- hydration to lower serum calcium levels
- loop diuretics to promote renal calcium secretion — furosemide (Lasix)
- medications that inhibit bone resorption — mithramycin (Mithracin), gallium nitrate (Ganite), phosphates, calcitonin

SURGICAL MANAGEMENT

- parathyroidectomy — removal of the gland or glands causing hypersecretion
  — if all four glands are hyperplastic, three and one-half glands are removed

NURSING MANAGEMENT

MEDICAL

- Monitor intake and output.
- Strain all urine for stones.

- Encourage fluid intake up to 3,000 ml/day unless contraindicated. Dehydration is dangerous for clients with hyperparathyroidism because it increases serum calcium level and promotes the formation of stones. Cranberry and prune juice make the urine more acidic and help prevent stone formation.
- Implement safety measures to prevent pathologic fractures.
- Encourage low calcium, low Vitamin D diet.
- Institute measures to prevent constipation and fecal impaction.
- Administer digitalis preparation cautiously, as hypercalcemia increases sensitivity to digitalis.

SURGICAL

Postoperative Care
In addition to routine postoperative care:
- Monitor for possible complications: airway obstruction, hemorrhage, injury to the recurrent laryngeal nerve, and hypocalcemia.
- Decrease strain on suture line by:
  — semi-Fowler's positioning.
  — supporting the head and neck with pillows and sandbags.
  — instructing the client not to extend or hyperextend the neck.
- Maintain airway patency by:
  — instructing client to cough and deep breathe.
  — gentle suctioning of the mouth and trachea.
  — humidified supplemental oxygen.
- Maintain tracheostomy set, endotracheal tube, and laryngoscope at bedside.
- Monitor intake and output.
- Reassure client that symptoms of mild tetany due to drop in serum calcium levels are temporary.
- Ensure that calcium gluconate is readily available.
- Encourage early ambulation as weight-bearing speeds the recalcification process.

FOCUSED DISCHARGE CARE

Instruct client regarding:
- dietary modifications - low calcium, low Vitamin D
- importance of adequate fluid intake

- importance of medications to control hyper-calcemia
- safety measures to reduce the risk of injury
- signs of hypocalcemia and hypercalcemia
- if postoperative:
  — wound care
  — importance of taking oral calcium prepara-tion (if prescribed)
- importance of follow-up appointments

(For more information, see pp. 1222-1226 of Polaski and Tatro, *Luckmann's Core Principles and Practice of Medical-Surgical Nursing.*)

Hypersensitivity Disorders

OVERVIEW

- Hypersensitivity is overreaction to a substance. Though widely referred to as allergic reaction, the word "hypersensitivity" is more appropriate as it denotes an increased immune response to the presence of an antigen (allergen) that results in tissue destruction.
- The occurrence and intensity of hypersensitivity responses depend on several factors: host defenses, the nature of the allergen, the concentration of the allergen, the route of allergen entrance into the body, and the exposure to the allergen.
- There are two general categories of hypersensitivity reactions based on the rapidity of the immune response: (1) immediate and (2) delayed. Immune globulins mediate immediate responses, whereas T cells govern delayed responses.
- Types of hypersensitivity reactions are:
  — **Type I Anaphylactic Hypersensitivity**
    — mediated by IgE antibodies that cause the release of histamine (causes vasodilation and fluid loss into interstitial space) and leuko-trienes (cause spasm of bronchial smooth muscles)

- forms of Type I:
  - anaphylactic shock—occurs within minutes
    - most severe form of Type I
    - clinical manifestations:
    - localized itching and edema
    - sneezing
    - wheezing, dyspnea
    - cyanosis
    - circulatory collapse
  - atopic allergies
    - include hay fever, some types of bronchial asthma, atopic dermatitis, some food and drug allergies
    - clinical manifestations:
      - rash
      - pruritus
      - nasal congestion
      - watery eyes
      - rhinorrhea
      - wheezing
      - urticaria

— **Type II Cytolytic or Cytotoxic Cell Hypersensitivity**
  - involves IgG or IgM antibodies that attach to antigens forming complexes that bind to cells, usually circulating blood cells, with resultant cell lysis
  - forms of Type II:
    - transfusion reactions (ABO incompatibility)
    - drug-induced hemolytic anemia
      - clinical manifestations:
        - headache and back pain (flank)
        - chest pain similar to angina
        - nausea and vomiting
        - tachycardia and hypotension
        - hematuria
        - urticaria
        - low hemoglobin

— **Type III Immune Complex Hypersensitivity**
  - results from the formation or deposit of antigen-antibody complexes in tissue. Inflammation results and leads to acute or chronic disease of the organ system in which the complexes are deposited.
  - forms of Type III:
    - rheumatoid arthritis
    - glomerulonephritis

- serum sickness (following injection of a foreign serum)
- systemic lupus erythematosus
— clinical manifestations:
- joint pain and tenderness
- urticaria
- hematuria
- decreased urinary output
- lymphadenopathy
- fever
— **Type IV Cell-Mediated or Delayed Hypersensitivity**
— sensitized T cells respond to antigens by releasing lymphokines which direct phagocytic cell activity
— forms of Type IV:
- intradermal injection of tuberculosis antigen in a client sensitized to tuberculosis
- graft-versus-host disease (GVHD) and transplant rejection
- contact dermatitis
— clinical manifestations:
- tuberculosis testing
  - edema and fibrin deposits that result in induration at the injection site
- GVHD
  - skin, gastrointestinal, and hepatic lesions
- contact dermatitis
  - itching
  - erythema
  - vesicular lesions

MEDICAL MANAGEMENT

- anaphylactic shock management:
  — oxygen
  — epinephrine
  — aminophylline
  — IV antihistamines
  — airway management
- transfusion reaction management:
  — immediate discontinuation of infusion
  — IV fluids
  — treat shock with epinephrine, fluids, and oxygen
  — mannitol for renal involvement

- allergy testing
- avoidance of allergens
- antihistamines
- decongestants
- corticosteroids
- anti-inflammatory agents
- immunosuppressant agents
- immunotherapy (desensitization)

NURSING MANAGEMENT

- Monitor client closely during blood administration for signs/symptoms of transfusion reaction.
- Assess for signs/symptoms of immediate or delayed response when administering the initial or test dose of a new medication.

FOCUSED DISCHARGE CARE

Instruct the client regarding:
- need to wear proper identification, identifying hypersensitivities
- importance of medication regime
- medication injection technique for client and/or household member for self-desensitization or epinephrine administration
- environmental control:
  — non-allergenic bed linens
  — replace carpets with throw rugs
  — launder bed linen frequently
  — use pull shades rather than venetian blinds
  — heating and cooling system that humidifies and filters the air
  — avoid smoking and smoke-filled areas
  — keep windows at home, in the car, and at work closed; use air conditioner if possible
  — stay indoors on windy days or when pollen count is high
  — avoid yardwork (mowing, raking)

(For more information, see pp. 192-196 of Polaski and Tatro, *Luckmann's Core Principles and Practice of Medical-Surgical Nursing.*)

Hypertension

OVERVIEW

- Arterial hypertension or high blood pressure is generally defined as a persistent elevation of systolic blood pressure above 140 mm Hg and diastolic pressure above 90 mm Hg.
- Arterial blood pressure is a product of cardiac output and total peripheral vascular resistance. Four control systems play a major role in maintaining blood pressure. These include the: (1) arterial baroreceptor system, (2) regulation of body fluid volume, (3) renin-angiotensin system, and (4) vascular autoregulation. Any factor producing an alteration of the above may affect systemic arterial blood pressure.
- Hypertension may be classified according to the following:
  — systolic hypertension
    - systolic pressure greater than 140 mm Hg (160 mm Hg over age 65)
  — diastolic hypertension
    - diastolic pressure greater than 90 mm Hg (95 mm Hg over age 65)
  — primary (essential, idiopathic) hypertension:
    - constitutes 90 to 95 per cent of all cases
    - etiology is multifactorial
    - characteristics include a gradual onset and prolonged course (benign hypertension) or an abrupt onset and a short dramatic course that proves fatal without swift intervention (malignant or accelerated hypertension).
  — secondary hypertension:
    - results from an identifiable cause (i.e., renal disease, endocrine disease, stress, exogenous hormones, etc.)
    - constitutes 5 to 10 per cent of the hypertensive population
  — borderline (labile) hypertension:
    - intermittent elevation of blood pressure, interspersed with normal readings
    - carry the risk of developing primary hypertension and cardiovascular disease

- white coat hypertension:
  - clients have normal readings except when blood pressure is taken by a health care professional
  - thought to be caused by anxiety related to health care visit
- malignant hypertension:
  - syndrome of markedly elevated blood pressure (diastolic pressure exceeds 140 mm Hg) associated with papilledema (edema and inflammation of the optic nerve at its point of entrance into the eye)
  - causes include: untreated hypertension, eclampsia, dissecting aortic aneurysm, drug or toxic substance ingestion
- benign hypertension:
  - uncomplicated hypertension usually of long duration and mild to moderate severity
  - may be primary or secondary
- Arterial hypertension affects nearly 50 million clients in the United States. It is the most common public health problem in the United States and the single most important predictor of cardiovascular risk.
- Risk factors include:
  - family history
  - age — incidence increases with age
  - gender - men experience hypertension at higher rates and at an earlier age
  - ethnic group — more prevalent in blacks
  - stress
  - obesity
  - nutrient imbalance (i.e., high sodium level, low potassium level)
  - cigarette smoking

CLINICAL MANIFESTATIONS

- elevation of blood pressure
- morning occipital headache
- fatigue
- dizziness
- palpitations
- flushing
- blurred vision

- epistaxis
- signs/symptoms of heart failure

MEDICAL MANAGEMENT

- Nonpharmacologic intervention is widely advocated as initial therapy for most clients, at least for the first three to six months after initial diagnosis.
  — weight reduction
  — sodium restricted, potassium supplemented diet
  — modification of dietary fat
  — exercise
  — restriction of alcohol
  — caffeine restriction
  — relaxation techniques
  — smoking cessation
  — exercise program
- Pharmacologic intervention
  — diuretics:
    - thiazide and sulfonamide diuretics—chlorothiazide (Diuril), hydrochlorothiazide (Esidrex), metolazone (Zaroxolyn)
    - loop diuretics—furosemide (Lasix), ethacrynic acid (Edecrin), bumetanide (Bumex)
    - potassium-sparing diuretics—spironolactone (Aldactone), triamterene (Dyrenium)
  — vasodilators:
    - hydralazine (Apresoline)
  — beta blockers:
    - propranolol (Inderal), metoprolol (Lopressor), atenolol (Tenormin)
  — alpha adrenergic inhibitors:
    - prazosin hydrochloride (Minipress), clonidine (Catapres)
  — calcium channel blocking agents:
    - nifedipine (Procardia), verapamil hydrochloride (Calan, Isoptin), diltiazem (Cardizem)
  — angiotensin-converting enzyme inhibitors:
    - captopril (Capoten), enalapril (Vasotec)

MALIGNANT HYPERTENSION

- parenteral administration of a combination of vasodilators (nitroprusside, nitroglycerin, hydralazine, enalaprilat) and adrenergic inhibitors (phentolamine, esmolol, propranolol)

- hemodynamic monitoring

NURSING MANAGEMENT

- Administer antihypertensives as prescribed.
- Monitor blood pressure to evaluate effectiveness of therapy.
- Monitor intake and output.
- Daily weights.
- Monitor laboratory results (serum sodium and potassium, BUN and creatinine, cholesterol)

FOCUSED DISCHARGE CARE

The long-term nature of intervention, high cost and untoward side effects of pharmacologic agents, and the lack of symptoms promote poor compliance with therapeutic regimen.

Instruct client regarding:
- disease process, factors contributing to its symptoms and risks, and prescribed medication therapy
- techniques for proper home blood pressure monitoring
- dietary modifications — low sodium, low fat, calorie restricted, low caffeine, low cholesterol
- importance of consistent exercise regime
- smoking cessation programs
- weight reduction
- importance of follow-up visits

(For more information, see pp. 781-795 of Polaski and Tatro, *Luckmann's Core Principles and Practice of Medical-Surgical Nursing.*)

Hyperthermia

OVERVIEW

- Hyperthermia is the term used to describe a client with an elevated body temperature.
- The anterior hypothalamus regulates body temperature by balancing heat gain and loss. The regulation

of body temperature is primarily through blood flow to the skin. When blood flow to the skin increases, heat is lost. If the body is too cold, cutaneous vessels constrict and metabolic heat production increases. The range for normal temperature is 96.8° to 100.4°F (36° to 38° C.). Central nervous system function is impaired when body temperature varies 4 degrees from this range. Seizures commonly occur when the body temperature exceeds 106° F. (41° C.). Irreversible changes occur with a temperature of 111° to 113° F. (44° to 45° C.).

- Causes of hyperthermia include malfunction of the thermoregulatory center (secondary to cerebral edema after a stroke, head injury, brain tumors, herniation syndrome), prolonged exposure to heat, loss of water, infection, cocaine toxicity, alcohol withdrawal and salicylate overdose.

CLINICAL MANIFESTATIONS

- visual disturbances
- headache
- nausea and vomiting
- rapid respirations
- rapid, bounding pulse
- muscle flaccidity
- delirium
- coma
- absence of sweating

MEDICAL MANAGEMENT

- cooling blanket
- antipyretics

NURSING MANAGEMENT

- Apply cooling blanket.
  — Monitor temperature closely, as rapid cooling may induce dysrhythmias and hypothermia.
  — Monitor skin condition.
- Administer antipyretics and monitor effectiveness.
- Monitor temperature frequently.
- Keep room temperature at 70° F.
- Remove excess blankets and clothing.

- Implement safety measures for possible seizure activity.

FOCUSED DISCHARGE CARE

Hyperthermia is resolved before discharge.

(For more information, see pp. 306-307 of Polaski and Tatro, *Luckmann's Core Principles and Practice of Medical-Surgical Nursing.*)

Hyperthyroidism

OVERVIEW

- Hyperthyroidism is the excessive secretion of thyroid hormone secondary to overfunctioning of the thyroid gland.
- The most common form of hyperthyroidism is Grave's Disease (toxic, diffuse goiter) which has three hallmarks: (1) hyperthyroidism, (2) thyroid enlargement secondary to hyperplasia, and (3) exophthalmus. Grave's disease is thought to be an autoimmune disorder.
- Grave's disease affects women four times as often as men and occurs between the ages of 20 and 40 years.
- Thyrotoxicosis (thyroid storm) is an acute exacerbation of thyrotoxic symptoms

CLINICAL MANIFESTATIONS

- tachycardia, palpitations, and elevated blood pressure
- increased respiratory rate and depth
- weight loss despite ravenous appetite
- diarrhea
- heat intolerance, profuse diaphoresis
- hand tremors at rest
- flushed, warm skin
- fine, soft hair
- mood swings ranging from mild euphoria to delirium
- agitation, restlessness, and irritability

- enlarged thyroid gland
- exophthalmus - protruding eyes and fixed stare secondary to fluid accumulation behind the eye
- fatigue and muscle weakness
- thyroid storm (thyroid crisis, thyrotoxicosis)—a medical emergency characterized by high fever, severe tachycardia, delirium, dehydration, and extreme irritability

MEDICAL MANAGEMENT

- antithyroid hormone medication—propylthiouracil (PTU), methimazole (Tapazole)
- radioiodine therapy with ^{131}I
- adrenergic blocking agents— as adjunctive therapy to control sympathetic nervous system activity

SURGICAL MANAGEMENT

- thyroidectomy — removal of the thyroid gland
- subtotal thyroidectomy — approximately 5/6 of the gland is removed

NURSING MANAGEMENT

MEDICAL

- Monitor vital signs.
- Daily weights, intake and output.
- Assess nutritional status, provide a high-calorie, low sodium (for exophthalmus), high protein, caffeine restricted diet.
- Monitor activity level; establish rest periods.
- For exophthalmus - provide eye moisturizers and eye patches as needed to prevent irritation, and elevate head of bed.
- Provide a cool environment.
- Assure client/significant other that behavioral manifestations should improve with intervention.
- Administer antithyroid hormone therapy.

SURGICAL
PREOPERATIVE CARE

In addition to routine preoperative care:

- Administer antithyroid and iodine preparations to attain an euthyroid state and decrease vascularity of the thyroid gland.
- Promote optimal nutritional balance.
- Promote rest.

Postoperative Care

In addition to routine postoperative care:
- Monitor for possible complications: respiratory obstruction, hemorrhage, hypocalcemia and tetany (resulting from accidental removal of one or more parathyroid glands), thyroid storm, and injury to the recurrent laryngeal nerve.
- Decrease strain on suture line by:
  — semi-Fowler's positioning
  — supporting the head and neck with pillows and sandbags
  — instructing the client not to extend or hyperextend the neck.
- Maintain airway patency by:
  — instructing the client to cough and deep breathe
  — gentle suctioning of mouth and trachea
  — humidified supplemental oxygen
- Maintain tracheostomy set, endotracheal tube, and laryngoscope at bedside for emergency treatment of airway obstruction.
- Monitor intake and output.
- Monitor rectal temperature at least every four hours (elevated temperature is one of the first signs of thyroid storm).

FOCUSED DISCHARGE CARE

Instruct client regarding:
- importance of taking antithyroid hormone medication daily
- symptoms of thyroid deficiency or excess
- measures to reduce eye discomfort and prevent corneal irritation:
  — wear dark glasses
  — avoid getting dust in eyes
  — wear eye patch(es) if irritated
  — elevate head of bed

- restrict salt intake
- if postoperative, include:
  - exercises to prevent contractures of the neck
  - wound care
  - for total thyroidectomy, importance of taking thyroid replacement medication
- importance of follow-up clinic/laboratory appointments

(For more information, see pp. 1213-1219 of Polaski and Tatro, *Luckmann's Core Principles and Practice of Medical-Surgical Nursing.*)

Hypocalcemia

OVERVIEW

- Hypocalcemia is a serum calcium level below 4.5 mEq/L.
- Hypocalcemia increases capillary permeability and causes neuromuscular excitability of skeletal, smooth and cardiac muscles. Severe hypocalcemia causes neuromuscular excitability that results in tetany. With hypocalcemia, the bone is stimulated to release calcium, which makes the bone osteoporotic and subject to fracture.
- The causes of hypocalcemia include:
  - inadequate dietary intake of calcium
  - Vitamin D deficiency (decreases calcium absorption from the GI tract)
  - excess intake of phosphorus (inhibits calcium absorption)
  - malabsorption of fat in the intestine (interferes with Vitamin D absorption)
  - metabolic alkalosis (decreases ionized calcium)
  - renal failure (increased loss of calcium)
  - Cushing's disease
  - hypoparathyroidism (decreased bone resorption)
  - inadvertent removal of the parathyroid gland with thyroidectomy
  - medications:

— magnesium sulfate, colchicine and neomycin — inhibit parathyroid hormone secretion
— aspirin, anticonvulsants and estrogen — alter Vitamin D metabolism
— phosphate preparations — decrease serum calcium levels
— steroids — decrease calcium mobilization
— loop diuretics — reduce calcium absorption
— antacids and laxatives — decrease calcium absorption

CLINICAL MANIFESTATIONS

- tetany symptoms — twitching around the mouth, tingling and numbness of the fingers, carpopedal spasms, facial spasms, laryngospasm and later convulsions
- Trousseau's sign — carpopedal spasm (contraction of the fingers and hand) elicited by inflating a blood pressure cuff on the upper arm for 1 to 5 minutes, constricting circulation
- Chvostek's sign — spasm of the muscles innervated by the facial nerve, elicited by tapping the client's face lightly (over the facial nerve) below the temple. Spasm of the face, lip or nose indicates a positive test.
- dyspnea, laryngeal spasm
- increased peristalsis, diarrhea
- prolonged QT interval
- dysrhythmias, palpitations
- pathologic fractures
- prolonged bleeding times (intrinsic pathway for coagulation is inhibited)
- serum calcium less than 4.5 mEq/L

MEDICAL MANAGEMENT

- determination/treatment of underlying cause
- calcium replacement therapy
- respiratory support
- cardiac monitoring
- dietary modifications — high calcium, low phosphate (if related to parathyroid deficiency)
- Vitamin D supplements

NURSING MANAGEMENT

- Administer calcium replacement therapy.
    — For oral preparations, give 30 minutes before meals for better absorption and with a glass of milk because Vitamin D is necessary in calcium absorption.
- Monitor for cardiac rhythm changes.
- Assess for signs of digitalis toxicity (bradycardia, nausea, vomiting, blurred vision), if administering a calcium supplement that enhances the action of digitalis.
- Monitor IV site if client is receiving intravenous calcium—is irritating to tissue and can cause sloughing if infiltration occurs.
- Assess for positive Chvostek's or Trousseau's signs and respiratory distress.
- Monitor laboratory findings — serum calcium, bleeding times.
- Institute appropriate safety measures.
- Monitor for any signs of bleeding.
- Use caution in turning or moving to prevent pathologic fractures.
- Maintain diet high in calcium, low in phosphorus (if related to parathyroid deficiency).

FOCUSED DISCHARGE CARE

Discharge care is based upon the etiologic factor(s) causing hypocalcemia.

(For more information, see pp. 60-63 of Polaski and Tatro, *Luckmann's Core Principles and Practice of Medical-Surgical Nursing.*)

Hypoglycemia (Insulin Reaction)

OVERVIEW

- Hypoglycemia is defined as a blood glucose level less than 60 mg/100 ml.
- Hypoglycemic reactions result from:
    — an overdose of insulin, or less commonly, a sulfonylurea

- — omitting a meal or eating less food than usual
  - — overexertion without additional carbohydrates to compensate
  - — nutritional and fluid imbalances due to nausea and vomiting
  - — alcohol intake.
- Untreated, prolonged hypoglycemia can result in coma. When the brain is deprived of glucose, brain cells are destroyed, which can cause permanent brain damage; memory loss, decreased learning ability. Paralysis also can result.

CLINICAL MANIFESTATIONS

It is important to realize that some medications, such as propranolol and sulfamethoxazole, can mask the symptoms of hypoglycemia, and clients may not know they are having a reaction.
- headache, weakness, irritability
- lack of muscular coordination
- apprehension
- diaphoresis
- combative behavior or behavior as if drunk or psychotic
- night hypoglycemia: bizarre nightmares, restlessness, diaphoresis, sleeplessness or confusion

NURSING MANAGEMENT

Treatment depends upon the severity of the reaction.
Mild Hypoglycemia
- Administer fast-acting sugar, such as orange juice or candy, such as lifesavers (instead of orange juice or candy, some clients prefer to purchase glucose tablets or a glucose gel). Follow this with a small snack of carbohydrate or graham crackers and milk. Perform a blood glucose test at the onset of symptoms. Retest the blood glucose in 15 to 30 minutes and treat again if the blood glucose is not over 100 mg/100 ml. Continue testing until the blood glucose is over 100 mg/100 ml.

Unconscious or semiconscious client:
- Glucagon may be administered intramuscularly or subcutaneously. Families should be instructed on how to do this at home. Unconscious or semicon-

scious clients must never be forced to drink fluids because aspiration may result.

- 20 to 50 mls of 50 per cent glucose by intravenous push may be given in the hospital setting.
- A longer acting carbohydrate and protein snack should follow either of the above treatments once the client regains consciousness.

FOCUSED DISCHARGE CARE

Instruct client/significant other regarding:
- signs/symptoms of hypoglycemia
- causes of hypoglycemia and preventive measures
- times of peak insulin action
- monitoring blood glucose
- always carrying fast-acting sugar
- following treatment of hypoglycemia with protein and carbohydrate snack
- monitoring blood glucose following hypoglycemic episode until value over 100 mg/100 ml
- administration of glucagon (by significant other)
- documentation of hypoglycemic episode in daily log
- importance of Medic Alert bracelet, necklace or identification card so that emergency care can be delivered if needed and client will not be mistaken for someone intoxicated or mentally ill

Also see, "Diabetes Mellitus", p. 208.

(For more information, see pp. 1192-1194 of Polaski and Tatro, *Luckmann's Core Principles and Practice of Medical-Surgical Nursing.*)

Hypokalemia

OVERVIEW

- Hypokalemia is a serum potassium level less than 3.5 mEq/L. It is a common electrolyte disorder.
- When serum potassium levels decrease, there is an increased potassium gradient between the cell and

the plasma, causing the resting membrane potential to increase, reducing excitability. Therefore, cell membranes are less responsive to stimuli. The respiratory system is profoundly affected through depression of nervous and muscle synapses.

- Causes of hypokalemia include:
  — gastrointestinal losses:
    — vomiting
    — diarrhea
    — nasogastric suctioning
    — laxative abuse
    — excessive tap water enemas
  — dietary changes:
    — malnutrition, starvation
    — potassium-free diet
    — potassium-free intravenous solutions when NPO
  — medications (which promote potassium loss):
    — potassium-wasting diuretics (thiazide, osmotic)
    — steroids
    — gentamicin
    — amphotericin B
    — digitalis preparations
  — redistribution of potassium
    — insulin moves potassium back into the cell
    — alkalosis causes potassium to shift into cells in exchange for hydrogen ions
  — disorders
    — Cushing's syndrome
    — acute renal failure (diuretic phase)
    — alcoholism

CLINICAL MANIFESTATIONS

- anorexia, vomiting, ileus, abdominal distention (slowed smooth muscle contraction)
- muscle weakness and paralysis
- leg cramps
- ECG changes — depressed ST segment, flat T wave and a prominent U wave (prolonged repolarization)
- vertigo, postural hypotension
- slow, weak pulse (cardiac arrest with severe hypokalemia)
- shallow respirations, shortness of breath

373

- fatigue, lethargy
- confusion, depression (slowed conduction of nerve impulses)
- polyuria
- decreased serum osmolality
- serum potassium less than 3.5 mEq/L

MEDICAL MANAGEMENT

- determination/management of underlying cause
- cardiac monitoring
- potassium replacement therapy
- dietary modifications — high potassium

NURSING MANAGEMENT

- Administer potassium replacement therapy.
  - — Potassium is *not* given intramuscularly and *never* given as an IV push (may cause cardiac arrest). Potassium given intravenously must always be diluted in intravenous fluids.
- Monitor IV sites closely as potassium is irritating to blood vessels.
- Monitor cardiac rhythm and assess for changes.
- Monitor respiratory status.
- Monitor bowel function.
- Monitor for signs of digitalis toxicity (bradycardia, nausea, vomiting, blurred vision), potentiated by hypokalemia.
- Implement appropriate safety measures.
- Monitor laboratory findings — serum potassium levels, digoxin levels.
- Encourage foods high in potassium.

FOCUSED DISCHARGE CARE

Discharge care is based on the etiologic factor(s) that caused hypokalemia.

(For more information, see p. 53-57 of Polaski and Tatro, *Luckmann's Core Principles and Practice of Medical-Surgical Nursing.*)

Hypomagnesemia

OVERVIEW

- Hypomagnesemia is a serum magnesium level below 1.5 mEq/L.
- Hypomagnesemia can lead to increased transmission of action potentials owing to an increased release of acetylcholine. A magnesium deficit also affects the potassium-sodium pump, causing hypokalemia and inhibits parathyroid hormone, so calcium levels may also be low.
- Factors causing hypomagnesemia include:
  — alcoholism — when accompanied by liver disease, due to decreased production of enzymes necessary for the intestinal absorption of magnesium
  — chronic malnutrition
  — prolonged hyperalimentation without magnesium replacement
  — excessive amounts of phosphorus in the intestine (usually from antacids) — will decrease magnesium absorption
  — prolonged loss of fluids from the gastrointestinal tract
  — hyperparathyroidism
  — prolonged diuretic therapy
  — medications:
    — furosemide, osmotic and thiazide diuretics, aminoglycoside antibiotics, amphotericin B, corticosteroids and digitalis — interfere with renal handling of magnesium

CLINICAL MANIFESTATIONS

- anorexia, nausea, abdominal distention
- cardiac dysrhythmias including premature ventricular contractions, atrial or ventricular fibrillation
- signs of digitalis toxicity (secondary to hypokalemia) (see below)
- tetany
- positive Chvostek's and Trousseau's signs, see "Hypocalcemia", p. 368.

- convulsions
- depression, psychosis and confusion
- serum magnesium below 1.5 mEq/L

MEDICAL MANAGEMENT

- determination/treatment of underlying cause
- magnesium replacement therapy
- cardiac monitoring
- dietary modification — high magnesium

NURSING MANAGEMENT

- Administer prescribed therapy.
- Assess cardiac rhythm for ECG changes.
- Monitor laboratory findings — magnesium, potassium, calcium.
- Monitor for signs of digitalis toxicity (bradycardia, nausea, vomiting, blurred vision).
- Assess neurological status.
- Institute appropriate safety measures

FOCUSED DISCHARGE CARE

Discharge care is based upon the etiologic factor(s) causing hypomagnesemia.

(For more information, see p. 66 of Polaski and Tatro, *Luckmann's Core Principles and Practice of Medical-Surgical Nursing.*)

Hyponatremia

OVERVIEW

- Hyponatremia is a serum sodium level below 135 mEq/L. It is one of the most common electrolyte disorders.
- As the extracellular fluid concentration of sodium decreases, the sodium concentration gradient between extracellular and intracellular fluids decreases. This hypo-osmolality can lead to intracellular edema.

These changes also mean that there is less sodium to move across the excitable membrane, which results in delayed membrane depolarization. Generally, the clinical manifestations reflect this decreased excitability.

- There are four types of hyponatremia:
  — hypovolemic hyponatremia — sodium loss is greater than water loss
    — causes:
      - diuretic use
      - diabetic glycosuria
      - aldosterone deficiency
      - renal disease
      - vomiting
      - diarrhea
      - excessive diaphoresis
      - burns
  — euvolemic hyponatremia — total body water is moderately increased and sodium remains at normal level
    — causes:
      - syndrome of inappropriate antidiuretic hormone (SIADH)
      - continuous secretion of ADH secondary to pain, medication or stress
  — hypervolemic hyponatremia — there is a greater increase in total body water than in sodium
    — causes:
      - congestive heart failure
      - liver cirrhosis
      - nephrotic syndrome
      - acute and chronic renal failure
  — redistributive hyponatremia — no change in total body water or sodium, but a water shift occurs between the intracellular and extracellular compartments
    — causes:
      - hyperglycemia
      - hyperlipidemia

CLINICAL MANIFESTATIONS

- nausea, vomiting, abdominal cramps
- hyperactive bowel sounds
- decreased blood pressure, orthostatic hypotension (hypovolemic hyponatremia)

- headache, apprehension
- lethargy
- confusion
- decreased muscle tone and deep tendon reflexes
- weakness
- serum sodium below 135 mEq/L

MEDICAL MANAGEMENT

- determination/management of underlying cause
- sodium replacement — 3 per cent saline solution
- fluid replacement (hypovolemic)
- fluid restriction (hypervolemic) — allows sodium balance to be regained
- normal saline in conjunction with furosemide (Lasix) — increases urinary sodium loss and reduces the risk of extracellular fluid volume expansion
- diuretic therapy
- dietary modifications - high sodium

NURSING MANAGEMENT

- Administer electrolyte and fluid replacement therapy as prescribed.
- Monitor vital signs.
- Monitor neurologic status.
- Monitor cardiac status.
- Daily weights.
- Monitor intake and output.
- Administer PRN antiemetics.
- Monitor laboratory findings—electrolytes, osmolality.
- Irrigate NG tube or wound sites with normal saline solution to prevent further sodium losses.
- Promote the intake of fluids containing sodium, such as broths or juices.
- Maintain fluid restriction (hypervolemic).
- Provide appropriate safety measures.

FOCUSED DISCHARGE CARE

Discharge care will be based on the etiologic factor(s) causing hyponatremia.

(For more information, see pp. 47-51 of Polaski and Tatro, *Luckmann's Core Principles and Practice of Medical-Surgical Nursing.*)

Hypoparathyroidism

OVERVIEW

- Hyposecretion of the parathyroid glands produces a syndrome opposite that of hyperparathyroidism. Serum calcium levels are low and serum phosphate levels are high.
- When parathyroid hormone (PTH) is reduced, bone resorption slows, serum calcium levels decrease, and phosphate levels rise.
- Causes are either:
  — iatrogenic - caused by (1) accidental removal of parathyroid glands during thyroidectomy, (2) infarction of the glands during surgery, or (3) strangulation of one or more glands by postoperative scar tissue
  — idiopathic - an autoimmune disorder with a genetic basis.
- Risk factors include thyroid and parathyroid surgery.

CLINICAL MANIFESTATIONS

The symptoms of hypoparathyroidism are mainly caused by low serum calcium levels. They are always more severe in clients who have elevated serum pH (alkalosis), as this decreases the amount of ionized calcium which worsens the symptoms.

- Acute hypoparathyroidism
  — increased neuromuscular irritability resulting in tetany (painful muscle spasms), irritability, grimacing, tingling of fingers and around the mouth, laryngospasm, and arrhythmias
  — positive Chvostek's and Trousseau's signs
  — convulsions
- Chronic hypoparathyroidism
  — lethargy
  — thin, patchy hair
  — brittle nails, dry, scaly skin
  — personality changes
  — cataract formation

MEDICAL MANAGEMENT

- Acute hypoparathyroidism:
  - IV calcium infusion - to elevate serum calcium as rapidly as possible
  - anticonvulsant therapy
  - respiratory support
- Chronic hypoparathyroidism:
  - oral calcium salts and Vitamin D

NURSING MANAGEMENT

- Assess client at risk for acute hypoparathyroidism (i.e., post thyroidectomy) for tetany, positive Chvostek's or Trousseau's sign, or respiratory distress.
- For acute hypoparathyroidism:
  - administer IV calcium as prescribed
  - monitor for respiratory distress, have emergency respiratory equipment at hand
  - monitor for convulsions and protect from injury
  - monitor for cardiac arrhythmias.
- Promote adequate rest.
- Administer calcium supplements and Vitamin D as prescribed.

FOCUSED DISCHARGE CARE

Instruct the client regarding:
- importance of medication regime
- dietary modifications - high in calcium, low in phosphorus
- signs of hypocalcemia and hypercalcemia
- follow-up appointments

(For more information, see pp. 1226-1229 of Polaski and Tatro, *Luckmann's Core Principles and Practice of Medical-Surgical Nursing.*)

Hypothermia

OVERVIEW

- Hypothermia is a condition of below normal body temperature.
- Hypothermia can occur accidentally through exposure to environmental cold, as a response to illness, or can be induced as a form of treatment. Hypothermia is induced during some surgical procedures to reduce blood flow to an area and blood loss. Hypothermia can also occur with central nervous system disorders, congestive heart failure, diabetes, or drug overdose.

CLINICAL MANIFESTATIONS

- below normal body temperature
- hypotension
- somnolence
- ventricular dysrhythmias

MEDICAL MANAGEMENT

- rewarming measures
- vasoactive therapy
- dysrhythmia management

NURSING MANAGEMENT

- Initiate warming blanket.
- Monitor temperature closely.
- Continuous cardiac/hemodynamic monitoring.
- Maintain warm room environment.
- Monitor pulmonary function.

FOCUSED DISCHARGE CARE

Hypothermia is resolved before discharge.

(For more information, see pp. 307-308 of Polaski and Tatro, *Luckmann's Core Principles and Practice of Medical-Surgical Nursing.*)

Hypothrombinemia

OVERVIEW

- Hypothrombinemia, a coagulation disorder, refers to a deficient amount of circulating prothrombin.
- Prothrombin is a protein produced in the liver and found in the blood. For prothrombin synthesis to take place, vitamin K must be present in the liver to act as a catalyst.
- Factors causing hypothrombinemia include:
  — vitamin K deficiency due to
    — liver failure
    — overdose of aspirin, coumarin or coumarin derivative (warfarin) which antagonize the action of vitamin K

CLINICAL MANIFESTATIONS

- ecchymosis after minimal trauma
- epistaxis
- hematuria
- gastrointestinal bleeding
- prolonged bleeding from a venipuncture site
- cerebral vascular hemorrhage

MEDICAL MANAGEMENT

- determination/treatment of underlying cause
- Vitamin K therapy
- infusion of prothrombin concentrates or prothrombin factors VII, IX and X
- dietary modification — high Vitamin K

NURSING MANAGEMENT

- Administer Vitamin K, prothrombin or factor therapy.
- Assess for signs of bleeding.
- Monitor laboratory findings — CBC, prothrombin time.
- Institute bleeding precautions:
  — soft toothbrush
  — electric razor

- hold pressure to venipuncture sites
- no intramuscular or subcutaneous injections
- no aspirin or non-steroidal anti-inflammatory drugs
- stress need to avoid blowing nose
- stress need to avoid straining with stool
- safety measures for ambulation

FOCUSED DISCHARGE CARE

Instruct client regarding:
- Vitamin K therapy
- signs/symptoms of complications and when to notify physician
- measures to prevent bleeding:
  - soft toothbrush, no flossing
  - electric razor
  - no aspirin or non-steroidal anti-inflammatory drugs
  - no contact sports
  - avoidance of constipation
- diet high in Vitamin K
- need for follow-up appointments

(For more information, see p. 869 of Polaski and Tatro, *Luckmann's Core Principles and Practice of Medical-Surgical Nursing.*)

Hypothyroidism

OVERVIEW

- Hypothyroidism refers to a deficiency of thyroid hormone resulting in slowed body metabolism. This hypometabolic state may lead to decreased oxygen consumption by the tissues and pronounced personality changes.
- Hypothyroidism occurs when there is insufficient release of thyroid hormone due to a problem within the hypothalamus, pituitary, or thyroid gland itself and results in a slowing of all body processes.

- Hypothyroidism affects women more than men (about 4 to 1). The highest incidence is between 30 and 60 years of age.
- The three types of hypothyroidism are:
  — Primary—caused by congenital defects of the thyroid (cretinism), defective hormone synthesis, iodine deficiency, surgery, or radioactive therapy for hyperthyroidism.
  — Secondary—caused by insufficient stimulation of a normal thyroid gland secondary to malfunction of the pituitary or hypothalamus.
  — Tertiary or Central—caused by failure of the hypothalamus to produce thyroid-releasing hormone (TRH), which stimulates the pituitary to secrete thyroid stimulating hormone (TSH).
- Risk factors include iodine deficient diet, radiation therapy to area of thyroid, and surgery for hyperthyroidism.

CLINICAL MANIFESTATIONS

There is a wide range of symptoms depending upon the severity of the disease:
- decreased heart rate, stroke volume, and cardiac output
- hyperlipidemia, hypercholesterolemia
- anemia, easy bruising
- dyspnea, fatigue, lethargy
- fluid retention and possible weight gain
- anorexia, constipation
- sensitivity to cold, decreased ability to sweat
- slowed physical and mental reactions
- forgetfulness, depression, apathy, paranoia
- dry, coarse skin and hair
- normal to enlarged thyroid gland
- expressionless face
- periorbital edema
- slow, deliberate speech
- myxedema—dry, waxy, non-pitting type of edema caused by abnormal deposits of mucin in skin and tissues. It is common in the pretibial and facial areas.
- myxedema coma—drastic decrease in metabolic rate, hypoventilation, hypotension, and hypothermia.

MEDICAL MANAGEMENT

- thyroid hormone preparation
- iodine preparation
- iodine enriched diet

NURSING MANAGEMENT

MEDICAL

- Monitor vital signs.
- Assess for signs/symptoms of decreased cardiac output.
- Daily weights.
- Assess nutritional status, encourage well balanced diet.
- Monitor intake and output.
- Administer thyroid preparations - assess for symptoms of thyrotoxicosis (tachycardia, diarrhea, sweating, agitation, tremors, shortness of breath).
- Establish a progressive exercise/activity program and monitor client tolerance.
- Implement measures to prevent constipation and fecal impaction. (Enemas should not be used for the client with cardiac problems due to the effect vagal stimulation may have.)
- Monitor pressure points for skin redness or breakdown.
- Provide measures to keep client comfortably warm.
- Assure client/significant other that client's appearance, energy level, affect, and mental capabilities will gradually improve with thyroid hormone therapy.
- Administer narcotics and sedatives judiciously due to decreased metabolic rate.

FOCUSED DISCHARGE CARE

Instruct client regarding:
- importance of taking thyroid hormone daily
- symptoms of thyroid deficiency or excess
- dietary management
- importance of follow-up appointments

(For more information, see pp. 1206-1213 of Polaski and Tatro, *Luckmann's Core Principles and Practice of Medical-Surgical Nursing*.)

Idiopathic Thrombocytopenic Purpura

OVERVIEW

- Idiopathic thrombocytopenic purpura (ITP) is the extravasation of small amounts of blood into the tissues and mucous membranes resulting from a platelet deficiency.
- The term thrombocytopenia means a reduction of platelets below 100,000/mm^3.
- ITP refers to thrombocytopenia caused by an unknown, possibly an autoimmune reaction. This disorder is characterized by the premature destruction of platelets. Normally, platelets survive 8 to 10 days. However, platelet survival in ITP is as brief as 1 to 3 days or less. ITP is characterized by the development of antibodies to one's own platelets, which are then destroyed by phagocytosis in the spleen and liver.
- Ninety per cent of adults with ITP are under 40 years of age; the ratio of women to men is 3 to 1.

CLINICAL MANIFESTATIONS

- petechiae
- ecchymosis
- epistaxis
- bleeding gums
- easy bruising
- heavy menses or bleeding between periods
- complications include:
  — cerebral hemorrhage
  — gastrointestinal bleeding
  — nerve pain or paralysis from pressure of hematomas on nerves

MEDICAL MANAGEMENT

- steroid therapy — to suppress phagocytic response of splenic macrophages (rarely produces a permanent cure)

- platelet transfusions
- plasmapheresis — to remove circulating antibodies

SURGICAL MANAGEMENT

- splenectomy — see "Splenectomy", p. 594
  - treatment of choice
  - 60 to 80 per cent of cases result in complete and permanent remission

NURSING MANAGEMENT

MEDICAL

- Administer steroids and platelet replacement therapy. See "Blood Component Transfusion", p. 88.
- Monitor laboratory findings — platelet count, CBC.
- Institute bleeding precautions:
  - soft toothbrush
  - electric razor
  - no intramuscular or subcutaneous injections
  - no aspirin or non-steroidal anti-inflammatory drugs
  - stress need to avoid blowing nose
  - stress need to avoid straining with stool
  - hold pressure to all venipuncture sites
  - safety measures for ambulation
- Assess for signs of bleeding into other tissues or organs.

SURGICAL

- See "Splenectomy", p. 594.

FOCUSED DISCHARGE CARE

Instruct client regarding:
- importance of long-term steroid therapy
- disease process, signs/symptoms of possible complications, and when to notifiy physician
- measures to prevent bleeding:
  - no aspirin or non-steroidal anti-inflammatory agents
  - no contact sports
  - avoid constipation

— soft toothbrush, no flossing
— electric razor
- need for follow-up clinic/laboratory appointments
- see "Splenectomy", p. 594

(For more information, see pp. 868–869 of Polaski and Tatro, *Luckmann's Core Principles and Practice of Medical-Surgical Nursing.*)

Incontinence, Urinary

OVERVIEW

- Incontinence is a condition in which involuntary loss of urine is a social or hygienic problem and is objectively demonstrable.
- There are six types of incontinence:
  — Stress — an immediate, involuntary loss of urine upon an increase in intra-abdominal pressure. Often associated with activities, such as laughing, sneezing, coughing or running.
  — Urge — inability to hold back the flow of urine when feeling the urge to void.
  — Overflow — urinary retention with overflow of small amounts of urine.
  — Reflex — abnormal activity of the spinal cord reflex leading to involuntary loss of urine. There is no sensation to void.
  — Psychological — incontinence due to altered mental state
  — Environmental — changes in mobility result in inability to reach toilet facilities before voiding occurs.
- Incontinence may be caused by:
  — sphincter weakness or damage
  — urethral deformity
  — alteration of the urethrovesical junction in women
  — weak abdominal and perineal muscle tone
  — dementia, confusion
  — certain medications
- Risk factors include:

- — **Stress incontinence**
  - — women and men — urethral irritation from infection, radiation damage to the bladder or after a prostatectomy
  - — women — loss of the urethrovesical junction angle
- — **Urge incontinence**
  - — multiple sclerosis (due to severe bladder spasms)
  - — urinary tract infection
  - — stroke
  - — medications interfering with mobility, such as hypnotics, tranquilizers, sedatives, and diuretics
- — **Overflow incontinence**— retention with bladder distention related to, for example, a nervous system lesion, fecal impaction or BPH.
- — **Reflex incontinence**— spinal cord injury resulting in complete loss of voluntary control of the bladder
- — **Psychological**— altered mental status
- — **Environmental**— changes in mobility

CLINICAL MANIFESTATIONS

- involuntary loss of control of voiding
- bladder spasms (associated with urge incontinence)

MEDICAL MANAGEMENT

Treatment for incontinence will depend upon the results of urodynamic evaluation, specific abnormalities identified for the client, environmental constraints, and informed choice for the client in treatment options.

- Pelvic muscle exercises (Kegel's) to strengthen the pubococcygeal muscle used for both males and females. Femina cones (weights placed in the vagina) may be used to enhance effectiveness of these exercises.
- Bladder training with the client voiding at short intervals (hourly or less) and gradually lengthening time between voidings to intervals up to 3 hours.
- Behavioral techniques and biofeedback for clients with stress or urge incontinence (may provide significant improvement but requires extensive training).

- Medications — used primarily with urge incontinence and sometimes stress incontinence.
- Psychotherapy and hypnosis also may help manage incontinence.

SURGICAL MANAGEMENT

- electrical stimulation devices — inhibit the micturition reflex. These include electrodes implanted within the pelvic muscles and intravaginal devices or anal plugs for indirect stimulation.
- Marshall-Marchetti-Krantz procedure — involves suturing the bladder neck and urethra to the perichondrium of the symphysis pubis or the periosteum of the superior pubic ramus.
- Raz procedure — done transvaginally and involves elevation and suspension of the bladder using tissue or inorganic materials for support.
- implantation of an artificial urinary sphincter — as a last resort measure.

NURSING MANAGEMENT

MEDICAL

- Instruct the client on Kegel exercises.
- Encourage adequate fluid intake up to 2,000 - 2,500 ml/day, instructing the client to avoid caffeine and alcohol, which stimulate the bladder.
- Develop a bladder training program and voiding schedule. Initially, the client should try to void every 30 minutes to 2 hours. As the program progresses, the voiding intervals are lengthened.
- Assist the client with a weight reduction and exercise program.
- Maintain integrity of the skin and instruct the client on the need for good skin care.
- Avoid use of adult diapers as this demeans the client and gives "permission" to be incontinent.
- If above measures fail, provide disposable pads or briefs to increase social mobility and protect the skin.
- External condom catheter — only needed if above measures fail.

In addition to routine postoperative care:
- Raz procedure
  — Maintain patency of suprapubic or urethral catheter for 5-8 days (the pressure of a filling bladder inhibits healing).
  — Encourage high fluid intake to prevent infection.
  — Initiate clamp and release program after healing occurs to help the detrusor muscle regain tone.
  — Obtain and measure residual urine as prescribed to determine the effectiveness of bladder emptying.

FOCUSED DISCHARGE CARE

- Instruct the client/family regarding:
  — removing barriers in the home that prevent easy access to toilet facilities
  — obtaining assistive devices or commode as needed.
  — providing good skin care.
- Instruct the client regarding:
  — Kegel exercises and use of Femina cones
  — bladder training routine.
  — symptoms of urinary tract infections.
  — how to maintain a toileting schedule.
  — fluid intake, and to decrease in evening.
- Refer to Continence Clinics and support groups.
- Discuss newsletters available from the Simon Foundation for Continence and Help for Incontinent Persons (HIP)

(For more information, see pp. 922-928 of Polaski and Tatro, *Luckmann's Core Principles and Practice of Medical-Surgical Nursing.*)

Increased Intracranial Pressure

OVERVIEW

- Intracranial pressure (ICP) is the pressure exerted in the cranium by its contents: the brain, blood and cerebrospinal fluid (CSF). The pressure is measured via the cerebrospinal fluid. Normal pressure of CSF is 5 to 10 mm Hg or 160 to 180 mm H_2O. Pressures over 250 mm H_2O are called increased ICP. If the pressure is recorded during a lumbar puncture, it may not reflect the ICP if CSF flow is obstructed between the brain and spinal cord.
- The skull is a hard bony container. Since the skull cannot expand, compensatory mechanisms come into play:
  (1) initial compensation — displacement of CSF into the spinal canal or into venous blood through the arachnoid mater.
  (2) secondary compensation — reduction of blood volume to the brain. This stage of compensation alters cerebral metabolism and eventually produces brain tissue hypoxia and necrosis.
  (3) final compensation — displacement of brain tissue (herniation).
- Increased ICP is most often associated with a rapidly expanding lesion (e.g., bleeding), an obstruction to the outflow of CSF (e.g., tumor), or increased CSF formation (e.g., cerebral edema).
- Clients at risk include those with expanding tumors in the brain, head injury, brain surgery, hydrocephalus, and bleeding (e.g., subarachnoid hemorrhage).

CLINICAL MANIFESTATIONS

- alteration in level of consciousness
- restlessness
- irritability
- confusion
- decrease in Glasgow coma score (see "Coma", p. 173).
- changes in speech
- pupillary reaction changes

- motor or sensory changes
- cardiac rate (bradycardia) and rhythm changes
- headache
- nausea and vomiting
- double vision (diplopia)
- hypertension with widened pulse pressure
- irregular respirations
- seizure activity

MEDICAL MANAGEMENT

- intracranial pressure monitoring — insertion of a subarachnoid or ventricular probe through a hole in the skull to measure ICP
- osmotic diuretics — Mannitol *remove fluid, ↓pressure*
- loop diuretics — furosemide *control edema* — *Lasix*
- steroid therapy — dexamethasone (Decadron) – to control edema *↑blood flow ↑reabsorb Na+Cl.*
- antacids and hydrogen blockers – stress ulcer prophylaxis
- barbiturate therapy — pentobarbital – to reduce ICP
- mechanical ventilation — hyperventilation induced by a ventilator or manual ventilation induces hypocapnia, which reduces cerebral blood volume and ICP
- anticonvulsant therapy

β-blockers – dilate arteries/veins to brain

SURGICAL MANAGEMENT

A craniotomy may be indicated to:
- place a shunt to allow drainage of CSF
- evacuate a subdural or epidural hematoma
- remove brain tissue (i.e., part of the temporal lobe) to give remaining structures room to expand. If compliance is low at the time of surgery, the bone flap used to gain access to the brain is not replaced or the dura may not be closed. Subsequent surgery is then required to repair the defect.

NURSING MANAGEMENT

MEDICAL

- Monitor for increased intracranial pressure readings and accompanying signs and symptoms (posturing or disorientation).

- Manually hyperventilate the client if ICP increases (hypocapnia decreases cerebral blood volume and ICP).
- Plan nursing interventions so that activities known to increase ICP are not performed when the ICP is elevated (e.g., suctioning, excessive hip flexion, repositioning).
- Monitor for other factors that may increase ICP:
  — excess water in ventilator tubing
  — excessive pulmonary secretions (increased pCO_2)
  — endotracheal tube taped too tightly against jugular vein, retarding venous circulation from the head
- Avoid ICP catheter infection by (1) keeping the area around catheter site clean, (2) reporting leakage from catheter, and (3) maintaining a closed system.
- Monitor respiratory status closely.
- Perform suctioning only when necessary to prevent increasing ICP.
  — never exceed 15 seconds in suctioning time (causes increased ICP)
  — never suction through the nose (may cause trauma and CSF leak)
- Monitor arterial blood gas results to correct acid-base imbalances promptly.
- Perform complete neurologic assessment using Glasgow coma scale (See "Coma", p. 173).
  — Even though the client may be in a coma, assessment of the pupils should continue as the pupils will dilate if the brain stem is compressed, and necessitate notification of the physician immediately.
- Prevent venous obstruction:
  — raise the head of the bed 30 degrees
  — avoid turning the head sharply to either side and keep head in alignment with the body
  — maintain regular bowel program (excessive strain can cause a Valsalva's maneuver resulting in venous back-up and increased ICP)
- Administer diuretics and steroids as prescribed.
- Monitor intake and output.
- Monitor parenteral fluid therapy closely administering only the minimal volumes prescribed.
  — IV solutions with dextrose are avoided as they move rapidly into the brain, causing edema.

- Monitor temperature closely.
  — Increased temperature will cause an increased metabolic rate and aggravates ICP. Hyperthermia requires vigorous treatment.
- Monitor hemodynamic parameters closely, if administering barbiturate therapy (may cause cardiac depression).
  — Monitor daily serum barbiturate level.
- Observe for and report any signs of increasing ICP (see "Clinical Manifestations" listed above).
- Maintain quiet, restful environment.
- Assess for complications of immobility (pulmonary embolism, deep vein thrombosis, skin breakdown).
- Administer stress ulcer prophylaxis.

SURGICAL

POSTOPERATIVE CARE

In addition to routine postoperative care and the above medical interventions:
- Assure patency of and record output of surgical drains placed.
- Monitor incision for CSF leak.
- Observe and report complications of craniotomy:
  — increased ICP
  — epidural or subdural hematoma (same symptoms as increased ICP with severe headach). Bleeding into posterior fossa may occur causing cardiac and respiratory arrest.
  — hydrocephalus — same symptoms as increased ICP with incontinence and sixth cranial nerve palsy

See "Intracranial Tumors", p. 403.

FOCUSED DISCHARGE CARE

Increased ICP is resolved before discharge.
Instruct the client regarding:
- wound care, if postoperative

(For more information, see pp. 302-306 of Polaski and Tatro, *Luckmann's Core Principles and Practice of Medical-Surgical Nursing.*)

Infectious Mononucleosis

OVERVIEW

- Infectious mononucleosis is a self-limiting condition characterized by painful enlargement of the lymph nodes.
- The cause of infectious mononucleosis is a herpes virus, the Epstein-Barr virus. The disease may be spread by the oropharyngeal route.
- Primarily a disease of the young, infectious mononucleosis usually strikes children between the ages of 3 and 5 years and young adults between the ages of 15 and 25 years.
- Fever typically lasts 4 to 6 weeks with a long convalescence until strength is regained.

CLINICAL MANIFESTATIONS

- fatigue
- headache
- malaise, myalgias
- fever
- pharyngitis
- lymphadenopathy
- maculopapular rash
- splenic enlargement with left upper quadrant pain

MEDICAL MANAGEMENT

No specific intervention mitigates or shortens the disease process.
- bedrest
- antipyretics

SURGICAL MANAGEMENT

- splenectomy

NURSING MANAGEMENT

MEDICAL

- Administer antipyretics and implement other cooling measures (tepid bath, light clothing).

- Monitor temperature.
- Monitor intake and output.
- Encourage rest.
- Administer PRN analgesics.

SURGICAL

- See "Splenectomy", p. 594.

FOCUSED DISCHARGE CARE

Instruct client regarding:
- need for adequate rest
- avoidance of contact sports for a period of at least one month (could result in splenic rupture)
- see "Splenectomy", p. 594

NO WAVE-RUNNING

(For more information, see p. 866 of Polaski and Tatro, *Luckmann's Core Principles and Practice of Medical-Surgical Nursing.*)

Infective Endocarditis

OVERVIEW

- Endocarditis is an inflammatory process of the endocardium, especially the valves. This disorder was once lethal, but morbidity and mortality have been reduced greatly with the use of antibiotics and advanced diagnostic procedures.
- Infective endocarditis may be classified as follows:
  — subacute bacterial endocarditis
    — develops gradually over weeks or months
    — common organism is Streptococcus viridans
    — most commonly diagnosed in clients with previously damaged hearts
  — acute bacterial endocarditis
    — develops over days or weeks with an erratic course and earlier development of complications
    — common organism is Staphylococcus aureus

　　　　— most often affects people with normal hearts
　　— native valve endocarditis
　　　　— infection of previously normal or damaged valve
　　— prosthetic valve endocarditis
　　　　— infection of an artificial valve
　　— nonbacterial thrombotic endocarditis
　　　　— caused by sterile thrombotic lesions (frequently aggregates of platelets) in clients with malignancies or other chronic diseases
- Circulating microorganisms in the bloodstream attach to the endocardial surface and multiply. Usually the multiplication of these organisms requires a rough or abnormal endocardium. Lesions (infective vegetation) form on the heart's valves causing valvular stenosis or insufficiency. The mitral and aortic valves are most often affected
- Risk factors include:
　　— rheumatic heart disease
　　— mitral valve prolapse
　　— invasive procedures (i.e., minor surgery, dental procedures, indwelling catheter)
　　— chronic debilitating disease
　　— intravenous drug abuse
　　— congenital heart disease
　　— heart valve replacement

CLINICAL MANIFESTATIONS

- fever, chills, rigors, sweats, malaise, weakness, anorexia, weight loss, backache, splenomegaly
- dyspnea, chest pain, murmur
- Roth's spots — visualized on fundoscopic examination as a white or yellow center surrounded by a red irregular halo
- Osler nodes — painful, erythematous nodules on the skin of the extremities, usually on the fingertips
- splinter hemorrhages — linear hemorrhages that appear similar to tiny splinters under the nail
- headaches and musculoskeletal complaints
- symptoms of cardiac failure

MEDICAL MANAGEMENT

- intravenous antibiotic therapy for 4-6 weeks

- antiinflammatory agents
- treatment of congestive heart failure

NURSING MANAGEMENT

- Maintain bedrest.
- Assess for rapid pulse, easy fatiguability, dyspnea, restlessness, signs of heart failure, and embolic manifestations.
- Administer antibiotics as prescribed.
- Treat fever with rest, cooling measures, forced fluids, and anti-pyretics.
- Encourage fluids and a well-balanced diet.
- Administer PRN analgesics.
- Provide rest periods.
- Implement progressive activity schedule.

FOCUSED DISCHARGE CARE

Instruct client regarding:
- cause of infective endocarditis
- purpose of long-term antibiotic administration and the need to comply with the entire course
- need for prophylactic antibiotics when undergoing dental procedures or surgical interventions
- good oral hygiene to prevent bacteremia
- signs/symptoms to report to physician:
  — fever, chills
  — malaise
  — anorexia
  — weight loss
  — increased fatigue
- activity restrictions
- importance of follow-up care. Recently there has been a trend to allow appropriate clients to complete the intravenous therapy at home with the assistance of home health agencies.

(For more information, see pp. 736-741 of Polaski and Tatro, *Luckmann's Core Principles and Practice of Medical-Surgical Nursing.*)

Intestinal Obstruction

OVERVIEW

- Intestinal obstruction is the partial or complete impairment of the forward flow of intestinal contents.
- Intestinal obstruction has a high mortality rate if not diagnosed and treated promptly.
- Obstruction of the small intestine may be caused by inflammation, neoplasms, adhesions, hernia, volvulus, intussusception, paralytic ileus, vascular problems, hypokalemia, food blockage or compression from outside the intestine.
- Obstruction of the large intestine usually is due to cancer but may be caused by diverticulitis and ulcerative colitis.
- Risk factors include: adhesions, hernia, volvulus, intussusception, tumors, neurogenic factors and obstruction of blood flow to the bowel.

CLINICAL MANIFESTATIONS

- nausea and vomiting (vomiting progresses from semi-digested food to watery material with bile and finally dark fecal material)
- abdominal pain in rhythmically recurring waves
- abdominal distention with high pitched bowel sounds
- visible peristaltic waves
- hypoxia (due to severe abdominal distention raising the diaphragm)

MEDICAL MANAGEMENT

- insertion of an intestinal tube
- gastric suction and rest for adynamic ileus

SURGICAL MANAGEMENT

Surgery is performed when medical management fails and is aimed at relieving the obstruction by elimination of the cause and removal of any ischemic bowel.

NURSING MANAGEMENT

- Assess presence and quality of bowel sounds.

- Assess for abdominal distention.
- Assess character, duration and quality of abdominal pain.
- Monitor for dehydration and electrolyte imbalance (especially note serum pH, potassium and sodium).
- Replace fluids and electrolytes as prescribed.
- Maintain intestinal tube to suction and monitor relief of distention and nausea.
- Monitor progression of weighted intestinal tube and maintain free loop for advancement.
- Monitor and document amount, color, odor and consistency of intestinal tube drainage or any emesis.
- Monitor intake and output.
- Monitor for signs/symptoms of bowel strangulation and report immediately to physician: emesis, increasing distention and pain, and fever.
- Prepare for emergency bowel resection if strangulation occurs.

FOCUSED DISCHARGE CARE

Postoperative discharge teaching depends upon the surgical procedure performed.
- Instruct client regarding:
  — ways to prevent recurrence and maintain bowel elimination
  — ways to regain nutritional status after weight loss

(For more information, see pp. 1079-1083 of Polaski and Tatro, *Luckmann's Core Principles and Practice of Medical-Surgical Nursing.*)

Intracellular Fluid Volume Excess

OVERVIEW

- Intracellular fluid volume excess (ICFVE) secondary to hypo-osmolar disorders results from either water excess or solute deficit. In water excess, the number of solutes is normal but diluted by excessive water. In solute deficit, the amount of water is normal, but there are too few particles per liter of water.

- Hypo-osmolar fluids move by osmosis to maintain fluid equilibrium, forcing fluids to move from lesser concentration (in the vessels) to the higher concentration (in the cells) in ICFVE. Too much fluid accumulates in the cell causing cellular edema.
- Causes of intracellular fluid volume excess include: administration of excessive amounts of hypo-osmolar intravenous fluids; brain injury or disease causing an increased antidiuretic hormone (ADH) production; consumption of excessive amounts of water; or increased secretion of antidiuretic hormone (SIADH) secondary to pain, narcotic use or stress.

CLINICAL MANIFESTATIONS

- headache, nausea, vomiting (cerebral cellular edema)
- apprehension, irritability, disorientation
- pupillary changes (pressure on third cranial nerve)
- decreased muscle strength
- unequal grasp
- weight gain
- bradycardia, widened pulse pressure (difference between systolic and diastolic pressure readings), increased respirations, muscle twitching, projectile vomiting, convulsions (increased intracranial pressure)
- low serum sodium level (hypo-osmolality)
- decreased hematocrit (hemodilution)

MEDICAL MANAGEMENT

- identification/management of underlying cause
- solute replacement therapy
- diuretic therapy

NURSING MANAGEMENT

- Administer solute replacement therapy.
- Monitor neurological status.
- Administer diuretic therapy.
- Monitor vital signs.
- Monitor intake and output.
- Daily weights.
- Institute appropriate safety measures.

FOCUSED DISCHARGE CARE

Discharge care is based upon the etiologic factor(s) causing the cellular fluid excess.

(For more information, see pp. 45-46 of Polaski and Tatro, *Luckmann's Core Principles and Practice of Medical-Surgical Nursing*.)

Intracranial Tumors

OVERVIEW

- Intracranial tumors may be benign or malignant, but both are potentially fatal. These tumors cause death by infiltration and compression of the brain tissue. The tumors occupy space and also produce cerebral edema. Because the skull is rigid, there is little room for expansion of contents. Brain tumors progressively increase intracranial pressure, which causes brain stem herniation and death.
- Intracranial tumors may be:
  — primary tumors which developed from central nervous system tissue
  — secondary tumors that have metastasized from other locations in the body
  — intra-axial tumors originating from glial cells within the cerebrum, cerebellum or brain stem. These tumors infiltrate and invade brain tissue.
  — extra-axial tumors originating from the skull, meninges, cranial nerves or pituitary gland. These tumors have a compressive effect on the brain.
- Primary brain tumors occur equally in males and in females of all age groups; 14,000 new cases are diagnosed yearly.
- There is no clear etiology for the development of primary tumors, and, therefore, no risk factors.
- Lung or breast cancer is a common primary site which metastasizes to the brain. Metastatic brain tumors are more frequent than primary tumors.
- Primary intracranial tumors do not metastasize to other sites in the body.

CLINICAL MANIFESTATIONS

Symptoms vary according to the area and extent of the brain involved.
- focal weaknesses
- sensory disturbances
- language disturbances
- coordination disturbances
- visual disturbances
- visual field deficits
- headaches (intermittent and of increasing duration)
- nausea and vomiting
- papilledema (edema of the optic disc)
- seizures
- dizziness and vertigo
- mental status changes (lethargy, drowsiness, confusion, disorientation and personality changes)

MEDICAL MANAGEMENT

Depends upon the type and location of the tumor and the client's condition
- intrathecal chemotherapy (placed within the cerebrospinal fluid via an intraventricular reservoir or lumbar puncture)
  — methotrexate currently is used
- systemic chemotherapy with lomustine (CCNU) or carmustine (BiCNU)
- direct administration of carmustine into the tumor with biodegradable, time-released wafers

SURGICAL MANAGEMENT

- radiation therapy via the Gamma Knife — low-dosage radiation sources are arranged around the client's head in a helmet device to focus on the tumor
- radiosurgery—a linear accelerator is used to deliver radiation
- brachytherapy — insertion of radioactive seeds through a catheter into the tumor. The seeds are left in place about two days.
- craniotomy—removal of the tumor through a surgical opening in the skull:
  (1) osteoplastic bone flap — the bone flap remains attached and hinged to other muscles and struc-

tures

(2) free-form flap - a section of cranium is cut away from its attachments and then replaced after the procedure

(3) enlarging burr hole — the bone is gradually is removed until enough brain is exposed for the procedure

- craniectomy — permanent removal of the cranium to relieve pressure on the brain by providing space for expansion

NURSING MANAGEMENT

MEDICAL

- Administer chemotherapy as prescribed and assess for side effects (see "Chemotherapy", p. 145).
- Assess neurological status.
- Maintain safety precautions.

SURGICAL

PREOPERATIVE CARE

In addition to routine preoperative care:
- Assess and document the following as a baseline for comparison with postoperative assessment findings:
  — vital signs; level of consciousness; orientation to person, place, and time; ability to follow instructions; pupil size, equality and reaction to light (Glasgow Coma Scale Score)
  — limb movements; limited or exaggerated movements; strength in extremities (grip); any paresis or paralysis; sensory abnormalities; edema
  — manifestations of increasing intracranial pressure
  — presence of aphasia, visual or auditory problems
- Provide emotional support to client and significant other.
- Administer parenteral corticosteroids as prescribed.
- Discuss scalp preparation (i.e., shaving) and reassurances that hair will grow back.
- Apply antiembolism stockings and sequential compression devices as prescribed, prior to transfer to the operating room.

In addition to routine postoperative care:
- Monitor and document the following, comparing to baseline assessment (report abnormals to the physician):
  — vital signs and neurologic function every hour until stable and then every two hours (include level of consciousness, ability to move extremities, speech, orientation and pupillary response)
- Monitor head dressing for any drainage.
- Assess intactness of head dressing — ensure it is not too tight.
- Obtain intake and output every hour.
- Monitor electrolyte levels, serum glucose, osmolarity and hematocrit.
- Assess for any signs of increasing intracranial pressure (headache, vomiting, seizures, visual or speech disturbances, widening pulse pressure, respiratory irregularity, muscle weakness or paralysis, pupillary changes, hypertension, bradycardia).
- Position as prescribed by physician to prevent increased intracranial pressure:
  — Supratentorial Surgery — elevate head of the bed 30 degrees; do not lower the head of the bed for any procedure without a written order from the neurosurgeon.
  — Infratentorial Surgery — keep client flat without head elevation, to prevent pressure on the brain stem. Turn every two hours, but *never* onto the back.
  — Posterior Fossa Surgery — position on either side but never on the back. A pillow may be placed under the head for support. Monitor for changes in vital signs because the surgery site is close to vital brain stem functions. Monitor for cardiac arrhythmias and air embolism related to positioning of the client during surgery.
  — Bone Flap (surgically removed for decompression) — place the client only on the unoperated side or back.
- Maintain ventilator function with hyperventilation to reduce intracranial pressure.
- Administer osmotic diuretic therapy and steroids as prescribed to prevent increased intracranial pressure.

- Monitor for cerebrospinal fluid leaks.
  — Place a gauze pad near the nose, ears or head dressing to absorb any drainage noted.
  — Test any blood or clear fluid for presence of glucose (the presence of glucose indicates cerebrospinal fluid [CSF]).

  Note if any drainage/fluid dries in concentric circles (indicates CSF).
- If CSF leak is present, notify physician and position with head of the bed elevated 20 degrees to prevent stasis of the CSF drainage.
- If CSF leak is present, administer prescribed antibiotics.
- Monitor for seizure activity; administer anti-convulsants as prescribed.
- Monitor for meningitis (may develop two to three days after surgery):
  — headache, nuchal rigidity, chills, fever, decreased level of consciousness, increased sensitivity to light
- Monitor for stress ulcer. Test gastric pH and administer antacids to maintain pH above 4.5.
- Apply cool, moist packs over the eyes or ecchymosis and periorbital edema. Administer prescribed artificial tears ointment.
- Use sterile technique for all dressing changes to prevent meningitis.
- Assess operative site and sites around drains or catheters for edema and signs of infection.
- As the wound heals, remove dry flaky scalp skin by softening the scalp with baby oil or glycerin and washing with soap and water.
- Administer prescribed medications for pain (such as acetaminophen or codeine).
- Keep the environment quiet, calm and dimly lit.
- Provide nasogastric feedings as prescribed, once the swallowing reflex and peristalsis are present.
- Monitor respiratory status and oxygenation to ensure cerebral oxygenation and avoid hypercapnia (hypercapnia increases intracranial pressure).
- Maintain patent airway.
- Do not suction through the nose (if the nasal membrane is torn, cerebrospinal fluid may leak, and an infection may result). Suction by other routes minimally (suctioning increases intracranial pressure).

- Provide method of communicating needs and facilitate communication (see "Communication" section in "Cerebrovascular Accident", p. 134).
- Prevent complications of immobility by providing frequent position changes (as prescribed).
- Begin range of motion exercises as prescribed.
- Encourage as much independence with self care as possible.
- Encourage client to discuss concerns or changes in body image or self esteem disturbances. Make referrals as necessary.
- Assist client/family to develop a plan for managing home care, if residual deficitspresent.
- Provide emotional support to family. Make referrals as necessary.

FOCUSED DISCHARGE CARE

Needs vary greatly depending upon the amount of brain damage, residual deficits and whether client is going home or to a long-term rehabilitation center. Referrals may be needed, especially to support groups for family members.

(For more information, see pp. 333-341 of Polaski and Tatro, *Luckmann's Core Principles and Practice of Medical-Surgical Nursing.*)

Irritable Bowel Syndrome (IBS)

OVERVIEW

- Irritable bowel syndrome (IBS) is a functional disorder of motility in the small and large intestines causing diarrhea, constipation or an alternation between the two. The motility can be altered by a number of factors including diet and emotions. It develops without organic disease or anatomic abnormality.
- IBS is the most common gastrointestinal disorder in Western society and is more common in women.
- IBS also is called spastic colon, irritable colon, nervous indigestion, pylorospasm and spastic colitis.

- Risk factors include:
  — diets high in rich foods such as creams and fats
  — stress
  — fresh fruits
  — gas producing foods
  — alcohol
  — cigarette smoking.

CLINICAL MANIFESTATIONS

- abdominal pain
- constipation or diarrhea
- hypersecretion of colonic mucous
- flatulence, nausea, anorexia
- left lower quadrant abdominal pain
- cramping in the morning or following eating

MEDICAL MANAGEMENT

Treatment is palliative and supportive.
- sedatives and antispasmodic medications
- vegetable mucilages, such as psyllium hydrophilic mucilloid (Metamucil)
- increased dietary fiber

NURSING MANAGEMENT

- Monitor number and characteristics of stools.
- Monitor intake and output.
- Maintain quiet environment.
- Administer antispasmodics as prescribed.

FOCUSED DISCHARGE CARE

Instruct client regarding:
- use of fiber to manage constipation and diarrhea
- adequate fluid intake (8 glasses of water daily)
- need for adequate sleep, exercise and nutrition
- diarrhea:
  — limit gas producing foods
  — avoid caffeine, alcohol and foods containing non-digestible carbohydrates (e.g., beans)
  — exclude milk and milk products

(For more information, see pp. 1083-1084 of Polaski and Tatro, *Luckmann's Core Principles and Practice of Medical-Surgical Nursing.*)

K

Kaposi's Sarcoma

- Kaposi's sarcoma is a vascular malignancy that presents as a skin disorder.
- Kaposi's sarcoma used to be a skin disease common in 50 to 60 year old men of Jewish or Mediterranean descent. Recently, Kaposi's sarcoma has been seen in many clients with acquired immunodeficiency syndrome (AIDS).
- The cause of Kaposi's sarcoma is not known, although the human immunodeficiency virus and cytomegalovirus have been suggested as the cofactors in its development. It is considered to be due to a failure in the immune system.
- Kaposi's sarcoma lesions begin as red, dark blue or purple macules on the lower legs that coalesce into larger plaques. These plaques frequently ulcerate or open and drain.
- The lesions spread by metastasis to the upper body, then to the face and oral mucosa. About 75 per cent of clients develop lesions of the lymph nodes, gastrointestinal tract and lungs.
- Clients report pain and itching in the lesions; as the disease progresses, the legs become edematous.
- Treatment involves excision of local lesions. Systemic lesions are treated with a combination of interferon-alpha, cytotoxic agents and radiation.

See also, "Human Immunodeficiency Virus (HIV) Infection", p. 334.

(For more information, see pp. 1360-1361 of Polaski and Tatro, *Luckmann's Core Principles and Practice of Medical-Surgical Nursing*.)

Laryngeal Cancer

OVERVIEW

- Cancer of the larynx or voice box is classified and treated by its anatomic site. Supraglottic tumors occur on the posterior surface of the epiglottis to the vocal cords, including the false vocal cords. Glottic tumors are tumors of the true vocal cords. Subglottic tumors occur on the under surface of the true vocal cords.
- Risk factors include cigarette smoking, alcohol abuse, voice abuse, chronic laryngitis, noxious fumes, and polluted air.

CLINICAL MANIFESTATIONS

- persistent cough, sore throat, or ear ache
- hoarseness that persists longer than two weeks
- neck masses
- difficulty swallowing or breathing
- hemoptysis

MEDICAL MANAGEMENT

Treatment depends upon the stage and site of the tumor.
- radiation therapy for glottic cancer limited to the true vocal cords or for supraglottic tumors that have not metastasized.
- chemotherapy generally is not performed except for prevention of new primary tumors.

SURGICAL MANAGEMENT

- Laser surgery with irradiation for small tumors.
- Partial laryngectomy is the removal of one-half or more of the larynx. It is performed for cancer involving one true vocal cord and sometimes a portion of

the other true vocal cord. A temporary tracheostomy is also performed.
- Supraglottic laryngectomy is a form of partial laryngectomy and is performed for cancer of the supraglottis. The surgeon removes the superior portion of the larynx from the false vocal cords to the epiglottis. Lymph node dissection and removal of a portion of the base of the tongue may or may not be performed, but the true vocal cords are preserved.
- Total laryngectomy is required for large glottic tumors with fixation of the vocal cords. The larynx is removed and the voice permanently lost. A permanent tracheostomy always is performed with this procedure.
- Radical neck dissection involves the above procedure for total laryngectomy plus removal of the lymphatic drainage channels and nodes, sternocleidmastoid muscle, spinal accessory nerve, jugular vein and submandibular area. It is performed when there is a risk of metastasis to the cervical lymph nodes.

NURSING MANAGEMENT

Surgical

Partial Laryngectomy

Preoperative Care
In addition to routine preoperative care:
- Assess the client's nutritional status, including usual caloric intake, lymphocyte levels, serum albumin, hemoglobin and hematocrit.
- Assess the oral mucosa and state of dentition.
- If the client is an active alcoholic, discuss with physician plans for support during the withdrawal period.
- Assess the client's usual coping strategies and available support systems (there will be some disfigurement after surgery).
- Discuss alternate means of communication to be used in the postoperative period.

Postoperative Care
In addition to routine postoperative care:
- Monitor closely for possible complications of airway obstruction, hemorrhage, fistula formation and tracheostomy stenosis.

- Monitor for carotid artery rupture— mild bleeding from the oral cavity, neck, or trachea may precede an impending rupture by 24 to 48 hours.
- Prevent aspiration by:
  — maintaining semi-Fowler to high-Fowler's position.
  — suctioning or instructing client to cough every hour to remove secretions.
  — instructing on swallowing technique (the epiglottis has been removed).
- Maintain a patent tracheostomy tube by cleaning the inner cannula to remove mucous as needed (at least 3 times/day).
- Prevent tracheostomy tube displacement or accidental decannulation by:
  — ensuring intactness of sutures
  — using two nurses to change tracheostomy ties
  — ensuring snugness of tracheostomy ties
  — keeping a tracheal dilator and emergency tracheostomy tray in the room
  — understanding use of stay sutures (if used)
- Reduce the risk of tracheal necrosis or stenosis by:
  — deflating the tracheostomy cuff (during exhalation) every shift to improve circulation and remove secretions
  — using the minimal *occlusion* volume technique to reinflate the cuff , never the minimal *leak* technique
- Monitor for and prevent infection by:
  — assessing the amount and color of drainage every 4 hours
  — assessing incisional site, noting any redness, swelling or tenderness
  — ensuring that supplemental oxygen is humidified
  — ensuring patency of wound drains
  — cleansing suture lines twice daily with hydrogen peroxide, followed by a saline rinse.
- Maintain NG tube to suction for removal of gastric secretions.
- Provide adequate nutrition through tube feedings when prescribed, using care to prevent aspiration.

FOCUSED DISCHARGE CARE

Instruct client regarding:

- wound care
- need for follow-up with speech and swallowing therapy
- need for follow-up of possible metastasis
- importance of good nutrition.

TOTAL LARYNGECTOMY

Preoperative Care
- Preoperative care is the same as for the partial laryngectomy client, except the tracheostomy is permanent, and the client will need to learn alternative methods to speak. Nasogastric feedings also will be started sooner.

Postoperative Care
Postoperative care is the same as for the partial laryngectomy client with the following added interventions:
- Provide nasogastric feedings when edema has subsided and the client can swallow his own secretions.
- Instruct on and provide an alternative means to communicate in the first few postoperative days, such as a writing board or picture boards where the patient can point to what he needs.
- Reinforce speech techniques taught by speech therapist:
  — use of an artificial larynx
  — esophageal speech
  — use of a voice button or trapdoor prosthesis.

FOCUSED DISCHARGE CARE

Instruct client regarding:
- tracheostomy care and dressing changes
- covering stoma lightly with bib, scarf, etc. to prevent entrance of foreign bodies
- need for smoking cessation program
- avoidance of water sports
- importance of wearing Medic-Alert bracelet (to identify need for mouth-stoma breathing if resuscitation needed)
- signs/symptoms to report to physician:
  — hemoptysis
  — difficulty swallowing/breathing

— change in voice quality
— persistent cough, sore throat
— lump in the neck or elsewhere in body.
- reinforce nutritional plan
- discuss follow-up with speech therapy.
- need for follow-up of possible metastasis

RADICAL NECK DISSECTION

Preoperative Care
In addition to routine preoperative care:
- Encourage the client to discuss fears and concerns, especially of deformity or diagnosis of cancer.
- Discuss what to expect after surgery (transfer to intensive care unit, drainage tubes, tracheostomy).
- Assess usual coping mechanisms/support systems.
- Discuss alternative means of communication (voice will be lost).

Postoperative Care
In addition to routine postoperative care:
- Monitor closely for patent airway (airway occlusion can occur due to bleeding or edema).
- If musculocutaneous flaps were used for repair, assess perfusion of the flap every hour for the first 24 hours, then every 4 hours.
- Place in semi-Fowler's to reduce edema.
- Monitor patency and drainage of neck catheters. Aspirate the drains or empty every 4 hours.
- Maintain pressure dressings (except on musculo-cutaneous flap) — reinforce as needed.
- Instruct on exercises to increase range of motion and muscle strength in affected shoulder.
- See also "Tracheostomy", p. 616.

FOCUSED DISCHARGE CARE

Instruct client regarding:
- increased risk of neck tissue injury because of lack of sensation
- avoidance of temperature extremes or use of heating pads
- wound care
- tracheostomy care
See also "Tracheostomy", p. 616.

(For more information, see pp. 548-560 of Polaski and Tatro, *Luckmann's Core Principles and Practice of Medical-Surgical Nursing.*)

Laryngeal Edema, Acute

- Laryngeal edema may be associated with inflammation, injury or anaphylaxis.
- Signs and symptoms are hoarseness and severe shortness of breath progressing to respiratory arrest.
- Emergency tracheostomy may be required because endotracheal intubation is difficult due to the edema.
- Subcutaneous epinephrine 1:1000 and intravenous corticosteroids are used if anaphylaxis is the cause.

(For more information, see p. 561 of Polaski and Tatro, *Luckmann's Core Principles and Practice of Medical-Surgical Nursing.*)

Laryngitis

- Laryngitis is an inflammation of the larynx or hoarseness. It may be due to an inflammatory process, voice abuse, gastroesophageal reflux, abnormal movements of the vocal cords, or a tumor of the vocal cords.
- Treatment of laryngitis is aimed at the causative factors, such as antibiotics for infection; voice rest for voice abuse; and antacids and histamine receptor antagonists for gastroesophageal reflux.
- Nursing care involves administration of supplemental humidification and mucolytic agents, voice rest and instructing the client to avoid whispering which strains the vocal cords.

(For more information, see p. 566 of Polaski and Tatro, *Luckmann's Core Principles and Practice of Medical-Surgical Nursing.*)

Laryngospasm

- Laryngospasm is a spasm of the laryngeal muscles due to:
  — administration of certain general anesthetic agents
  — repeat and/or traumatic endotracheal intubation attempts
  — inhaled agents or foreign material
  — hypocalcemia.
- Treatment is administration of 100 per cent oxygen until the laryngeal spasm stops. If the laryngospasm continues, paralysis with neuromuscular blocking agents may be necessary to allow intubation. Mechanical ventilation follows.
- Emergency cricothyroidotomy or tracheostomy may be required.

(For more information, see pp. 561-562 of Polaski and Tatro, *Luckmann's Core Principles and Practice of Medical-Surgical Nursing.*)

Leukemia

OVERVIEW

- Leukemia is a malignant disease of the blood-forming organs. Leukemia accounts for 8 per cent of all human cancers and is the most common malignancy in children and young adults. One-half of all leukemias are classified as acute with rapid onset and progression. The remaining are classified as chronic and have a more indolent course.

- Acute leukemia is caused by neoplastic proliferation of large numbers of abnormal immature leukocytes in the bone marrow that infiltrate the lymph nodes, liver, spleen and eventually all body systems. In addition, the production of other blood cells (i.e., red blood cells, platelets, and neutrophils) is inhibited and results in inadequate oxygen transport, thrombocytopenia and immune system malfunction.
- Chronic leukemias have a gradual onset and a more protracted course. The white cells produced are more mature and can better defend the body against infection. Chronic leukemia occurs in clients between the ages of 25 and 60 years.
- There are two major forms of acute leukemia: (1) lymphocytic (ALL) — involves the lymphocytes and lymphoid organs, and (2) nonlymphocytic (ANLL) — involves the hematopoietic stem cells that differentiate into myeloid cells (monocytes, granulocytes, erythrocytes and platelets). ALL presents most often in children 2 to 10 years of age. Acute nonlymphocytic leukemia (ANLL), formerly known as acute myelogenous leukemia (AML), is characterized by aberrations in the growth of megakaryocytes, monocytes, granulocytes and erythrocytes.
- Chronic leukemia is classified as chronic myelogenous leukemia (CML) or chronic lymphocytic leukemia (CLL).
  - CML originates in the stem cells. After a relatively slow course for a median of 4 years, the CML client invariably enters a blast crisis that resembles acute leukemia. During this phase, increasing numbers of blasts (immature myeloid precursor cells, especially myeloblasts) proliferate in the blood and bone marrow.
  - CLL is characterized by the proliferation of early B lymphocytes. CLL is an indolent form of leukemia most often seen in men over 50 years of age. As the disease progresses, lymphocytes infiltrate the lymph nodes, liver, spleen and bone marrow. Progression of the disease may take as long as 15 years. Blast crisis results in the death of more than 70 per cent of the clients.
- Overexposure to radiation is a major risk factor for the development of leukemia, often years after the initial exposure. Alkylating agents used to treat other

cancers, especially in combination with radiation therapy, also increase the risk for developing leukemia.

CLINICAL MANIFESTATIONS

The signs and symptoms of all types of leukemia are similar. The clinical history will usually reveal symptoms characteristic of anemia, thrombocytopenia, and leukopenia.
- fatigue, weakness
- easy bruising
- bleeding gums
- epistaxis
- fever
- headache and generalized pain
- feeling of abdominal fullness and early satiety (as a result of splenomegaly)
- pallor
- scattered petechiae and ecchymosis
- generalized lymphadenopathy
- hepatosplenomegaly
- bone and joint pain
- CBC values:
  — WBC may be normal, abnormally low or extremely high. The differential may reveal that one type of leukocyte is predominant.
  — Platelet count — usually low.
  — Hemoglobin — usually low.

MEDICAL MANAGEMENT

Acute Leukemia

- chemotherapy
  — protocol involves three phases:
    — induction—client receives an intensive course of chemotherapy designed to induce a complete remission.
    — consolidation phase — modified courses of intensive chemotherapy are given to eradicate the disease.
    — maintenance phase — small doses of different combinations of chemotherapeutic agents are given every 3 to 4 weeks and continued for a year or more.

　　　　— agents used:
　　　　　　— ANLL:
　　　　　　　　• cytarabine
　　　　　　　　• 6-thioguanine
　　　　　　　　• mercaptopurine
　　　　　　　　• vincristine
　　　　　　　　• prednisone
　　　　　　　　• cyclophosphamide
　　　　　　　　• daunorubicin
　　　　　　　　• doxorubicin
　　　　　　— ALL:
　　　　　　　　• vincristine
　　　　　　　　• daunorubicin
　　　　　　　　• prednisone
　　　　　　　　• cyclophosphamide
　　　　　　　　• L-asparaginase
　• radiation therapy
　• bone marrow transplantation — see "Bone Marrow Transplantation", p. 92
　• blood component replacement therapy
　• broad spectrum antibiotics and antifungals for signs/symptoms of infection

CHRONIC MYELOGENOUS LEUKEMIA (CML)

　• leukopheresis — temporary lowering of the white cell count using an automated blood cell separator that returns red cells and plasma to the client
　• plateletpheresis — operates on same principle as leukopheresis but removes platelets
　• chemotherapy
　　— busulfan
　　— hydroxyurea
　　— cytosine arabinoside
　　— methotrexate
　　— daunorubicin
　　— prednisone
　　— vincristine
　• blood component replacement therapy
　• bone marrow transplantation — see "Bone Marrow Transplantation", p. 92
　• antibiotic therapy
　• allopurinol (Zyloprim) therapy — used to prevent cell lysis syndrome caused by rapid cell lysis, which increases uric acid in the blood, and can lead to renal failure; increased levels of serum phosphate,

uric acid and potassium; and decreased serum calcium

Chronic Lymphocytic Leukemia (CLL)

- radiation therapy
- chemotherapy
  — chlorambucil
  — prednisone
  — vincristine
  — cyclophosphamide
- blood component therapy
- antibiotic therapy

SURGICAL MANAGEMENT

Chronic Lymphocytic Leukemia

- splenectomy

NURSING MANAGEMENT

Medical

- Administer prescribed chemotherapy. See "Chemotherapy", p. 145.
- Administer blood component replacement therapy. See "Blood Component Transfusion", p. 88.
- See "Radiation Therapy", p. 543.
- Monitor temperature and assess for any signs/symptoms of infection.
- Maintain protective isolation or laminar flow if neutrophil count is less than 500/mm³.
- Restrict visitors with possible communicable diseases.
- Provide meticulous oral and physical care.
- Maintain a low-bacteria diet excluding raw fruits and vegetables.
- Avoid rectal suppositories and rectal temperatures (may seed the bloodstream with microorganisms).
- Obtain cultures as ordered.
- Administer antibiotics as prescribed.
- Monitor the client for signs/symptoms of bleeding: ecchymosis, petechiae, epistaxis, heme-positive stools, disorientation.
- Test all urine, stool and emesis for blood.

- Monitor vital signs, noting symptoms of altered tissue perfusion.
- Institute bleeding precautions:
  — soft toothbrushes
  — avoid blowing nose
  — avoid straining with stool
  — electric razor
  — no intramuscular or subcutaneous injections
  — no aspirin products
  — pad side rails and maintain uncluttered environment
  — use paper tape only
- Monitor laboratory findings — CBC, platelet count, culture reports.
- Administer antiemetics as prescribed.
- Daily weights.
- Encourage small, frequent feedings.
- Administer analgesics to relieve the pain of mucositis.
- Encourage the client to balance rest with exercise.
- Provide emotional support and referrals to assist the client/family in dealing with a potentially fatal prognosis.

Surgical

- See "Bone Marrow Transplantation", p. 88.
- See "Splenectomy", p. 594.

FOCUSED DISCHARGE CARE

- Instruct client regarding:
  — disease process and treatment regime
  — signs/symptoms to report to physician
  — measures to prevent infection:
    - avoid large crowds and wear a mask in public
    - good personal hygiene
    - female clients should douche only per physician order and avoid the use of tampons
    - maintain a balance between exercise and rest
    - maintain a well-balanced diet
    - avoid fresh fruits and vegetables and raw meat
    - avoid anyone with an infectious disease
    - change air conditioner and furnace filters weekly

- remove additional sources of bacteria found in standing water: fish tanks, flower vases, humidifiers
— measures to reduce risk of bleeding:
  - soft toothbrush
  - electric razor
  - avoid blowing nose or straining with stool
  - safety precautions
— see "Chemotherapy", p. 145
— see "Radiation Therapy", p. 543
— see "Bone Marrow Transplantation", p. 88
— importance of follow-up clinic and laboratory visits
- Refer to available community resources.

(For more information, see pp. 854-859 of Polaski and Tatro, *Luckmann's Core Principles and Practice of Medical-Surgical Nursing.*)

Leukoplakia

- Leukoplakia is a potentially precancerous yellow-white or gray-white lesion occurring in the oral mucous membranes. It results from chronic irritation of the mucosa by physical, thermal or chemical factors. Men are twice as affected as women.
- Treatment is aimed at elimination of the cause.

(For more information, see p. 1012 of Polaski and Tatro, *Luckmann's Core Principles and Practice of Medical-Surgical Nursing.*)

Liver Neoplasms (Primary)

- Primary liver neoplasms may be adenomas or hepatocellular carcinoma.

- Adenomas are benign hepatic cell tumors. They may be related to oral contraceptive use by women or androgen use by men. They may be dangerous due to their vascularity. Treatment may be discontinuation of the hormone if the tumor is hormone dependent. Surgical excision may be necessary in some cases.
- Primary hepatocellular carcinoma (malignant hepatoma) may be caused by hepatitis B, chronic liver disease, nitrosamines, polyvinylchloride, anabolic steroid use or long-term androgen therapy. Resections or liver transplants are performed for some cases.
- See "Chemotherapy," p. 145, and "Radiation Therapy," p.543.

(For more information, see pp. 1133-1134 of Polaski and Tatro, *Luckmann's Core Principles and Practice of Medical-Surgical Nursing.*)

Liver Transplant

- Liver transplant is now considered a feasible intervention for end-stage liver diseases including:
  — primary biliary cirrhosis (adult)
  — hepatitis — chronic or fulminant (usually adult)
  — sclerosing cholangitis (adult)
  — biliary atresia (pediatrics)
  — Alpha-1 antitrypsin deficiency (usually pediatric)
  — confined hepatic malignancy (adult or pediatric)
  — Wilson's disease
  — Budd-Chiari syndrome
- The transplant may be orthotopic (the diseased liver is removed and the new liver implanted in the same location) or heterotopic (the diseased liver is not removed during transplant). Heterotopic transplants are rarely performed.
- The criteria for matching donors and recipients for liver transplantation include compatible blood type and liver size.
- The major postoperative complications specific to liver transplantation include infection, hypertension

and rejection. Symptoms of acute rejection include: fever, flu-like symptoms, increasing liver function enzymes and right upper quadrant pain.
- There are several drugs available to treat rejection and new antirejection drugs are currently under investigation.

NURSING MANAGEMENT

POSTOPERATIVE CARE

In addition to routine postoperative care:
- Observe for signs/symptoms of respiratory compromise.
- Monitor fluid and electrolyte status.
- Monitor for signs/symptoms of bleeding.
- Monitor blood pressure, pulse, central venous pressure and pulmonary artery pressures.
- Follow immunosuppressive protocols.
- Monitor wound drains and bile drains for patency.

FOCUSED DISCHARGE CARE

- Instruct client/significant other regarding:
  — signs/symptoms of rejection
  — prevention of and signs/symptoms of infection
  — immunosuppressive therapy and possible side effects
  — avoidance of over the counter medications unless physician approves
  — diet (usually no added salt), exercise and activity
  — care of lines, wound or T-tube
  — follow-up laboratory studies
  — cancer prevention (no smoking, use of sunscreen — emphasized due to immunosuppression)
  — avoidance of alcohol
  — when to call the local physician and/or the transplant team
  — need for Medic-Alert bracelet
- Refer to home health care agency/support groups as needed.

(For more information, see pp. 1135 of Polaski and Tatro, *Luckmann's Core Principles and Practice of Medical-Surgical Nursing*

Liver Tumors (Metastatic)

OVERVIEW

- Metastatic tumors of the liver are tumors that began elsewhere in the body and have spread to the liver.
- The liver is one of the most common sites of metastasis due to the liver's high rate of blood flow, size and portal drainage from the major abdominal organs.
- Metastatic tumors spread to the liver by:
  (1) direct extension from adjacent organs
  (2) the hepatic arterial system
  (3) the portal venous system
- Unfortunately, these tumors may be far advanced before clinical manifestations are present, and this condition usually carries a poor prognosis.

CLINICAL MANIFESTATIONS

Manifestations may be vague until the tumor is advanced.
- minor temperature elevation
- gastrointestinal symptoms
- back pain
- right upper quadrant distress
- tenderness
- abdominal distention
- diarrhea or constipation
- nausea
- hepatomegaly
- jaundice

Some clients also may develop polycythemia, blood sugar disorders and hypercalcemia.

MEDICAL MANAGEMENT

- dearterialization of the liver by hepatic artery ligation to decrease oxygen supply to the liver and reduce number and activity of tumor cells
- irradiation

- percutaneous biliary drainage or internal placement of a biliary drain to help pass bile into the duodenum and decrease jaundice and discomfort
- regional perfusion of the liver via the hepatic artery to relieve pain and slow tumor growth
- chemotherapy — systemic or via an implanted pump

SURGICAL MANAGEMENT

- resection may be an option if the tumor is small and confined to one segment or lobe and if the client can withstand the surgery

NURSING MANAGEMENT

Varies according to the procedures performed and the amount of liver dysfunction.
- Assess for metabolic dysfunctions, bleeding problems, ascites, edema, inability to metabolize drugs, hypoproteinemia, jaundice and endocrine complications.
- Prepare the client for all procedures and assess for post procedure complications.
- Provide emotional support to the family and client.
- See also "Chemotherapy", p. 145.
- See also "Radiation Therapy", p. 543.

FOCUSED DISCHARGE CARE

- Instruct client/significant other regarding:
  - side effects of chemotherapy
  - skin care of irradiated areas
  - pain management
  - signs/symptoms to report to physician
  - importance of follow-up care
- Refer to home health care agency, hospice and cancer support groups as needed.

(For more information, see pp. 1134-1135 of Polaski and Tatro, *Luckmann's Core Principles and Practice of Medical-Surgical Nursing.*)

Low Back Pain

OVERVIEW

- Low back pain occurs in the lower lumbar, lumbosacral or sacroiliac areas. It often relates to degenerative processes or musculotendinous strain.
- Other causes of low back pain include: (1) ruptured vertebral disc or herniation of the nucleus pulposus, (2) back or pelvic fracture, (3) tumor, (4) infection (osteomyelitis), (5) congenital back deformity, (6) muscle spasm, and (7) strain from stretched abdominal muscles secondary to obesity or pregnancy.

CLINICAL MANIFESTATIONS

- low back pain worsened by sitting or standing
- early morning stiffness
- sciatic radiation

MEDICAL MANAGEMENT

- bedrest
- local heat, local ice
- analgesics
- muscle relaxants
- anti-inflammatories
- traction
- lumbosacral corset
- muscle-strengthening exercises

SURGICAL MANAGEMENT

- Depends upon underlying problem.

NURSING MANAGEMENT

- Administer analgesics, muscle relaxants, and anti-inflammatories as prescribed.
- Maintain bedrest.
- Apply local heat and/or ice.
- Collaborate with physical therapy for prescribed exercises and adaptive devices.
- See "Traction", p. 622.

FOCUSED DISCHARGE CARE

Instruct client regarding:
- lengthy rehabilitation
- treatment regime
- use of adaptive devices
- techniques for managing chronic back pain:
  — maintain erect posture
  — avoid prolonged standing or sitting
  — when sitting, use a footstool to keep knees level with hips
  — avoid bending, lifting, twisting at waist level
  — squat with straight lower back
  — alternate activity with rest
  — begin a fitness program with physician approval

(For more information, see pp. 1319-1321 of Polaski and Tatro, *Luckmann's Core Principles and Practice of Medical-Surgical Nursing.*)

Lung Cancer

OVERVIEW

- Lung cancer is malignancy in the epithelium of the respiratory tract. There are four major types of lung cancer:
  - (1) small cell carcinoma (oat cell) — usually presents as a hilar or central mass; rapid growth with early metastasis to mediastinum, thoracic and extrathoracic structures
  - (2) squamous cell cancer — arises from bronchial epithelium; slow growth, metastasis not common. If metastasis occurs, it is usually to the lymphatic system, adrenals and liver.
  - (3) adenocarcinoma — arises from the bronchial mucus gland; grows slowly; metastasizes to lung or other organs
  - (4) large cell carcinoma — arises peripherally in the lung as single or multiple masses; grows slowly with metastasis to the kidney, liver and adrenals.

- Survival from lung cancer remains low, especially for clients with small cell carcinomas.
- Lung cancer is the leading cause of death from cancer in the United States. The incidence of lung cancer is rising at a faster rate than any other cancer type.
- Risk factors include: cigarette smoking; passive smoke (inhaling smoke from the environment surrounding an active smoker); exposure to radioactive isotopes, polycyclic hydrocarbons, vinyl chloride, mustard gas, metallurgical ores, asbestos fibers and air pollution.

CLINICAL MANIFESTATIONS

Symptoms vary according to tumor type, location and extent and previous pulmonary health.
- Centrally located pulmonary tumors
  — coughing, wheezing, stridor, dyspnea
  — chest, shoulder, back pain
  — hemoptysis
  — pericardial effusion, cardiac tamponade and rhythm disturbances, if extends to pericardium
- Peripheral pulmonary tumors
  — sharp, severe pleural pain that worsens on inspiration
  — signs/symptoms of pleural effusion
- Apical pulmonary tumors (Pancoast's tumors)
  — no symptoms until tumor extends into surrounding structures
  — arm and shoulder pain from tumor involvement of the first thoracic and eighth cervical nerves of the brachial plexus
  — rib pain
  — Horner's syndrome (due to sympathetic nerve ganglia involvement)
    — pupil contraction on affected side of face
    — partial eyelid ptosis on affected side of face
    — absence of sweating on affected side of the face
- warning signs of lung cancer:
  — any change in respiratory pattern
  — persistent cough
  — sputum streaked with blood
  — hemoptysis
  — rust-colored or purulent sputum

- chest, shoulder or arm pain
- dyspnea
- recurrent episodes of pleural effusion, pneumonia or bronchitis

MEDICAL MANAGEMENT

Treatment depends upon tumor type, stage and underlying health status.

- radiation therapy — used alone or in combination with chemotherapy or surgery; may also be used for palliation of symptoms
- chemotherapy — small cell lung cancer responds well; use of chemotherapy for non-small cell lung cancer is controversial

SURGICAL MANAGEMENT

- pulmonary resection is the treatment of choice for early stage non-small cell lung cancer:
  - wedge resection — removal of a small, localized area of diseased tissue. Pulmonary structure and function are relatively unchanged.
  - segmental resection — removal of one or more lung segments (a bronchiole and its alveoli)
  - lobectomy — removal of an entire lobe of the lung. The remaining lung overexpands to fill in the thoracic space previously occupied by the resected tissue.
  - pneumonectomy — removal of an entire lung. Once the lung is removed, the involved side is an empty space. The phrenic nerve is severed on the affected side to paralyze the diaphragm in an elevated position to reduce the size of this cavity.
- laser therapy - palliative for the relief of endobronchial obstructions caused by nonresectable lung tumors

NURSING MANAGEMENT

MEDICAL

- See "Chemotherapy", p. 145, and "Radiation Therapy", p. 543.

PREOPERATIVE CARE

In addition to routine preoperative care:
- Provide emotional support and facilitate discussion of fears and concerns of client and significant other.
- Instruct client and significant other regarding:
  — anticipated surgical procedure
  — early postoperative period and presence of chest tubes (except with pneumonectomy), drainage tubes, intubation, mechanical ventilation and oxygen therapy
  — postoperative exercises
    — respiratory exercises and splinting
    — leg exercises
    — arm/shoulder exercises

POSTOPERATIVE CARE

In addition to routine postoperative care:
- Monitor for potential postoperative complications and report to physician immediately.
  — respiratory failure
  — tension pneumothorax
  — pulmonary embolus
  — pulmonary edema
  — cardiac dysrhythmias
  — hemorrhage, hemothorax, hypovolemic shock
  — thrombophlebitis
  — subcutaneous emphysema around incision and in the chest and neck
- Monitor breath sounds.
- Monitor dressing and incisional area for bleeding.
- Position client in side-lying position on non-operative side in immediate postoperative period, until consciousness regained.
- Place client in semi-Fowler's position once vital signs are stable and turn every 1 to 2 hours as appropriate (head of bed up 30 to 45 degrees).
- Avoid positioning on operative side if wedge resection or segmentectomy performed (hinders expansion of remaining lung tissue).
- Avoid complete lateral positioning after pneumonectomy (may cause mediastinal shift and compression of remaining lung).
- Assist with coughing and deep breathing every 1 to 2 hours during the first 24 to 48 hours.

432

- Evaluate need for suctioning.
- Administer analgesics, assess effectiveness and schedule pulmonary and leg exercises when medication is at maximal effectiveness.
- Maintain closed chest tube drainage (usually not used after pneumonectomy).
- Monitor amount and type of chest tube drainage.
- Begin passive range of motion exercises of arm and affected shoulder on affected side 4 hours after recovery following anesthesia. Perform twice every 4 to 6 hours for the first 24 hours. Progress to 10 to 20 times every 2 hours, eventually progress to active range of motion.
- Encourage ambulation when condition permits.
- Assess client's tolerance of activity.
- Provide emotional support and facilitate discussion of fears and concerns.
- Encourage use of previously successful coping strategies.

FOCUSED DISCHARGE CARE

- Instruct client regarding:
  — wound care
  — continuation of exercise program
  — avoidance of environmental irritants
  — activity limitations and avoidance of heavy lifting
  — signs/symptoms to report to physician (e.g., infection, deteriorating respiratory status)
  — importance of follow-up to detect complications, recurrence of malignancy or metastasis
- Refer to cancer support groups as appropriate.
- Refer to home health care agency as appropriate.

(For more information, see pp. 603-613 of Polaski and Tatro, *Luckmann's Core Principles and Practice of Medical-Surgical Nursing.*)

Lymphadenitis

- Lymph nodes act as defense barriers and are secondarily involved in virtually all systemic infections and in many neoplastic disorders.
- Generalized lymphadenopathy (enlargement of two or three regionally separated lymph node groups) is usually due to inflammation, neoplasm or immunologic reaction.
- In acute lymphadenitis, the inflamed nodes are most commonly located in the cervical region in association with infections of the teeth or tonsils or in the axillary or inguinal regions secondary to infections in the extremities. The lymph nodes are enlarged, tender, warm and reddened.
- Chronic lymphadenitis occurs in the course of a longstanding infection. The lymph nodes become scarred with fibrous tissue. Clinically, the nodes are enlarged, firm to palpation and not tender or warm.
- The management of lymphadenitis is treatment of the underlying cause.

(For more information, see p. 820 of Polaski and Tatro, *Luckmann's Core Principles and Practice of Medical-Surgical Nursing*.)

Lymphedema

OVERVIEW

- Lymphedema is swelling due to impaired transcapillary fluid transport and transportation of lymph.
- Failure of lymph transport allows plasma proteins in the interstitial fluid to accumulate. As the lymph channels dilate, valves become incompetent. The osmotic pressure is reduced by drawing water into interstitial areas. The fluid seeks pathways through the tissues, which causes inflammation, lymphatic thrombosis and eventually fibrosis.

- Primary lymphedema is an inherited trait that results in abnormal development of lymph vessels.
- Secondary lymphedema occurs because of damage or obstruction of the lymph system by another disease process or procedure. Examples include:
  — neoplasms
  — trauma
  — surgical excision of axillary, inguinal or iliac nodes
  — irradiation

CLINICAL MANIFESTATIONS

- bilateral mild edema of ankles and legs in women at puberty
- unilateral edema of the entire leg
- bilateral edema present at birth or an early age
- skin vesicles filled with lymph
- dull, heavy sensation in affected limb(s)
- reduction but not disappearance of swelling when legs are elevated
- rough skin

MEDICAL MANAGEMENT

There is no cure once swelling occurs.
- physical therapy — manual squeezing of the tissue to press stagnant lymphatic fluid to the proximal part of the limb, followed by active and passive exercises to transport the lymph further into the lymphatic system and bloodstream
- pneumatic pumping device
- diuretics
- elastic stockings or arm sleeves

SURGICAL MANAGEMENT

Surgery is used only if medical management is not beneficial. Though not curable, the final appearance may be more acceptable.
- all skin, subcutaneous tissue and deep fascia are removed and the extremity is covered with a skin graft

NURSING MANAGEMENT

- Monitor extremity for signs of infection.

- Provide meticulous skin care.
- Keep extremity elevated above right atrium.
- Apply elastic stockings or sleeves as prescribed.
- Apply and monitor pneumatic compression device.
- Encourage activity and exercises.

FOCUSED DISCHARGE CARE

Instruct client regarding:
- operation of pneumatic compression device
- application of elastic stocking or arm sleeve
- measures to prevent infection
- signs/symptoms of infection to report
- prescribed exercises
- importance of elevating limb above the heart whenever possible

(For more information, see pp. 819-820 of Polaski and Tatro, *Luckmann's Core Principles and Practice of Medical-Surgical Nursing.*)

Mechanical Ventilation

OVERVIEW

- Mechanical ventilation is the use of a positive-pressure ventilator with an artificial airway (either tracheostomy or endotracheal tube).
- Indications for mechanical ventilation include inadequate ventilation and hypoxemia.
- Common disorders that may require mechanical ventilation include: pneumonia, adult respiratory distress syndrome (ARDS), rib fractures, cardiogenic shock, Guillian-Barré syndrome, myasthenia gravis, head injury and airway obstruction.
- Positive-pressure ventilators may be categorized as: (1) those for short-term use (intermittent positive-pressure breathing [IPPB]) and (2) those for continuous use (continuous mechanical ventilation).
  - (1) IPPB is use of a pressure-cycled ventilator to deliver pressurized breaths to a spontaneously breathing client in ten to twenty minute treatments. It is infrequently prescribed.
  - (2) Continuous mechanical ventilation (CMV) is used to: maintain adequate ventilation; deliver precise concentrations of FIO_2; deliver adequate tidal volumes; and to decrease the work of breathing in clients who cannot sustain adequate ventilation on their own.
- Continuous mechanical ventilators may be pressure-cycled (delivers a volume of gas using positive pressure during inspiration until a preselected pressure has been reached) or volume-cycled (delivers a pre-set tidal volume of inspired gas regardless of the pressure required to deliver this volume). A pressure limit can be set to prevent dangerously high pressures from occurring.
- Adverse physiologic effects of positive pressure delivered via a mechanical ventilator include:

- — decreased cardiac output
- — possible ischemia of the gastric mucosa, leading to bleeding and stress ulceration (due to decreased blood flow to the splanchic area resulting from descent of the diaphragm into the abdomen during the inspiratory phase)
- — water retention (due to an increase in anti-diuretic hormone)
- — possible cerebral edema if severe alkalosis occurs.
- Ventilation may be assisted or controlled.
  - — Assisted ventilation is person-cycled. The client's own inspiratory effort turns on ("trips") the ventilator, initiating the mechanical inspiratory phase.
  - — Controlled ventilation governs a client's rate of ventilation by automatically cycling the ventilator at a predetermined number of cycles per minute; the ventilator does all of the work of breathing, the client does none.
- Clients who are on controlled ventilation and have spontaneous respirations may "fight" or "buck" the ventilator because they cannot synchronize their own respirations with the machine's cycle. If the nurse is unable to help them relax and breathe with the ventilator, sedatives and possibly neuromuscular blocking agents may be indicated, such as pancuronium bromide (Pavulon), curare or vercuronium bromide (Norcuron). Neuromuscular blocking agents block the transmission of nerve impulses and result in muscle paralysis. They do not affect sensorium or perception of pain and always should be used in conjunction with sedation or analgesics.
- Positive end-expiratory pressure (PEEP) and continuous positive airway pressure (CPAP) are ventilator techniques applied during expiration, whereby intrathoracic pressures are not allowed to return to ambient pressure. This helps keep the alveoli open, increases functional residual capacity (FRC) and enhances oxygenation as a result of the enlarged surface area that is available for diffusion.
- The adverse physiologic effects of positive airway pressure (i.e., CPAP and PEEP) are basically the same as those discussed for mechanical ventilation. There are also the following risks:

- — rupture of the lungs (barotrauma)
- — pneumothorax
- — subcutaneous emphysema
- — pneumomediastinum
- — cardiovascular embarrassment (decreased cardiac output)
- — increased intracranial pressure
- Intermittent mandatory ventilation (IMV) is the setting of a ventilator to deliver a specific respiratory rate. If the client breathes at a rate higher than the machine rate, these breaths will not be positive-pressure ventilations.
- Pressure support ventilation (PSV) is a recent ventilation method that augments spontaneous inspiratory effort with a preset level of positive airway pressure. When the client on PSV initiates a breath, the machine is triggered and delivers a flow of gas at the preset pressure.

NURSING MANAGEMENT

Promote respiratory function.
- Auscultate lungs frequently to assess for adventitious sounds, to validate endotracheal tube placement, and to ensure bilateral ventilation of the lungs.
- Suction as needed, providing pre- and post-hyperinflation and hyperoxygenation.
- Do not instill normal saline into airway prior to suctioning to loosen secretions and promote coughing as research has shown this practice to be unsafe (1995).
- Turn and reposition every two hours.
- Position on unaffected side.
- Secure endotracheal tube (ETT) properly.
- Use a bite block or oral airway, if needed.
- Monitor arterial blood gas values and pulse oximetry.
- Check the machine and alarms frequently to ensure proper functioning.
- Always have a self-inflating resuscitation bag readily available.
- Use a manual resuscitation bag if the alarm sounds and you cannot quickly correct the problem.
- Monitor peak inspiratory pressures and ventilatory parameters hourly.

- Assess if the client's breathing rate is greater than the mechanical ventilatory rate.
- Maintain patency of endotracheal tube or tracheostomy.
- Prevent loose connections or kinks in the tubing.

Provide a communication method and assist to decrease anxiety.
- Explain all procedures.
- Explain purpose of ventilator to client and family; discuss how it helps breathing, how it feels, how to cooperate with the machine and different types of alarms.
- Develop a means of communication, via writing or picture board.
- Place call light within reach and be sure all staff know that client cannot speak.
- Encourage significant others to talk to client.
- Provide distractions (e.g., TV and radio).
- Medicate with antianxiety medication and sedatives as prescribed.
- If client is on neuromuscular blocking agents:
  — Be sure other staff know the client is on a neuromuscular blocking agent and can still feel pain and hear.
  — Be sure that client receives sedation in conjunction with neuromuscular blocking agents.
  — Explain to the client the cause of paralysis and provide reassurance.

Monitor for complications.
- Assess for possible early complications due to mechanical ventilation:
  — rapid electrolyte changes
  — severe alkalosis
  — hypotension secondary to changes in cardiac output.
- Monitor for signs of respiratory distress: restlessness, apprehension, irritability, use of accessory muscles and increased heart rate.
- Assess for signs/symptoms of barotrauma: increasing dyspnea; agitation; decreased or absent breath sounds; tracheal deviation away from the affected side; subcutaneous emphysema; and decreasing PaO_2 levels.

- Assess for cardiovascular depression: hypotension, tachycardia, bradycardia, dysrhythmias, weak peripheral pulses, increases in pulmonary wedge pressure or signs of increased heart failure.
- Monitor for signs of inadvertent extubation: vocalization, low-pressure alarm, bilateral decrease in upper lobe airway sounds, gastric distention and clinical manifestations of inadequate ventilation.
- If inadvertent extubation occurs, manually ventilate with a self-inflating resuscitation bag and notify physician for reintubation.
- Prevent endotracheal tube pressure on nares or oral mucosa.
- Provide good oral care.
- If client is on PEEP or CPAP, assess:
  — blood pressure and heart rate
  — breath sounds
  — urinary output
  — signs of increased heart failure
  — subcutaneous emphysema

Prevent infection.
- Maintain sterile technique when suctioning.
- Monitor color, amount and consistency of sputum.
- Drain water from tubing; do not drain it back into the humidifier.

Provide adequate nutrition.
- Begin tube feeding as soon as it is evident the client will remain on the ventilator for a long time.
- Weigh daily.
- Monitor intake and output.

Monitor for gastrointestinal bleeding.
- Monitor bowel sounds.
- Monitor gastric pH and hematest gastric secretions every shift.

Maintain muscle strength.
- Perform range of motion exercises and ambulate to chair when able.
- Encourage client to perform exercises in bed, if able.

(For more information, see pp. 533-538 of Polaski and Tatro, *Luckmann's Core Principles and Practice of Medical-Surgical Nursing.*)

Meningitis (Bacterial)

OVERVIEW

- Bacterial meningitis is an inflammation of the arachnoid, pia and intervening cerebrospinal fluid. The infection spreads throughout the subarachnoid space around the brain and spinal cord and usually involves the ventricles.
- The most common bacteria causing meningitis are Neisseria meningitidis, Streptococcus pneumoniae and Haemophilus influenzae. These organisms are often present in the nasopharynx. It is not known how they enter the bloodstream and the subarachnoid space.
- Twenty to twenty-five thousand cases occur yearly in the United States.
- The mortality rate is less than five per cent, if treated. Residual neurological deficits are rare.

CLINICAL MANIFESTATIONS

- headache
- chills
- fever
- nausea
- vomiting
- back pain
- stiff neck
- generalized seizures
- signs of meningeal irritation also occur:
  — nuchal (neck) rigidity
  — positive Brudzinski's sign (forward neck flexion with the client supine, produces flexion of both thighs at the hips and flexion movements of the ankles and knees)
  — positive Kernig's sign (pain, hamstring muscle spasm and resistance to further leg extension at the knee occurs when the thigh is flexed at a right angle to the abdomen, the knee is flexed 90 degrees to the thigh and then the lower leg is extended)

MEDICAL MANAGEMENT

Bacterial meningitis is a medical emergency. Treatment must be instituted immediately, or death can result in hours or days.

- large doses of the appropriate antibiotic intravenously four to six times daily for ten days (high doses are required to reach the cerebrospinal fluid)
- analgesics for pain (used with caution so as not to mask signs of neurologic deterioration)

NURSING MANAGEMENT

- Monitor fluid and electrolyte imbalance.
- Perform hourly neurological checks to detect early signs of increasing intracranial pressure or seizures.
- Administer antibiotic therapy as prescribed.
- Maintain strict isolation.
- Maintain safety precautions.

FOCUSED DISCHARGE CARE

Instruct client/significant other regarding:
- antibiotic therapy
- use of analgesics
- follow-up care

(For more information, see pp. 360-362 of Polaski and Tatro, *Luckmann's Core Principles and Practice of Medical-Surgical Nursing.*)

Meningitis (Viral)

- Acute viral meningitis (aseptic meningitis) is usually due to mumps virus or one of the picornaviruses.
- Aseptic meningitis involving the subarachnoid space usually resolves within two weeks.
- Clinical manifestations include: drowsiness; photophobia; headache; pain when moving the eyes; neck and spine stiffness with flexion; weakness; rash; fever; and positive Brudzinski's and Kernig's signs (for definitions, see "Meningitis [Bacterial]" p. 442).

- Treatment is symptomatic and involves bedrest and control of fever, headache, pain and seizures.

(For more information, see p. 362 of Polaski and Tatro, *Luckmann's Core Principles and Practice of Medical-Surgical Nursing.*)

Multiple Myeloma

OVERVIEW

- Multiple myeloma is an abnormal proliferation of plasma cells.
- With this overproduction, bone destruction also occurs. In addition, multiple myeloma is characterized by disruption of red blood cell, leukocyte and platelet production, secondary to crowding of the bone marrow by plasma cells.
- Complications of multiple myeloma include hypercalcemia (from release of calcium with bone destruction), renal failure (from particles of coagulated protein that block the tubules) and neurological disorders (secondary to spinal cord compression).
- This condition commonly occurs in clients over 40 years of age. It is more common in men and blacks.

CLINICAL MANIFESTATIONS

Onset is insidious and gradual. Most clients pass through a long presymptomatic period that lasts from 5 to 20 years.
- backache or bone pain that worsens with movement
- presence of pathologic fractures
- hypercalcemia — anorexia, nausea, vomiting, constipation, confusion, abdominal pain
- renal failure
- paresthesia, paralysis

MEDICAL MANAGEMENT

- chemotherapy — melphalan and prednisone or a combination of alkylating agents — cyclophosphamide, carmustine, vincristine

- radiation therapy
- hypercalcemia management

SURGICAL MANAGEMENT

- laminectomy (the excision of a vertebral posterior arch to relieve spinal cord compression)

NURSING MANAGEMENT

MEDICAL

- Administer ordered chemotherapy. See "Chemotherapy", p. 145.
- Assess for signs of hypercalcemia and administer prescribed therapy.
- Encourage fluids to 3 liters/day.
- Monitor intake and output.
- Daily weights.
- Monitor laboratory findings — CBC, BUN, creatinine, serum calcium.
- Administer antiemetics.
- Administer analgesics.
- Institute appropriate safety measures.

SURGICAL

- See "Herniated Intervertebral Disc", p. 323, for care of the laminectomy client.

FOCUSED DISCHARGE CARE

- Instruct client regarding:
  — disease process and treatment regime
  — potential chemotherapy side effects and interventions – see "Chemotherapy", p. 145
  — signs/symptoms of hypercalcemia
  — importance of adequate fluids, low calcium diet
  — household safety measures
  — importance of follow-up visits
- Refer to available community resources.

(For more information, see pp. 862-863 of Polaski and Tatro, *Luckmann's Core Principles and Practice of Medical-Surgical Nursing.*)

Multiple Sclerosis

OVERVIEW

- Multiple sclerosis (MS) is a progressive degenerative disease that affects the myelin sheath of neurons in the central nervous system (CNS).
- The myelin sheath is essential for normal conduction of nerve impulses to and from the brain and spinal cord. In MS, patches of myelin deteriorate at irregular intervals along the nerve axon causing slowing of nerve conduction. Although this may occur anywhere in the central nervous system, the areas most commonly involved are the optic nerves, cerebrum, and cervical spinal cord. The exact cause of MS is unknown.
- Precipitating factors that can precede the onset or an exacerbation of MS include: infection, physical injury, emotional stress, pregnancy, and fatigue.
- MS has two major courses: (1) exacerbating remitting — client has episodes of neurologic dysfunction (exacerbations) from which he or she recovers and is able to function normally (remission), and (2) chronic progressive — client experiences a steady decline in neurologic function that can occur over several years.
- The onset of MS usually occurs between the ages of 20 and 40 years old, and it affects women twice as often as men.
- Life expectancy is about 85 per cent of the general population. The usual cause of death is bacterial infection of the lungs, bladder, or pressure ulcers.

CLINICAL MANIFESTATIONS

- weakness or tingling sensations (paresthesias) of one or more extremities
- vision loss
- loss of coordination
- bowel and bladder dysfunction
- seizures
- fatigue that worsens as the day progresses
- muscle spasticity
- depression

- cognitive and psychosocial problems
- emotional lability

MEDICAL MANAGEMENT

- corticosteroid therapy — adrenocorticotropic hormone, prednisone
- immunosuppressant therapy — Cytoxan
- seizure control — Dilantin
- antidepressant therapy — Elavil
- antispasmodic therapy — Lioresal, Valium, Dantrium

NURSING MANAGEMENT

- Institute measures for neurogenic bladder:
  — maintain fluid intake at 2000 ml/24 hours
  — avoid fluid intake after the evening meal
  — encourage to attempt voiding every three hours
  — intermittent catheterization if indicated.
- Encourage high fiber diet.
- Administer stool softeners as prescribed.
- Institute a bowel training program.
- Assess ability to perform activities of daily living.
- Provide adequate rest periods.
- Plan activities at client's peak energy level (usually in morning).
- Collaborate with physical and occupational therapy for methods to reduce energy consumption and adaptive devices for ambulation and self-care.
- Encourage and promote range of motion and muscle strengthening exercises.
- Determine areas of numbness and intervene to prevent injury and development of pressure ulcers.
- Provide emotional support to client and family.

FOCUSED DISCHARGE CARE

- Instruct client/family regarding:
  — disease process and prognosis
  — avoidance of physical and emotional stressors that may precipitate an exacerbation
  — skin care measures
  — bowel/bladder training regime
  — intermittent catheterization technique
  — importance of adequate rest

— exercise regime
— use of adaptive devices
— importance of follow-up appointments
- Refer to community resources — support groups, respite care, Home Health Care.

(For more information, see pp. 375-378 of Polaski and Tatro, *Luckmann's Core Principles and Practice of Medical-Surgical Nursing.*)

Musculoskeletal Surgical Procedures

OVERVIEW

- Arthroscopy — an endoscopic procedure that allows direct visualization of joint structures. It may be used for diagnosis, removal of torn meniscus, removal of foreign bodies and adhesions, patellar shavings, and biopsy of synovial disorders.
- Arthroplasty — the surgical replacement or reconstruction of a joint to relieve pain, improve or maintain range of motion or correct deformity.
- Osteotomy — a surgical procedure used to realign the bone by removing a wedge from it.
- Tenotomy — cutting of a tendon, used to release contracture related to spasticity.
- Bone grafting — transplanting pieces of cancellous or compact bone to new locations.

POSTOPERATIVE NURSING MANAGEMENT

- Monitor amount of drainage on dressings or casts.
- Elevate the extremity, supporting along the entire length.
- Position, turn and exercise the client as prescribed.
- Reinforce information taught by physical therapy and occupational therapy.
- Reinforce range of motion, resistive and isometric exercises as taught by physical therapy.
- Refer to home health care as necessary.
- Discuss complications to report to physician.
- Discuss follow-up care.

(For more information, see pp. 1285-1287 of Polaski and Tatro, *Luckmann's Core Principles and Practice of Medical-Surgical Nursing.*)

Myasthenia Gravis

OVERVIEW

- Myasthenia gravis (MG) is an autoimmune disease that presents as muscular weakness and fatigue that worsens with exercise and improves with rest.
- Myasthenia gravis is caused by loss of acetylcholine receptors in the post-synaptic neurons of the neuromuscular junction. The cause of myasthenia gravis is unknown.
- Myasthenia gravis may occur at any age, although there are two peaks of onset. In early-onset myasthenia gravis, at age 20 to 30 years, women are more often affected than men. In late-onset, after age 50, men are more often affected.
- The course of myasthenia gravis varies, with remissions and exacerbations. Signs and symptoms may progress quickly or slowly and fluctuate from day to day.

CLINICAL MANIFESTATIONS

- increasing weakness with sustained muscle contraction. (If client is asked to hold arms up, the power of muscle contraction diminishes, and arms drift downward. After a period of rest, the muscles regain their strength.)
- muscle weakness increased at end of day
- ptosis (drooping of upper eyelid)
- diplopia (double vision)
- expressionless face and tendency for mouth to hang open due to weakness of the facial muscles
- dysphagia (muscles of chewing and swallowing in-

volved)
- nasal quality to speech
- respiratory distress (respiratory muscle involvement)

MEDICAL MANAGEMENT

- short-acting anticholinesterase compounds — pyridostigmine (Mestinon), neostigmine (Prostigmin)
- corticosteroids — prednisone (reduces level of serum acetylcholine receptor antibodies)
- plasmapheresis — to remove plasma proteins containing antibodies believed to cause myasthenia gravis

SURGICAL MANAGEMENT

- thymectomy — removal of thymus gland that may alter some immunological control mechanism that affects the production of antibodies to the anticholinesterase receptor

NURSING MANAGEMENT

- Administer anticholinesterase drugs precisely on time to maintain blood levels.
- Ensure suctioning equipment is maintained at bedside and instruct client on self-suctioning.
- Initiate aspiration precautions.
- Plan activities at time of client's highest energy level and allow for rest periods.
- Assess muscle strength before and after activity.
- Observe for myasthenia crisis (an exacerbation of myasthenic symptoms caused by under-medication with anticholinesterase drugs):
    — increased pulse and respirations
    — increased blood pressure
    — severe respiratory distress and cyanosis
    — bowel and bladder incontinence
    — absence of cough and swallow reflex
    — increased secretions, increased lacrimation
    — restlessness.
- Intervene in myasthenia crisis:
    — support respiratory function – suction excess secretions, administer supplemental oxygen and assisted ventilation

       — administer additional anticholinesterase medication if responds to Tensilon treatment.
- Observe for cholinergic crisis (an acute exacerbation of muscle weakness caused by over-medication with anticholinesterase (cholinergic) drugs):
  — nausea, vomiting, diarrhea
  — abdominal cramps
  — blurred vision
  — facial muscle twitching
  — excessive pulmonary secretions
  — weakness with difficulty swallowing, chewing, speaking, and breathing
  — apprehension.
- Intervene in cholinergic crisis:
  — support respiratory function – suction, administer supplemental oxygen and assisted ventilation
  — hold cholinergic drugs until cholinergic effects decrease.
- Collaborate with physical and occupational therapy for exercises and adaptive devices.

FOCUSED DISCHARGE CARE

- Instruct the client regarding:
  — disease process and prognosis
  — importance of medication regime
    - timing of doses is critical to maintain a chemical balance at the neuromuscular junction
    - no omission of doses.
  — importance of available suctioning equipment in the home
  — self-suctioning technique or teaching household members suctioning technique
  — symptoms of myasthenia crisis and cholinergic crisis and crisis intervention
  — factors that may predispose client to an exacerbation — infection, emotional stress, surgery, physical stress
  — need for adequate rest periods
  — use of adaptive devices and exercises
  — importance of wearing medical alert identification
  — importance of follow-up appointments
- Refer to available community resources.

(For more information, see pp. 379-382 of Polaski and Tatro, *Luckmann's Core Principles and Practice of Medical-Surgical Nursing.*)

Myocarditis

OVERVIEW

- Myocarditis is an inflammation of the myocardial wall.
- Myocardial damage from acute myocarditis typically results from the direct invasion by or the toxic effects of the microorganism in cardiac myocytes.
- It can be caused by almost any bacterial, viral, or parasitic organism, as well as radiation, toxic agents, and certain drugs.
- Myocarditis affects clients of all ages and may be acute or chronic.
- In most cases, myocarditis is self-limiting and uncomplicated.

CLINICAL MANIFESTATIONS

- may be asymptomatic
- fatigue, dyspnea, palpitations
- chest pain experienced as a mild continuous pressure distinguishable from effort-induced angina
- fever
- dysrhythmias

MEDICAL MANAGEMENT

- specific therapy for underlying infection
- bedrest to decrease cardiac workload
- supplemental oxygen
- dysrhythmia management

NURSING MANAGEMENT

- Assess for changes in cardiac or respiratory status.
- Treat fever with rest, cooling measures, forced flu-

ids, and anti-pyretics.
- Administer antimicrobial therapy as prescribed.
- Encourage fluids and a well balanced diet.
- Administer PRN analgesics.
- Provide adequate rest periods.
- Implement progressive activity schedule.

FOCUSED DISCHARGE CARE

Instruct client regarding:
- disease process and treatment regimen
- need to monitor pulse rate and rhythm and report any sudden changes
- need to continue self-monitoring after the infectious process resolves
- need to keep all follow-up appointments
- avoidance of exposure to risks

(For more information, see pp. 741-742 of Polaski and Tatro, *Luckmann's Core Principles and Practice of Medical-Surgical Nursing.*)

Nasal Fracture

OVERVIEW

- Simple nasal fractures may be reduced in an emergency facility. For more extensive fractures, surgery may be performed under local anesthesia with mild sedation.
- Intranasal packing, internal or external splints, and an external dressing may be applied

NURSING MANAGEMENT

- See "Nasal Septoplasty", p. 454.

(For more information, see p. 562 of Polaski and Tatro, *Luckmann's Core Principles and Practice of Medical-Surgical Nursing.*)

Nasal Septoplasty

OVERVIEW

- Nasal septoplasty is performed for a deviated nasal septum when the deviation is causing obstruction to nasal breathing, dryness of the nasal mucosa causing bleeding, or a cosmetic deformity. An incision is made on either side of the septum; the mucous membrane is elevated, and the offending portion of cartilage is straightened or removed. A local anesthetic with mild sedation commonly is used.
- Intranasal packing and internal splints may be used to control bleeding and prevent hematoma formation.

NURSING MANAGEMENT

In addition to routine postoperative care:
- Maintain patent airway.
- Assess for edema and hemorrhage.
- Provide analgesics as prescribed and assess for adequate pain relief.

(For more information, see p. 562 of Polaski and Tatro, *Luckmann's Core Principles and Practice of Medical-Surgical Nursing.*)

Near Drowning Accidents

OVERVIEW

- Near-drowning or immersion syndrome is a diagnosis given to clients who initially survive suffocation after submersion in water or a fluid medium.
- Fresh water drowning is more common than salt water drowning.
- Common risk factors for near drowning include alcohol or drug ingestion, overestimation of swimming skills, hypothermia, hyperventilation and hypoglycemia.
- Fresh water and salt water wash out alveolar surfactant. Fresh water also changes the surface tension of surfactant. The loss of surfactant leads to alveolar collapse, intrapulmonary shunting and hypoxemia. Poor perfusion and hypoxemia result in acidosis and eventual pulmonary edema. Alterations in fluid-electrolyte balance often are seen.

NURSING MANAGEMENT

- Obtain a history of the submersion. Include the length of submersion, temperature of the water, type of water and any associated injuries (such as spinal cord injuries).
- Maintain airway, breathing and circulation (ABC's).

- Assess for any signs of hypoxia (confusion, irritability, lethargy or unconsciousness).
- Assist with intubation and ventilate with 100% oxygen and 5 to 10 cm of positive end-expiratory pressure (PEEP) to prevent the alveoli from collapsing.
- Remove wet clothing and wrap in a warm blanket.
- Rewarm the client slowly.
- Correct acid-base or electrolyte abnormalities as prescribed.
- Monitor diagnostic studies.
- Observe client for at least 24 hours for any complications, especially pulmonary edema.

(For more information, see pp. 1572-1573 of Polaski and Tatro, *Luckmann's Core Principles and Practice of Medical-Surgical Nursing.*)

Nephrotic Syndrome

OVERVIEW

- Nephrotic syndrome is a set of clinical symptoms arising from protein-wasting secondary to diffuse glomerular damage. The glomerular basement membrane becomes abnormally permeable to protein molecules, particularly albumin. Proteins are excessively filtered into the tubules and excreted into the urine.
- The causes of nephrotic syndrome are numerous; the most common is glomerulonephritis.
- Predisposing factors include allergic reaction; medication and drug reactions; renal vein thrombosis; sickle cell disease; and congestive heart failure.

CLINICAL MANIFESTATIONS

- proteinuria, hypoalbuminemia, and edema
- waxy pallor of the skin
- anorexia, malaise, irritability
- anemia

MEDICAL MANAGEMENT

- steroids, loop diuretics, and plasma volume expanders
- cytotoxic agents, indomethacin, and antiplatelet agents
- long-term anticoagulant therapy to prevent renal vein thrombosis.
- diet of adequate carbohydrate and adequate calories with a mild sodium restriction, and protein intake 1 to 15 g/kg daily
- fluid restriction if client is hyponatremic

NURSING MANAGEMENT

- Assess for signs/symptoms of complications:
  — renal failure
  — hypovolemia
  — thromboembolism
  — abnormal thyroid function
  — increased susceptibility to infections
- Discuss ways to reduce edema and prevent skin breakdown.
- Assess for signs/symptoms of electrolyte imbalance from diuresis.
- Strict intake and output.
- Daily weights.
- Measure edematous areas daily.

FOCUSED DISCHARGE CARE

- Instruct the client regarding:
  — long-term anticoagulant therapy and safety precautions
  — need for meticulous skin care
  — dietary restrictions
  — activity restrictions
- Discuss with the client/significant other coping with long-term illness; make referrals as needed.

(For more information, see pp. 956-957 of Polaski and Tatro, *Luckmann's Core Principles and Practice of Medical-Surgical Nursing.*)

Neurogenic Bladder Dysfunction

OVERVIEW

- There are 5 major types of neurogenic bladder dysfunction:
    - Uninhibited — the urge to void causes urine excretion.
    - Sensory Paralytic — the client cannot perceive bladder fullness which leads to retention with overflow incontinence.
    - Motor Paralytic — the client perceives the bladder filling but is unable to initiate micturition.
    - Autonomous — the client cannot perceive bladder fullness nor initiate or maintain urination without "assistance".
    - Reflex — the client has no sensation and the bladder contracts reflexively but does not empty completely.
- All types are caused by central or peripheral nervous system lesions.

CLINICAL MANIFESTATIONS

- urine retention or incontinence depending upon the type of dysfunction

MEDICAL MANAGEMENT

- bladder training is attempted with or without intermittent catheterization or pharmacologic therapy

SURGICAL MANAGEMENT

- external sphincterotomy (incision of the bladder neck) to restore normal emptying.
- for uninhibited bladder dysfunction, injection of alcohol into the subarachnoid space or cutting of the sacral nerves may inhibit reflex bladder contractions. Electrodes implanted in the epidural space also serve this purpose.

NURSING MANAGEMENT

- Instruct the client/significant other regarding:
  - methods to apply external pressure on the abdomen to help control the detrusor muscle
  - the Credé maneuver
  - methods to stimulate trigger points on lower abdomen, inner thighs, and pubic area to initiate micturition (i.e., stroking, pinching, applying ice)
  - intermittent self catheterization
  - amounts of fluid to drink.
- Monitor and instruct patient/significant other on signs and symptoms of autonomic dysreflexia, which can occur from bladder distention. This is a medical emergency and must be treated immediately. (See "Spinal Cord Injury", p. 586.)

FOCUSED DISCHARGE CARE

- Determine client's ability to function in the home setting and significant others available for assistance.
- Include significant others in all teaching.
- Assess need for home health care follow-up.
- Instruct the client/significant other regarding:
  - signs/symptoms of urinary tract infection and to report to physician
  - self catheterization technique
  - bladder training program

(For more information, see pp. 940-943 of Polaski and Tatro, *Luckmann's Core Principles and Practice of Medical-Surgical Nursing.*)

Non-Hodgkin's Lymphoma

OVERVIEW

- Non-Hodgkin's disease is a lymphoma that results in uncontrolled proliferation of lymphocytes.

- Involvement of the disease generally starts in the lymph nodes and progresses to extralymphatic sites.
- Lymphomas are classified as either (1) Hodgkin's - contains Reed-Sternberg cell or (2) non-Hodgkin's - without the Reed-Sternberg cell.
- There are many classification systems used to differentiate non-Hodgkin's lymphoma based on histology and cytologic characteristics.
- Overall, the prognosis of non-Hodgkin's lymphoma is poorer than that of Hodgkin's disease.
- Non-Hodgkin's lymphoma is more common in adults in their middle and older years, and is more common in males than females.

CLINICAL MANIFESTATIONS

- painless, enlarged lymph nodes
- fevers and night sweats
- weight loss
- hepatosplenomegaly
- nonproductive cough, dyspnea (mediastinal involvement)
- edema of the face, neck, right arm (superior vena cava syndrome secondary to compression by enlarged lymph nodes)
- jaundice (bile duct obstruction)
- renal failure (ureteral obstruction)
- progressive anemia with fatigue and malaise

MEDICAL MANAGEMENT

- chemotherapy
- radiation therapy

SURGICAL MANAGEMENT

- tumor debulking prior to radiation or chemotherapy

NURSING MANAGEMENT

- Administer prescribed chemotherapy.
- See "Chemotherapy", p. 145.
- See "Radiation Therapy", p. 543.
- Monitor laboratory findings — CBC, platelet count, renal profile.

- Encourage balanced diet.
- Encourage rest.

FOCUSED DISCHARGE CARE

- Instruct client regarding:
  — disease process and treatment regime
  — see "Chemotherapy", p. 145
  — see "Radiation Therapy", p. 543
  — signs/symptoms to report to physician
  — importance of follow-up visits
- Refer to available community resources (cancer support groups).

(For more information, see pp. 864-865 of Polaski and Tatro, *Luckmann's Core Principles and Practice of Medical-Surgical Nursing.*)

Obesity

OVERVIEW

- Obesity is weight 20 percent or greater than the desirable weight for adults of a given sex and height.
- It is caused by a caloric intake that exceeds energy expenditure.
- Complications include: atherosclerosis, ischemic heart disease, hypertension and diabetes mellitus.

CLINICAL MANIFESTATIONS

- weight as defined above

MEDICAL MANAGEMENT

- caloric restriction with an exercise program
- use of support groups (TOPS, Overeaters Anonymous, Weight Watchers) for appetite re-education in which the client learns to eat and be satisfied with nutritious, well-balanced foods that are low in calories

SURGICAL MANAGEMENT

- jaw wiring to reduce food intake
- gastric stapling (gastroplasty)—involves stapling the top part of the stomach. A small opening in the line of staples allows food to enter the rest of the stomach slowly. The client can eat only about 30 ml of food every 5 minutes.

NURSING MANAGEMENT

MEDICAL

- Instruct on healthy diet with correct portion size.
- Assist to develop a regular exercise program.

- Assist to develop other ways to deal with stress, boredom and anxiety.
- Obtain weights at regular intervals.
- Assist to develop improved self esteem.

FOCUSED DISCHARGE CARE

- Instruct client regarding:
  — reinforcement of nutritional plan and exercise program
- Refer to support groups (TOPS, Overeaters Anonymous, Weight Watchers).

(For more information, see pp. 1036-1037 of Polaski and Tatro, *Luckmann's Core Principles and Practice of Medical-Surgical Nursing*.)

Osteoarthritis

- Osteoarthritis (OA) is a noninflammatory joint disease characterized by a degeneration and loss of articular cartilage in synovial joints.
- OA was previously called degenerative joint disease (DJD), but the term DJD is generally considered inaccurate because there is no biochemical or metabolic degeneration.
- OA is classified as:
  — Primary (idiopathic)
    — associated with aging
    — most common type existing in about 60 million people in the United States. It occurs in about 50 per cent of the people by the age of 16 years.
    — weight bearing joints are the most commonly affected
  — Secondary
    — caused by conditions that lead to damage to joint surfaces (repetitive strain and sprains, joint dislocation, etc)
- The pathophysiology of OA is loss of articular cartilage due to enzymatic destruction. Layers of the cartilage loosen and eventually the subchronal bone becomes unprotected and dense.

CLINICAL MANIFESTATIONS

- aching pain
- crepitation
- stiffness
- enlarged joints
- contractures
- muscle spasms

MEDICAL MANAGEMENT

- pain management — nonsteroidal anti-inflammatory agents, steroid injections (for acute pain into a single joint), heat therapy, skin traction or cervical collars may be used for OA of the vertebrae.
- weight reduction
- daily exercise regime

SURGICAL MANAGEMENT

- osteotomy — removal of a section of bone to realign a joint
- total hip and knee replacements

NURSING MANAGEMENT

MEDICAL

- Administer anti-inflammatory and pain medications as ordered.
- Apply ice/heat therapy as ordered
- Consult physical/occupational therapy for assistive devices
- Encourage activity — self-care, ambulation, etc.

(For more information, see p. 230 of Polaski and Tatro, *Luckmann's Core Principles and Practice of Medical-Surgical Nursing.*)

Osteomalacia

OVERVIEW

- Osteomalacia is a disease in which the bone becomes abnormally soft because of a disturbed calcium and phosphorus balance secondary to a vitamin D deficiency, which results in marked deformities of the weight-bearing bones and pathologic fractures.
- Osteomalacia occurs mainly in the spine, pelvis and lower extremities.
- Osteomalacia is similar to rickets, which occurs in children; therefore, the condition is called adult rickets.
- Osteomalacia mainly affects women.
- Risk factors include:
  — hypoparathyroidism
  — renal tubular disorders
  — hepatobiliary disease
  — small intestine disease
  — use of long-term anticonvulsants, tranquilizers, sedatives and muscle relaxants

CLINICAL MANIFESTATIONS

- scoliotic or kyphotic deformities of the spine
- bone pain
- muscle cramps
- bowing and bending deformities of the long bones
- decreased serum calcium and phosphorus

MEDICAL MANAGEMENT

- vitamin D replacement
- supplemental calcium
- pain management
- dietary modifications — high calcium, high phosphorus
- management of fractures, if present

SURGICAL MANAGEMENT

- repair of fractures

NURSING MANAGEMENT

- Administer vitamin and mineral supplements as prescribed.
- Administer analgesics.
- Consult physical therapy for adaptive devices for ambulation or activities of daily living and strengthening exercises.
- Monitor laboratory findings — calcium and phosphorus levels.
- Encourage diet high in calcium and phosphorus.

FOCUSED DISCHARGE CARE

Instruct client regarding:
- disease process and treatment regime
- use of adaptive devices
- use of PRN analgesics
- dietary modifications — high calcium, high phosphorus

(For more information, see pp. 1297-1298 of Polaski and Tatro, *Luckmann's Core Principles and Practice of Medical-Surgical Nursing.*)

Osteomyelitis

OVERVIEW

- Osteomyelitis is a term used to describe any infection of the bone. Acute osteomyelitis responds to a four to six week course of intravenous antibiotics, whereas chronic osteomyelitis persists longer than four weeks and involves sequestered (necrotic bone that has separated from living tissue) areas of infection.
- Osteomyelitis is generally bacterial in origin, but may also be caused by viral or fungal infections. Staphylococcus aureus is the most common organism, but Escherichia coli, Klebsiella, Proteus, Pseudomonas and Salmonella may also cause osteomyelitis. These organisms may be directly

introduced into the bone, may be spread from adjacent soft tissue infection or travel through the blood to the site. The bacteria are able to multiply readily in bone because bone has a slow circulatory system.
- Early diagnosis is important to prevent progression of the infection.

CLINICAL MANIFESTATIONS

- fever (usually above 101° F. (38° C.))
- localized pain or tenderness
- erythema (redness)
- heat and swelling around the infected bone
- elevated WBC and ESR (erythrocyte sedimentation rate)
- positive blood cultures

MEDICAL MANAGEMENT

- needle aspiration (to relieve pressure within the bone)
- antibiotic therapy for four to six weeks

SURGICAL MANAGEMENT

Chronic Osteomyelitis
- sequestrectomy (removal of the dead bone) and cauterization (removal of scar tissue, infected tissue, sequestra and necrotic bone, leaving a saucer-like depression)
    — surgery is followed by a four to six week course of IV antibiotics, followed by a course of oral antibiotics

NURSING MANAGEMENT

MEDICAL

- Administer antibiotics as prescribed.
- Monitor temperature and administer PRN antipyretics.
- Administer PRN analgesics and anti-inflammatory agents and assess effectiveness.
- Provide wound care as indicated.
- Encourage progressive exercise/ambulation program.

- Monitor laboratory findings — WBC, ESR, blood culture reports.

POSTOPERATIVE CARE

In addition to routine postoperative care:
- Administer antibiotics as prescribed.

FOCUSED DISCHARGE CARE

Because of the extended IV antibiotic regime for both acute and chronic osteomyelitis, the client is often sent home with IV access in place and a referral made to a home health care agency to complete antibiotic therapy.

Instruct client regarding:
- disease process and need for long-term antibiotic therapy
- care of IV access catheter and site
- wound/incision care
- signs/symptoms to report (fever, increased wound drainage, increased pain)
- use of PRN analgesics
- importance of follow-up appointments

(For more information, see pp. 1298-1299 of Polaski and Tatro, *Luckmann's Core Principles and Practice of Medical-Surgical Nursing*.)

Osteoporosis

OVERVIEW

- Osteoporosis is a common age-related metabolic bone disease in which there is a severe general reduction in the skeletal bone mass and an increased susceptibility to fractures, especially in the wrist, hip and vertebral column. Bone resorption occurs faster than bone formation.

- The exact pathophysiology of the development of osteoporosis is unknown.
- Osteoporosis can be classified as:
  — primary — not associated with an underlying medical condition
  — secondary — results from an associated condition such as hyperparathyroidism, long-term corticosteroid or heparin administration
- In the United States alone, osteoporosis affects 25 million individuals and is responsible for 1.3 million fractures each year. One-third of American women over age fifty will eventually have a compression or vertebral fracture of the spine related to osteoporosis.
- Risk factors include:
  — female gender — bone loss related to menopause is considered to be the most important reason for this difference. In postmenopausal women, estrogen production and bone calcium storage decrease. Estrogen appears to protect against bone loss.
  — northern European descent
  — petite, thin women with sedentary lifestyles
  — small-framed thin men
  — inadequate dietary intake of calcium
  — lactose intolerance
  — Vitamin D deficiency
  — bedridden status
  — use of antacids
  — use of laxatives
  — Cushing's disease
  — heavy cigarette smoking
  — heavy caffeine intake

CLINICAL MANIFESTATIONS

Osteoporosis often is not diagnosed until the client presents with a fracture.
- shortened stature
- difficulty bending over
- marked kyphosis of the thoracic spine (dowager hump)
- impaired breathing (due to deformities of the spine and rib cage)
- back pain
- pain at the site of fracture

MEDICAL MANAGEMENT

- management of fractures, if present
- vitamin D therapy
- calcium supplements
- calcitonin therapy — inhibits bone loss
- estrogen or estrogen combined with progesterone
- sodium fluoride given with calcium and vitamin D to stimulate bone growth
- brace for vertebral fracture
- pain management
- dietary modification — high calcium

SURGICAL MANAGEMENT

- repair of fractures

NURSING MANAGEMENT

- Administer vitamin D and calcium supplements, calcitonin and estrogen therapy as prescribed.
  - Administer calcium supplements one hour after meals and at bedtime.
  - Common side effects include constipation, gastric distention, flatulence, hypercalcemia and hypophosphatemia.
- Administer analgesics as prescribed.
- Consult with physical therapy for muscle strengthening exercises and adaptive devices for ambulation and activities of daily living.
- Encourage high calcium diet.
- Institute appropriate safety measures.
- Monitor laboratory findings — calcium and phosphorus levels.

FOCUSED DISCHARGE CARE

Instruct client regarding:
- disease process and treatment regime
- dietary modifications — high calcium, avoidance of beverages with caffeine
- limiting alcohol intake and avoidance of smoking
- importance of weight-bearing exercises (walking, tennis, stair climbing) to increase bone mass
- use of PRN analgesics

- use of adaptive devices and muscle strengthening exercises
- safety measures in the home environment

(For more information, see pp. 1292-1295 of Polaski and Tatro, *Luckmann's Core Principles and Practice of Medical-Surgical Nursing.*)

Otitis Media

- Otitis media is infection of the middle ear. It may be acute (sudden in onset and short in duration) or chronic (repeated infections usually associated with drainage). Repeated infections can cause perforation and hearing loss.
- Serous otitis media is fluid in the middle ear and may be found in conjunction with upper respiratory infections or allergies.
- The treatment for otitis media is antibiotic therapy.
- A surgical procedure called a myringotomy may be performed for recurrent otitis media. An incision is made into the tympanic membrane through which fluid is removed and a transtympanic tube inserted. This tube normally extrudes by itself in three to twelve months.
- The nurse instructs the client to:
  — obtain prompt treatment for allergic or upper respiratory infections
  — avoid getting water in the ear (by using cotton balls)
  — seek medical attention for decreased hearing, pain in the ear or drainage from the ear.
- Following surgery, the nurse instructs the client to:
  — blow the nose gently, one side at a time
  — sneeze or cough with mouth open for one week after surgery
  — avoid physical activity for one week and exercises or sports for three weeks after surgery
  — avoid heavy lifting
  — keep ear dry for four to six weeks after surgery
  — not shampoo for one week after surgery

— protect ear when necessary with two pieces of cotton (outer piece saturated with petroleum jelly)
— avoid airplane flights for the first week after surgery
— report any drainage other than slight bleeding

(For more information, see pp. 463-464 of Polaski and Tatro, *Luckmann's Core Principles and Practice of Medical-Surgical Nursing.*)

Ovarian Cancer

OVERVIEW

- Ovarian cancer is the leading cause of death from reproductive malignancies.
- The exact etiology is unknown, although there does appear to be a familial association.
- Risk factors include: family history, age over 40 years, multiparity, infertility, history of heavy menstrual bleeding, dysmenorrhea and possibly obesity with a diet high in animal fat.
- Ovarian cancer tends to grow and spread silently without symptoms until pressure is placed on other organs or metastasis occurs. Because it is so difficult to detect, early diagnosis generally is not made and thus, the long-term survival rate is poor.

CLINICAL MANIFESTATIONS

- abdominal distention
- urinary frequency and urgency
- pleural effusion
- malnutrition
- pain from pressure of the growing tumor
- constipation
- ascites
- urinary or bowel obstruction

MEDICAL MANAGEMENT

- irradiation or chemotherapy following surgery for ovarian cancer

SURGICAL MANAGEMENT

- total abdominal hysterectomy with bilateral salpingo-oophorectomy (TAH-BSO), omentectomy and removal of all visible tumor is the surgery of choice

NURSING MANAGEMENT

See sections on "Chemotherapy", p. 145, "Radiation Therapy", p. 543, and "Uterine Tumors, Benign", p. 646 (for care following TAH-BSO).

(For more information, see p. 1491 of Polaski and Tatro, *Luckmann's Core Principles and Practice of Medical-Surgical Nursing.*)

Pacemakers

OVERVIEW

- A pacemaker is a device that delivers electrical stimuli to the heart through electrodes that have been implanted in the heart muscle. A pacemaker initiates the heart beat when the heart's intrinsic conduction system fails or is unreliable.

- Problems with the conduction system develop when (1) the SA node is damaged and unable to promote a reliable rhythm, (2) impulses from the SA node and atria are not transmitted through the AV junction to the ventricles, or (3) dysrhythmias from ectopic foci are present.

- Pacemakers consist of a pulse generator (the pacemaker's power source) responsible for sending out appropriately timed signals, and a lead-electrode system (the sensory circuit) responsible for identifying and analyzing intrinsic activity and responding appropriately. The lead delivers the electrical impulse from the pulse generator to the myocardium. The lead is a flexible conductive wire encased by insulating material. The electrode is at the end of the lead and delivers the impulse directly to the myocardium. Not only does this system deliver electrical impulses, but it relays information about spontaneous intracardiac signals back to the sensing circuit in the pulse generator.

- Pacemakers are classified according to a five-letter code: the first letter denotes the cardiac chamber to be paced (the atrium [A], the ventricle [V], or both [dual] chambers [D]); the second letter denotes the chamber to be sensed (the atrium [A], the ventricle [V], dual [D] or none [O]; the third letter, the type of response, that is, sensed intrinsic activity will cause the pacemaker's impulse to be "triggered" [T] (to pace) or "inhibited" [I] (not to pace) or both [D]. For example, a VVI pacemaker paces in the ventricle, senses in the ventricle and will inhibit pacing if the client's intrinsic rhythm is sensed. Letter four, rate adaptiveness and programmability, and letter five, antitachydysrhythmic functions are infrequently seen in practice.

- The ECG of a paced rhythm appears different from that of a normal sinus rhythm. A pacing artifact is seen. With atrial pacing, a P wave follows the artifact. The QRS complex appears normal with atrial pacing; the impulse travels through usual conduction systems. The ECG with ventricular pacing shows an abnormal QRS because the impulse begins in the ventricle.

- Pacing modes:
  (1) Asynchronous (fixed rate) Pacing
    — Pacing mode delivers an electrical impulse to the heart at a preset fixed rate regardless of intrinsic cardiac activity.
    — There is no sensory mechanism; the pacing mechanism ignores the client's intrinsic rhythm.
    — Major disadvantages:
      — potential tachycardia when both the pacemaker and SA node fire.
      — atrial and ventricular synchrony do not occur.
      — risk that a ventricular pacemaker stimulus may occur during the vulnerable period producing ventricular tachycardia or ventricular fibrillation.
      — the heart is not allowed to vary its rate to accommodate changes in client's activity level.
  (2) Noncompetitive (demand) Pacing
    — Pacemaker fires only on demand or when needed to stimulate atrial or ventricular contraction.
    — If intrinsic beats are sensed, the pacemaker is inhibited. If a spontaneous P wave or QRS does not occur, the pacemaker discharges at a preset delay interval to either the atria (atrial demand pacing) or ventricle (ventricular demand pacing).
  (3) Synchronous Pacing

- The sensing electrode is placed in the atrium and the pacing electrode in the ventricle. Thus, the pacemaker unit senses atrial activity and elicits a stimulus to prompt ventricular depolarization.
- Allows the heart rate to vary, and atrial-ventricular synchrony occurs.
- A built-in safety mechanism causes ventricular depolarizations to occur at a fixed rate should atrial rates become too fast.

(4) Atrioventricular Sequential Pacing
- The ventricle is sensed and the atria paced. If the ventricle does not depolarize after a preset interval, it is also paced. If the ventricle depolarizes on its own, ventricular output through the pacemaker is inhibited.
- The atria is paced regardless of its own intrinsic activity; therefore, competition may occur, leading to atrial fibrillation.

(5) Universal Atrioventricular Pacing
- Pacemakers consist of both atrial and ventricular circuits that sense and pace their respective chambers. If spontaneous atrial activity does not occur, the atrium is paced. Any sensed atrial activity inhibits pacing function. If ventricular depolarization does not occur in the preset time interval, the ventricle is paced.
- The advantage of this mode is that it more closely mimics the normal heart. Atrial-ventricular synchrony is maintained, and the heart rate can change to meet metabolic demands.

- Methods of pacing:
  - Temporary Pacing:
    - used in short term pacing
    - the pulse generator is external
    - pacing electrodes are inserted via the transvenous route (antecubital, femoral, jugular, or subclavian veins) and threaded into the right atrium or right ventricle.
  - Permanent Pacing:
    - indicated in long-term management of symptomatic or life-threatening dysrhythmias
    - pacing electrode is inserted either via transvenous route or by direct application to the epicardial surface during thoracotomy

— the pulse generator is implanted in the subcutaneous tissue below the clavicle

NURSING MANAGEMENT (POST PERMANENT PACEMAKER PLACEMENT)

Temporary Pacemaker Placement

- Monitor cardiac rhythm continuously.
- Secure connections.
- Monitor control settings.
- Perform dressing changes according to institutional policy.
- Protect client from electromicroshocks:
  - cover exposed wires with rubber gloves or electrical tape
  - enclose pulse generator in a rubber glove to keep dry
  - assure electrical equipment is grounded
- Monitor pacemaker function. The location and type of pacing lead is documented.
- Assess for potential complications:
  - phlebitis at the site
  - pneumothorax
  - atelectasis
  - diaphragmatic stimulation (seen as hiccupping or twitching at the the pacemaker site)

Permanent Pacemaker Placement

- Monitor client's cardiac rhythm continuously.
- Instruct client to avoid excessive extension or abduction of the arm on the operative side.
- Assess for possible complications: wound infection, phlebitis at the insertion site, pneumothorax, atelectasis, pericardial fluid accumulation, diaphragmatic stimulation (seen as twitching at the pacemaker site or hiccupping) and dysrhythmias.
- Evaluate rhythm strip for possible signs of pacemaker malfunction:
  - failure to pace properly — intermittent absence of pacing artifact or rapid, inappropriate firing
  - failure to capture — pacing artifact present but not followed by a QRS complex or P wave
  - failure to sense:

— pacing artifact present despite presence of QRS complexes and P waves

— oversensing — pacemaker senses electrical activity within the myocardium that should be ignored

— symptoms of pacemaker malfunction include syncope, bradycardia or tachycardia, and palpitations.

- Monitor activity tolerance.

FOCUSED DISCHARGE CARE

Instruct the client regarding:
- wound care — assess wound daily; report signs of inflammation. Avoid constrictive clothing that puts excessive pressure on wound and generator.
- importance of taking pulse daily and to notify physician if pulse slower than set rate
- when to seek medical attention — if experiencing palpitations, vertigo, or syncope
- avoidance of areas with high voltage, magnetic force fields, or radiation:
  — large running motors
  — power plants
  — arc welding machines
  — microwave ovens (maintain 5 feet distance)
- need to inform airport security of pacemaker. Metal detectors may be triggered by the pacemaker's metal casing but the detector itself will not harm the pacemaker.
- importance of carrying identification card
- avoidance of activity that can cause blunt trauma to the pulse generator
- avoidance of vigorous movement of the arms and shoulders and lifting weights greater than 5 to 10 pounds for first 6 weeks
- importance of regular physician visits
- need for regular telephone monitoring of the client's electrocardiogram
- indications of battery depletion — pulse rate below set rate, syncope, shortness of breath

(For more information, see pp. 723-728 of Polaski and Tatro, *Luckmann's Core Principles and Practice of Medical-Surgical Nursing.*)

Paget's Disease

OVERVIEW

- Paget's disease is defined as a disorder of bone architecture characterized by an initial phase of increased rate of bone tissue breakdown by osteoclasts, followed by excessive abnormal bone formation by osteoblasts. The diseased bone is structurally weak and prone to fracture. Paget's disease most frequently affects the femur, tibia, lower spine, pelvis and cranium.
- The exact cause of Paget's disease is unknown.

CLINICAL MANIFESTATIONS

- may be asymptomatic
- bone pain
- skeletal deformity (barrel-shaped chest, bowing of the tibia/femur or kyphosis)
- changes in skin temperature (warm and flushed)
- pathologic fractures
- cranial nerve compression (vertigo, hearing loss, blindness)
- cranial changes — skull is soft, thick and enlarged

MEDICAL MANAGEMENT

- pain management—aspirin, indomethacin, ibuprofen
- management of fractures
- calcitonin administration — decreases bone resorption
- mithramycin administration—decreases serum calcium

SURGICAL MANAGEMENT

- repair of fractures

NURSING MANAGEMENT

- Administer prescribed medications.
- Administer PRN analgesics.

- Consult physical therapy for adaptive devices for ambulation and activities of daily living.
- Institute safety measures.

FOCUSED DISCHARGE CARE

Instruct client regarding:
- disease process and treatment regime
- use of PRN analgesics
- use of adaptive devices
- safety measures
- signs/symptoms of hypo- or hypercalcemia

(For more information, see pp. 1295-1297 of Polaski and Tatro, *Luckmann's Core Principles and Practice of Medical-Surgical Nursing.*)

Pancreatic Cancer

OVERVIEW

- Pancreatic cancer is the fifth most common cause of cancer death. Ninety per cent of pancreatic cancer clients die within the first year after diagnosis.
- Pancreatic cancer appears to be linked to diabetes mellitus, alcohol use, history of previous pancreatitis and the ingestion of a high fat diet.

CLINICAL MANIFESTATIONS

- jaundice
- weight loss
- abdominal pain

MEDICAL MANAGEMENT

- palliative based on symptoms:
  — analgesics
  — nutritional supplements

SURGICAL MANAGEMENT

- pancreatic resection — removal of tumor-involved area of the pancreas
- palliative — to remove obstruction

NURSING MANAGEMENT

MEDICAL

- Administer analgesics and assess effectiveness.
- Encourage a well-balanced diet.

SURGICAL—PANCREATIC RESECTION

POSTOPERATIVE CARE

In addition to routine postoperative care:
- Monitor proper functioning and output of drains.
- Monitor for hyperglycemia.
- Administer pancreatic enzyme replacement therapy (Pancrease) when taking food by mouth.

FOCUSED DISCHARGE CARE

- Instruct client regarding:
  — if postoperative:
    — wound care
    — signs/symptoms of infection
    — pancreatic enzyme replacement therapy
    — insulin therapy
- Refer to available community resources (home health care, hospice).

(For more information, see p. 1155 of Polaski and Tatro, *Luckmann's Core Principles and Practice of Medical-Surgical Nursing.*)

Pancreatitis, Acute

OVERVIEW

- Acute pancreatitis is an inflammation of the pancreas that may result in autodigestion of the pancreas by its own enzymes.
- The precise mechanism causing pancreatic damage is unclear. The pathologic changes may be due to premature activation of proteolytic and lipolytic pancreatic enzymes (these enzymes are normally activated in the duodenum). This causes tissue damage in the pancreas. Exactly how the enzymes are activated is unknown, but they may be triggered by reflux of bile from the duodenum into the pancreatic duct or by pancreatic duct obstruction. The net effect is autodigestion of the pancreas.
- In 90 per cent of the cases of acute pancreatitis, the cause is related to excessive alcohol intake or biliary tract disease.
- Acute pancreatitis is a fairly common, but potentially lethal inflammatory process that results in varying degrees of pancreatic edema, fat necrosis, and hemorrhage. Typically, the manifestations disappear once the causative factors are eliminated. Nine out of ten clients experience the disease with mild or moderate symptoms and improve with supportive care.

CLINICAL MANIFESTATIONS

- abdominal pain — begins in mid-epigastrium and reaches maximal intensity several hours into the illness and may radiate to the back
- nausea and vomiting
- fever
- tachycardia
- epigastric tenderness, abdominal distention
- jaundice
- hypotension, hypovolemia, hypoperfusion
- hyperglycemia (as a result of damage to the islets)
- hypocalcemia
- elevated white blood count
- elevated serum amylase and lipase levels

MEDICAL MANAGEMENT

- parenteral fluid and electrolyte replacement
- pancreatic enzymes
- antacids — to neutralize gastric secretions
- nasogastric tube placement to suppress pancreatic stimulation
- histamine hydrogen-receptor blocking drugs
- anticholinergics
- narcotic analgesics — meperidine (morphine is contraindicated because it may cause spasm of the sphincter of Oddi, which could potentiate pancreatic injury)
- NPO status initially with total parenteral nutrition (hyperalimentation) and lipid administration

SURGICAL MANAGEMENT

- pancreatic excision
- correction of associated biliary tract disease

NURSING MANAGEMENT

- Maintain NG tube and NPO status.
- Monitor intake and output.
- Administer PRN analgesics and assess effectiveness.
- Administer antacids, anticholinergics and histamine hydrogen-receptor blocking agents as prescribed.
- Monitor pulse, blood pressure, and hemodynamic parameters for fluid volume changes.
- Monitor heart rhythm for dysrhythmias secondary to electrolyte imbalance.
- Monitor laboratory values — electrolytes, blood sugars, arterial blood gases.
- Encourage prophylactic pulmonary hygiene measures.
- Daily weights.
- Monitor response to oral intake when taking liquids (if oral intake is resumed too soon, re-exacerbation of symptoms may occur).
- Administer pancreatic enzymes (if pancreas severely damaged) as prescribed to replace enzyme deficit and aid in digestion.

FOCUSED DISCHARGE CARE

Instruct client regarding:

- medication regime — pancreatic enzyme replacement, insulin replacement (both dependent upon degree of pancreatic damage)
- glucose monitoring, if indicated
- dietary restrictions:
  — restricting alcohol, tea, coffee, spicy foods and heavy meals that stimulate pancreatic secretion
  — eating small, frequent meals
  — maintaining high protein, low-fat and moderate- to high-carbohydrate diet
- symptoms that may indicate recurrence — steatorrhea (fatty-looking stools), severe back or epigastric pain, persistent gastritis, weight loss, symptoms of hyperglycemia
- if alcohol-related, the importance of alcohol abstinence and available community resources
- importance of follow-up visits

(For more information, see pp. 1149-1154 of Polaski and Tatro, *Luckmann's Core Principles and Practice of Medical-Surgical Nursing.*)

Pancreatitis, Chronic

OVERVIEW

- Chronic pancreatitis is a progressive, inflammatory, destructive disease of the pancreas. It involves progressive fibrosis and degeneration of the pancreas.
- Characteristically, the pancreas is progressively destroyed by repeated exacerbations of usually mild attacks of pancreatitis. This results in scarring and calcification of pancreatic tissue with irreversible damage, affecting both endocrine and exocrine functions.
- Chronic alcoholism is the most frequent cause of chronic pancreatitis.

CLINICAL MANIFESTATIONS

- abdominal pain — dull alternating with severe
- vomiting
- fever
- jaundice
- weight loss (client decreases food intake because food aggravates the pain)
- hyperglycemia (involvement of islet tissue)
- abdominal distention and flatus
- passage of foul, fatty stools (steatorrhea)

MEDICAL MANAGEMENT

- analgesics
- dietary restrictions — low fat, low caffeine, no spicy foods
- insulin therapy, if indicated
- pancreatic enzyme replacement — Pancrease
- histamine hydrogen-receptor blocking drugs — ranitidine (Zantac), cimetidine (Tagamet)
- antacids

SURGICAL MANAGEMENT

Several surgical approaches are available. The goals of surgical intervention are to: (1) correct the primary tract disease, (2) relieve ductal obstruction, and (3) relieve pain.

NURSING MANAGEMENT

MEDICAL

- Administer analgesics and monitor effectiveness.
- Maintain patent NG tube.
- Monitor blood glucose levels.
- Daily weights.
- Monitor intake and output.
- Monitor for signs of delirium tremors, if alcohol-related.
- Administer pancreatic replacement therapy.
- Administer hyperalimentation and lipid therapy.

In addition to routine postoperative care:
- Monitor for signs of hyperglycemia.
- Monitor proper function and placement of T-tube, NG tube, etc.
- Administer pancreatic replacement therapy when no longer NPO.

FOCUSED DISCHARGE CARE

Instruct client regarding:
- dietary restrictions
- insulin therapy (if indicated)
- signs of hypoglycemia and hyperglycemia
- pancreatic enzyme replacement therapy
- wound care (if postoperative)
- if alcohol-related, the importance of abstinence and available community resources
- importance of follow-up laboratory and clinic visits

(For more information, see pp. 1154-1155 of Polaski and Tatro, *Luckmann's Core Principles and Practice of Medical-Surgical Nursing.*)

Parkinson's Disease

OVERVIEW

- Parkinson's disease is an idiopathic syndrome characterized by tremor and rigidity.
- Parkinson's disease involves degeneration of dopamine-producing cells in the substantia nigra, which leads to degeneration of neurons in the basal ganglia. Once cell loss in the substantia nigra reaches 80 per cent, symptoms appear. The cause of nigral cell degeneration is unknown.
- Parkinson's disease often develops in clients after age 60.

- The three cardinal features of Parkinson's disease are tremor, rigidity, and bradykinesia (slowing of the ability to initiate voluntary movement).

CLINICAL MANIFESTATIONS

- generalized feeling of stiffness
- mild, diffuse muscular pain
- hand tremor at rest ("pill-rolling" movement of the thumb against the fingers)
- difficulty initiating voluntary movements (bradykinesia)
- inability to initiate movement (akinesia)
- gait changes:
  — initially – slight stiffness of one leg while walking with corresponding arm held flexed at elbow and abducted at the shoulder; client may drag one foot
  — later – typical shuffling gait with short steps and lack of associated swinging of the arms while walking
- characteristic stance — head, shoulders, and spine flexed forward, giving the appearance of stooped posture
- characteristic facial expression — masklike without expression
- speech pattern — slow, low-volumed, and monotonous in tone with poor articulation
- involuntary drooling
- intellectual ability is usually unimpaired
- decreased lacrimation (tearing)
- constipation
- incontinence
- heat intolerance, excessive perspiration
- lack of spontaneous swallowing

MEDICAL MANAGEMENT

- levodopa therapy — synthetic precursor of dopamine, delivers dopamine to the basal ganglia - Sinemet, Symmetral
- anticholinergics to control symptoms — Cogentin, Artane, Kemadrin

NURSING MANAGEMENT

- Maintain fluid intake of at least 2000 ml/24 hours.
- Establish bowel training program.
- Initiate appropriate safety measures.
- Assess ability to perform activities of daily living.
- Collaborate with physical and occupational therapy for adaptive devices for ambulation and self-care activities.
- Allow plenty of time to complete activities.
- Establish a progressive activity/exercise program with adequate rest periods.

FOCUSED DISCHARGE CARE

- Instruct client regarding:
  — disease process and prognosis
  — bowel regime:
    — regular time for bowel movement
    — fluid intake to 2000 ml/day
    — high fiber diet
    — stool softeners
  — techniques to enhance voluntary movement:
    — to reduce hand tremors — hold small objects in hand, grip arms of chair when seated, etc.
    — to initiate movement — rock back and forth
  — daily range of motion exercises
  — importance of good posture to prevent flexion of the neck and shoulders
  — importance of adequate rest
  — home safety measures:
    — remove loose carpeting and throw rugs
    — place grab bars in bathroom
    — obtain elevated toilet seat
  — use of adaptive devices for walking and to perform self-care activities
  — importance of follow-up appointments
- Refer to available community resources.

(For more information, see pp. 378-379 of Polaski and Tatro, *Luckmann's Core Principles and Practice of Medical-Surgical Nursing*.)

Parotitis (Surgical Mumps)

OVERVIEW

- Parotitis is inflammation of the parotid (salivary) glands. It results from inactivity of the gland due to lack of oral intake or certain medications, such as diuretics. As secretions of the glands diminish, oral bacteria can invade and multiply.

NURSING MANAGEMENT

- Provide frequent oral hygiene.
- Ensure adequate hydration.
- Encourage use of sugarless gum or hard candies to stimulate gland secretion.

(For more information, see p. 1016 of Polaski and Tatro, *Luckmann's Core Principles and Practice of Medical-Surgical Nursing.*)

Pelvic Inflammatory Disease (PID)

OVERVIEW

- PID refers to ascending pelvic infections, that is, those involving the upper genital tract (beyond the cervix).
- Causative organisms include gonococci, streptococci, staphylococci and other pus-producing organisms. Infection may spread:
  — from the endometrium to the fallopian tubes and to the pelvic cavity;
  — via lymphatics across the parametrium to the tubes or ovaries;
  — or from the pelvic cavity itself.
- Complications include: pelvic abscess, septic shock and sterility.

- Chronic PID can occur if treatment is inadequate or the illness did not respond to treatment. Irreversible sterility may result.

CLINICAL MANIFESTATIONS

- malaise, fever, chills, general aching, tachycardia
- anorexia, nausea, vomiting
- sharp, severe aching on both sides of the abdomen or pelvis (pain is worse with defecation)
- heavy, purulent, odoriferous discharge
- chronic PID:
  — chronic pelvic discomfort, menstrual disturbances
  — dysfunctional uterine bleeding
  — constipation
  — malaise
  — periodic return of acute symptoms

MEDICAL MANAGEMENT

- antibiotic therapy for acute or chronic PID

SURGICAL MANAGEMENT

- laparotomy with removal of infection for acute or chronic PID
- removal of uterus, ovaries and tubes may be necessary in some cases of acute or chronic PID

NURSING MANAGEMENT

MEDICAL

- Administer antibiotics as prescribed.
- Administer analgesics and assess effectiveness.
- Document amount, color, odor and appearance of the drainage.

FOCUSED DISCHARGE CARE

- Provide support (client may feel guilty if disease was sexually transmitted).
- Encourage ventilation of feelings over loss of fertility, if appropriate.
- Instruct client regarding:

- source of infection, need to have partner treated
- avoidance of sexual activity and douching
- how to identify recurrences
- general hygienic measures to prevent recurrences
    - washing perineal area regularly with soap and water
    - wiping front to back
    - changing tampons or pads several times a day during menses
    - washing hands before and after changing tampons and pads and after wiping perineal area
- maintaining adequate rest, sleep, nutrition
- when sexual activity can be resumed

(For more information, see pp. 1477-1479 of Polaski and Tatro, *Luckmann's Core Principles and Practice of Medical-Surgical Nursing.*)

Penile Disorders

URETHRAL STRICTURE

- Stricture is caused by urethral scarring or narrowing.
- Urethral stricture may be congenital or caused by untreated urethritis (inflammation of the urethra) or urethral injury (due to urologic instrumentation, e.g., cystoscopy).
- Clinical Manifestations:
    - narrowed urinary stream
    - over-distended bladder
    - signs of infection
    - dysuria
- Treatment:
    - surgically released by urethral dilation or urethroplasty

PHIMOSIS

- In phimosis, the penile foreskin (prepuce) is constricted at the opening, making retraction difficult or impossible.

- Clinical Manifestations:
  — edema, erythema
  — tenderness
  — purulent drainage
- Treatment:
  — control infection, if present, with local treatment and broad-spectrum antimicrobial agents

PARAPHIMOSIS

- Paraphimosis occurs when tight foreskin, once retracted, cannot return to its normal position. Circulation is impeded, and the glans swells rapidly.
- Treatment:
  — manual reduction
  — surgical incision

PRIAPISM

- Priapism is prolonged, persistent erection without sexual desire.
- Priapism can last hours or days and is usually very painful.
- There is no known cause, although it is sometimes associated with leukemia or sickle cell anemia.
- It is considered an emergency situation because circulation is compromised, and client may not be able to void.
- Treatment:
  — conservative:
    — bedrest
    — prostatic massage
    — sedation
    — analgesics
    — warm blankets
    — catheterization if unable to void
  — surgical:
    — aspiration with a large bore needle or incision of the corpus cavernosa

(For more information, see pp. 1463-1465 of Polaski and Tatro, *Luckmann's Core Principles and Practice of Medical-Surgical Nursing.*)

Peptic Ulcer Disease

OVERVIEW

- Peptic ulceration is a break in continuity of esophageal, gastric or duodenal mucosa.
- Peptic ulcers may form when aggressive factors exceed the defensive resistance of the mucosa. Aggressive factors may be the result of hypersecretion of gastric juices, increased stimulation of the vagus, decreased inhibition of gastric secretions, increased capacity or number of the parietal cells to secrete acid, or increased response of the parietal cells to the stimulator.
- There are 3 types of ulcers:
  (1) Duodenal Ulcers—occur within 1.5 cm of the pylorus. They are characterized by high gastric acid secretion.
  (2) Gastric Ulcers — occur within one inch of the pylorus of the stomach in an area of gastritis. They are most likely caused by a break in the "mucosal barrier" and tend to heal within a few weeks.
  (3) Stress Ulcers — usually occur after an acute medical crisis. They may be caused by:
     — severe trauma or major illness
     — severe burns (sometimes called Curling's ulcers)
     — head injury or intracranial disease (often called Cushing's ulcers)
     — drug ingestion
     — shock
     — sepsis
- Risk factors include: smoking, steroids, aspirin, caffeine, alcohol, Crohn's disease, Zollinger-Ellison syndrome, an infection with H. pylori, chemotherapeutic agents, hepatic disease and biliary disease.

CLINICAL MANIFESTATIONS

- aching, burning, cramplike, gnawing pain
- pain in upper epigastrium with localization to the left of the midline (gastric ulcers)
- pain in right epigastrium (duodenal ulcers)

- pain associated with food intake and relieved by vomiting (gastric ulcers)
- pain when stomach is empty, relieved by food or antacids (duodenal ulcers)
- gastrointestinal bleeding
- nausea, vomiting

MEDICAL MANAGEMENT

- hyposecretory agents (cause reduction in acid secretion):
  — H_2 receptor antagonists—block histamine-stimulated gastric secretion (e.g., ranitidine [Zantac], famotidine [Pepcid], cimetidine [Tagamet])
  — prostaglandin analogs — inhibit gastric acid secretion (misoprostal [Cytotec])
  — anticholinergics — decrease gastrointestinal motility and inhibit gastric acid secretion by blocking the action of acetylcholine on smooth muscles (e.g., dicyclomine [Bentyl])
  — antacids — generally increase gastric pH to reduce pepsin activity and strengthen the mucosal barrier and esophageal sphincter tone
- mucosal barrier fortifiers (e.g., sucralfate)
  — prevent hydrogen ion back diffusion into the mucosa and stimulate mucous production
- avoidance of coffee, alcohol and milk
- physical and emotional rest
- stress reduction
- **medical management of complications due to ulcers; hemorrhage**
  — nasogastric tube to prevent gastric dilation, to administer saline lavage, and to check gastric pH.
  — arterial administration of vasopressin
  — arterial embolization via angiography
  — ranitidine and antacids
  — replacement of fluid, blood and electrolytes
  perforation
  — nasogastric tube to suction
  — antibiotics
  — replacement of fluid, blood and electrolytes
  — surgical intervention, see "Surgical Management" on next page

SURGICAL MANAGEMENT

- **subtotal gastrectomy** — a term referring to any surgery that involves partial removal of the stomach:
  (1) Billroth I — removal of a part of the distal portion of the stomach, including the antrum. The remainder of the stomach is anastomosed to the duodenum (combined procedure called gastroduoden-ostomy). It decreases the incidence of dumping syn- drome that often occurs after a Billroth II procedure.
  (2) Billroth II — reanastomosis of the proximal remnant of the stomach to the proximal jejunum (gastrojejunostomy). The duodenum is preserved because pancreatic secretions and bile necessary for digestion continue to be secreted into the duodenum even after gastrectomy, and a route to the intestine must be preserved for them.

- **total gastrectomy** — removal of the stomach with anastomosis of the esophagus to the jejunum (esophagojejunostomy). The thoracic approach is used. Principal intervention for stomach cancer.

- **pyloroplasty** — widening of the existing exit of the stomach at the pylorus. May be indicated for obstruction due to scarring from repeated ulcerations and healing.

- **potential complications following gastric surgery:**
  — marginal ulcers — ulcers at operative site
  — hemorrhage
  — alkaline reflux gastritis — due to reflux of duodenal contents when the pylorus is bypassed or removed
  — acute gastric dilation — postoperative distention of the stomach
  — vitamin B_{12} and folic acid deficiency
  — reduced absorption of calcium and vitamin D
  — "dumping syndrome" — due to rapid entry of food into the jejunum without proper mixing or duodenal digestive processing. Usually subsides in 6 to 12 months. See "Nursing Management" p. 497, for signs/symptoms.
  — gastrojejunocolic fistula — characterized by fecal vomiting, diarrhea, weight loss and anorexia
  — pyloric obstruction — manifested by vomiting

NURSING MANAGEMENT

MEDICAL

- Administer medications as ordered and assess effectiveness of medication for the client's pain.
- Monitor gastric pH.
- Encourage rest to reduce peristalsis and gastric secretions.
- Administer antacids with small amounts of water to assure passage beyond the esophagus and into the stomach.
- Monitor for signs/symptoms of bleeding/hemorrhage and report to physician: dark, tarry stools (melena) or coffee ground emesis (hematemesis).
- Monitor intake and output.
- Monitor for signs/symptoms of hypovolemia.
- Maintain nasogastric tube to suction.
- Hematest nasogastric drainage and stools.
- If bleeding occurs:
  — monitor vital signs
  — administer fluids, electrolytes and blood products
  — perform saline lavage (do not use iced saline
    — it causes mucosal damage due to decreased tissue perfusion).
- Monitor for signs/symptoms of perforation and report to physician immediately:
  — sudden, sharp, severe pain beginning in the mid-epigastrium, then spreading over entire abdomen
  — abdominal tenderness, hardness and rigidity
  — client bending over or drawing up knees to decrease tension
- If perforation occurs, prepare for surgery.
- Monitor for signs/symptoms of obstruction and report to physician:
  — vomiting
  — feeling of fullness
  — abdominal distention
  — pain at night
- Instruct on small frequent meals and bland diet.
- Instruct on avoidance of milk, alcohol, tobacco and caffeine.
- Discuss stress reduction, possible alterations in lifestyle and relaxation techniques.
- Discuss ulcer development, rationale for treatment and ways to prevent recurrence.

In addition to routine postoperative care:
- Maintain patent nasogastric or gastrostomy tube to suction to prevent retention of gastric secretions.
- Assess for abdominal distention and report to physician — do not reposition tubes. Irrigate *gently* only if ordered.
- Assess amount and color of nasogastric drainage (should be bright red in immediate postoperative period, but dark red by the end of 24 hours).
- Administer pain medications and assess effectiveness.
- Assess the operative site for excessive drainage — too much fluid in the gastric stump may cause pressure and injury. Report bleeding or hemorrhaging.
- Assess for and report to physician signs/symptoms of gastric dilation (may occur in immediate postoperative period):
  — epigastric pain, tachycardia, hypotension
  — hiccups, complaints of fullness, gagging.
- Assess for alkaline reflux gastritis.
- Assess for gastrojejunocolic fistula (fecal vomiting, diarrhea, weight loss, anorexia).
- Assess for signs/symptoms of pyloric obstruction — vomiting.
- Maintain patency of chest tubes (following total gastrectomy) and monitor output.
- Assist with turning, coughing, deep breathing and incentive spirometry (pulmonary hygiene is painful due to high abdominal incision).
- Start diet by beginning clear water, 30 ml at a time.
  — Aspirate tube approximately one hour later, to see if fluid retained.
  — Progress to soft foods and eventually to regular diet of 5 to 6 meals/day.
  — Discuss that progress will be slow — may take up to a year to eat 3 normal meals daily.
- Discuss nutritionally balanced diet.
- Assess for signs/symptoms of dumping syndrome:
  — vertigo, tachycardia, syncope, sweating, pallor, palpitations, diarrhea and nausea 5 to 30 minutes after eating

— epigastric fullness, abdominal cramping, stomach rumbling, distention, nausea and desire to defecate 2 to 3 hours after eating.
- Instruct client on management of dumping syndrome:
  — eat in recumbent or semi-recumbent position
  — lie down after meals
  — increase fat content in diet
  — no fluids 1 hour before, 2 hours after, or with meals
  — take medications as ordered to delay gastric emptying

FOCUSED DISCHARGE CARE

MEDICAL

- Instruct client regarding:
  — need for compliance with therapy (recurrence rate is over 50 percent if maintenance therapy stopped)
  — need to continue medical regimen even though pain may be gone
  — factors that cause pain and ways to eliminate
  — stress reduction, coping and relaxation techniques
  — diet and foods/beverages to avoid
  — signs/symptoms of complications and to report these to physician
  — signs/symptoms of recurrence and to report these to physician
  — avoidance of aspirin, aspirin-containing products and non-steroidal anti-inflammatory agents as these are ulcerogenic
  — smoking cessation program

SURGICAL

- In addition to the above interventions under "Medical", instruct the client regarding:
  — signs/symptoms of infection
  — wound care
  — adequate nutrition, progression of diet
  — need for follow-up for pernicious anemia for clients who had gastric resection
  — management of dumping syndrome
  — signs/symptoms of complications and to report these to physician

(For more information, see pp. 1039-1048 of Polaski and Tatro, *Luckmann's Core Principles and Practice of Medical-Surgical Nursing.*)

Pericarditis

OVERVIEW

- Pericarditis is a syndrome caused by inflammation of the parietal and visceral pericardium. Causes include: infections, myocardial injury, hypersensitivity, and collagen disease.
- This inflammatory process may develop either as a primary condition, or secondary to a number of diseases. It may be acute or chronic (constrictive pericarditis).
- Pericarditis may be either exudative or dry (fibrinous). With the exudative type, the exudate can accumulate in the pericardial sac causing a tamponade that restricts cardiac filling and emptying. In dry pericarditis, adhesions form within the pericardial space, along with deposits of serous fibrin and calcification.

CLINICAL MANIFESTATIONS

- chest pain similar to myocardial infarction; at other times mimics pleurisy. Pain is exacerbated with respirations and rotating the trunk but does not radiate. Sitting up frequently relieves the pain.
- pericardial friction rub
- fever, chills, malaise, joint pain, anorexia
- dyspnea
- S-T segment elevation

MEDICAL MANAGEMENT

- specific treatment for underlying causes
- non-steroidal anti-inflammatory agents
- analgesia

NURSING MANAGEMENT

- Assess for changes in cardiac or respiratory status.
- Assess for cardiac tamponade (paradoxical pulse greater than 10 mm Hg, muffled heart sounds, distended neck veins, hypotension, narrowed pulse pressure). See "Cardiac Tamponade", p. 123.
- Treat fever with rest, cooling measures, forced fluids, and anti-pyretics.
- Administer antimicrobial therapy as prescribed.
- Encourage fluids and well balanced diet.
- Administer PRN analgesics.
- Provide adequate rest periods.
- Implement progressive activity schedule.

FOCUSED DISCHARGE CARE

Instruct client regarding:
- how to monitor pulse and rhythm and to report any sudden changes
- disease process and treatment regimen
- need for follow-up care

(For more information, see pp. 742-743 of Polaski and Tatro, *Luckmann's Core Principles and Practice of Medical-Surgical Nursing*.)

Perioperative Nursing Care

OVERVIEW

- Perioperative refers to events during the entire surgical period from preparation for surgery to recovery from the temporary effects of surgery and anesthesia.
- Perioperative nursing practice consists of three phases: preoperative, intraoperative and postoperative.

- Preoperative Phase—this phase begins when the decision for surgical intervention is made and ends with transfer of the client to the operating room bed.
- Intraoperative Phase — begins when the client is transferred to the operating room bed and ends when the client is admitted to the postanesthesia care unit (PACU).
- Postoperative Phase — this period begins with admission to the postanesthesia recovery area and ends with the resolution of surgical sequelae.

PREOPERATIVE PHASE - NURSING CARE

- Preoperative preparation may take place in: (1) the physician's office or outpatient center before admission to the health care facility, (2) on admission and during the days before the operation, (3) the night before surgery if the client is hospitalized, or (4) the morning of surgery on admission.
- Obtain a preoperative history and perform a physical assessment, gathering information about:
  (1) age — older adults have the lowest tolerance to the stressful effects of surgery
  (2) presence of pain
  (3) nutritional status — nutritional status directly correlates with intraoperative success and postoperative recovery. Both nutritional deficiencies and excess (obesity) place the client at increased risk
  (4) fluid and electrolyte balance — imbalances should be corrected before surgery
  (5) presence of infection
  (6) cardiovascular function
  (7) pulmonary function
  (8) renal function
  (9) gastrointestinal function
  (10) liver function — liver disease increases risk because a client is unable to detoxify medications and anesthetic agents or to metabolize carbohydrates, fats and amino acids
  (11) endocrine function
  (12) neurologic function
  (13) hematologic function

(14) medication history — some medications may increase operative risk by increasing coagulation time or by interacting unfavorably with the anesthetic

(15) presence of trauma

(16) health habits — clients who smoke or abuse drugs or alcohol have an increased surgical risk. Smokers have reduced hemoglobin levels, are more likely to have damaged lung tissue and are more susceptible to thrombus formation. Clients who use alcohol or drugs may experience withdrawal symptoms.

(17) previous surgery and anesthesia

(18) responses of family members to surgery and anesthesia

(19) allergies and reactions; any dietary restrictions

(20) any serious or chronic illnesses

(21) current symptoms or discomforts

(22) religious affiliation

(23) social history — the client's marital status, significant others, support systems and occupation all should be explored. It is also important to determine whether the client has insurance or whether the surgery will cause financial hardship. Any of these factors can cause increased stress and delayed healing.

- Perform a psychosocial assessment of the client and assess level and cause of anxiety (fear of the unknown is generally the greatest fear).
- Reassure the client and significant others. Provide information about the surgery, health care facility and answer all questions. If possible, introduce the client or family to others who have successfully undergone similar surgery. A visit by a volunteer from a local support group (e.g., local laryngectomy or colostomy organization) also may be arranged.
- Arrange for a visit from clergy, if the client desires.
- Explain and prepare for diagnostic tests.
- Ensure that informed consent is obtained (generally, the surgeon explains the surgical procedure, possible risks, complications and alternatives.
- Provide individualized preoperative teaching (preoperative instruction decreases anxiety, decreases postoperative complications and decreases the length of stay). Include:

- deep breathing and coughing exercises (encourage the client to perform deep breathing exercises before coughing to stimulate the cough reflex)
- turning and extremity exercises
- pain control methods
- postoperative equipment (i.e., tubes, drains, intravenous infusion devices)
- preoperative preparation.
- Cleanse the operative area the night prior to surgery with an antiseptic, such as povidone-iodine, or Hibiclens as prescribed.
- Maintain NPO status after midnight as prescribed.
- Perform enemas as prescribed (usually for procedures involving the gastrointestinal tract, perianal or perineal areas and pelvic cavity).
- Provide measures to promote sleep the night before surgery.

Interventions on the Day of Surgery

- Take and record vital signs (report significant changes from baseline to physician).
- Check identification band to ensure it is accurate, legible and securely fastened to the client.
- Check for and carry out any special orders.
- Verify that the client has not eaten for the last eight hours (however, the physician may occasionally order scheduled oral medications to be taken with a small sip of water).
- Ask the client to void. Record the time and amount voided.
- Assist with oral hygiene as necessary.
- Remove dentures and bridgework and store in a secure place.
- Have the client remove jewelry.
- Assist the client with putting on a hospital gown, antiembolic hose or ace wraps, if prescribed.
- Remove colored nail polish and all skin make-up.
- Notify operating room nurse if client has hearing aid — leave it in place, so that the client can hear when awakening from anesthesia.
- Administer preoperative medications as prescribed. If sedatives are given, initiate safety precautions. The operative permit and transfusion permit (if required)

must be signed and witnessed before the client receives any medication that will alter his or her consciousness (such as narcotics or tranquilizers).

- Complete the preoperative checklist as per health care facility policy.
- Assist with transporting the client to surgery.
- Direct significant others to the designated surgical lounge — ask them to leave a phone number where they can be reached if they leave the facility for any reason.

INTRAOPERATIVE NURSING CARE

The nurse works in collaboration with the surgical team during the intraoperative phase. This team is highly trained and specialized. General nursing interventions include:

- assisting with client positioning
- maintaining surgical asepsis
- preventing client heat loss
- assisting with surgical wound closure
- assessing drainage
- transporting the client to the postanesthesia or intensive care unit

POSTOPERATIVE NURSING CARE

Postanesthesia Care Unit (PACU)

- The PACU nurse monitors and documents:
  — absence of and return of reflexes (such as the pharyngeal [gag] reflex). The nurse stays at the bedside until the client's gag reflex returns.
  — level of consciousness
  — temperature and vital signs
  — skin color and dryness
  — condition of the dressing
  — drainage tubes and output
  — intravenous infusions
  — infusion of blood products or colloids
  — renal function and fluid and electrolyte balance
  — client's comfort and safety
  — pain
  — anesthetic, respiratory, cardiovascular or other possible complications

- After transfer from the PACU, the nurse on the unit makes an initial assessment of the client after the transfer, including:
  — respiratory status
  — cardiovascular status
  — neurological status
  — surgical wound
  — intravenous lines
  — tubes (e.g., catheters, NG tube, hemovac, Jackson-Pratt drains, etc)
  — positioning
  — pain
- Goals and interventions for the postoperative period are to:
  (1) Restore optimal functioning.
    — Monitor vital signs — follow protocol as defined by your institution.
    — Monitor wound for signs/symptoms of bleeding.
    — Monitor for shock.
    — Monitor for complications specific to type of procedure performed.
  (2) Maintain and promote adequate airway and respiratory function.
    — Monitor for signs/symptoms of pulmonary complications (such as atelectasis, pneumonia and pulmonary emboli): increased temperature, restlessness, dyspnea, tachycardia, hemoptysis, pulmonary edema, altered breath sounds and thick viscous sputum.
    — Assist with turning, coughing and deep breathing every one to two hours.
    — Encourage use of incentive spirometry.
    — Encourage and assist with early ambulation.
    — Monitor color, consistency and odor of any sputum production — thick, odorous, colored sputum indicates infection.
  (3) Maintain adequate cardiac function and promote tissue perfusion.
    — Monitor for thrombophlebitis — redness, swelling or tenderness of an extremity and the presence of Homan's sign.
    — Prevent thrombophlebitis through postoperative leg exercises, early ambulation, antiem-

505

bolic support stockings, adequate hydration and low-dose heparin.

— Monitor for signs/symptoms of myocardial infarction: dyspnea, chest pain, shoulder or jaw pain, tachycardia, diaphoresis, cyanosis or dysrhythmias.

— Monitor for signs/symptoms of blood loss: postural hypotension, tachycardia, tachypnea, decreased urine output, cool, clammy skin and decreased level of consciousness.

(4) Maintain adequate fluid and electrolyte balance and adequate renal function.

— Monitor intake and output.

— Assess serum electrolyte values and report abnormal findings to the physician immediately.

— Maintain patency of nasogastric tubes.

— Obtain an order for an antiemetic if the client develops nausea and vomiting.

— Administer replacement fluids as prescribed.

— Monitor patency of urinary catheter.

— Monitor for signs/symptoms of urinary tract infection.

— Monitor for bladder distention if urinary catheter is not present: fullness above symphysis pubis or voiding 30 to 60 ml of urine every 20 to 30 minutes.

— If bladder distention occurs:
  • run tap water so the client hears it
  • pour warm water over the female perineum
  • assist male clients to sit or stand (if not contraindicated)
  • administer pain medication as prescribed
  • insert a straight or indwelling catheter as prescribed.

(5) Promote comfort and rest.

— Change client's position, straighten bed linens or give a back rub.

— Provide prescribed analgesics and assess effectiveness. Narcotics should be given routinely during the first 24 hours after surgery and as needed up to 72 hours. There is little danger of overmedication as long as careful assessment is performed. The client will recover faster if comfortable and able to comply with breathing and ambulation.

— Provide and explain use of patient controlled analgesia (PCA) pump as prescribed.

(6) Promote adequate nutrition and elimination.

— Assess for return of bowel sounds (usually within 24 to 48 hours after surgery).
— Advance prescribed diet as tolerated.
— Monitor for paralytic ileus and notify physician if the following occur: diminished or absent bowel sounds, abdominal distention and feeling of fullness.

(7) Promote wound healing.

— Assess the wound for signs of infection, such as redness, drainage, odor, pain and induration.
— Observe the wound for edema, bleeding or change in color.
— Observe the wound for approximation of the suture line.
— Monitor drains and assess the color, consistency and amount of drainage.
— Maintain strict asepsis when coming in contact with the wound.
— Monitor for wound dehiscence (opening of the wound edges) or wound evisceration (protrusion of internal organs, such as bowel, through the incision). Other signs/symptoms that occur include the client feeling that something "gave way" or sudden, profuse pink serous drainage from the wound. These complications generally develop on the sixth to seventh day after surgery.
— Interventions for wound dehiscence or evisceration include:
  • Remain calm.
  • Place the client in semi-Fowler's position with the knees slightly bent.
  • Stay with the client and have someone notify the surgeon immediately.
  • Cover any protruding coils of intestine with sterile dressings moistened with sterile saline.
  • Moisten dressings frequently with sterile normal saline.
  • Monitor the client's vital signs because shock may ensue.

- Reassure the client that the physician is on the way.
- Prepare the client for return to the operating room.

(8) Promote and maintain activity and mobility.
— Have client flex the ankles and legs and reposition in bed if not contraindicated.
— Encourage and assist with early ambulation as prescribed.

(9) Provide emotional support and foster positive body image.
— Provide empathetic listening and encourage expression of feelings.
— Encourage discussion between client and significant others of anticipated changes due to surgery and how this will affect their lives.
— Arrange support group and community referrals for the client and significant others.

(10) Plan for discharge.
— Provide specific written instructions regarding:
  - wound care (signs of infection)
  - activity restrictions
  - dietary instructions
  - postoperative medication instruction
  - personal hygiene
  - follow-up appointments with surgeon or clinic
— Provide referrals to home health care agency as appropriate.

(For more information, see pp. 82-114 of Polaski and Tatro, *Luckmann's Core Principles and Practice of Medical-Surgical Nursing.*)

Peritonitis

OVERVIEW

- Peritonitis is inflammation of the peritoneal membrane which is normally sterile.
- Sources of inflammation may be through the bloodstream, the external environment or through the gastrointestinal tract. Normal flora of the intestine becomes a source of infection if it enters the sterile peritoneal cavity.

CLINICAL MANIFESTATIONS

- pain, usually localized but may be generalized
- abdominal rigidity
- increase in pain with any pressure or motion of the abdomen
- nausea, vomiting, low grade fever
- shallow respirations
- absence of bowel sounds

MEDICAL MANAGEMENT

- fluid, electrolyte and protein replacement
- long intestinal tube to suction (such as Miller-Abbott, Cantor or Harris tube)
- intravenous antibiotic therapy

SURGICAL MANAGEMENT

- incision and drainage of the abscess once it is walled off

NURSING MANAGEMENT

MEDICAL

- Monitor intake and output.
- Assess for adequate hydration:
  — moist mucous membranes
  — good skin turgor.
- Daily weights.
- Maintain NPO status and administer intravenous fluids.

- Assess for signs/symptoms of sepsis.
- Maintain nasogastric tube to suction.

POSTOPERATIVE CARE

In addition to routine postoperative care:
- Monitor for complications of adult respiratory distress syndrome, sepsis or shock.

FOCUSED DISCHARGE CARE

Instruct client regarding:
- signs/symptoms of infection and to report to physician
- wound care
- activity restrictions
- need to finish full course of antibiotics

(For more information, see pp. 1060-1061 of Polaski and Tatro, *Luckmann's Core Principles and Practice of Medical-Surgical Nursing*.)

Pheochromocytoma

OVERVIEW

- Pheochromocytoma is a catecholamine-secreting tumor of the adrenal medulla. Excessive secretion of epinephrine and norepinephrine by the tumor can produce severe symptoms and death.
- Pheochromocytoma is more common in women than men, and most commonly occurs in middle age.
- Tumors are typically benign.

CLINICAL MANIFESTATIONS

- hypertension (persistent, fluctuating, intermittent, or paroxysmal in nature)
- pounding headache
- diaphoresis

- apprehension
- palpitations
- nausea and vomiting
- hyperglycemia and glucosuria (excessive catecholamine release results in increased conversion of glycogen to glucose)
- acute attacks are associated with profuse diaphoresis, dilated pupils, and cold extremities
- severe hypertension can precipitate cerebral vascular accident or sudden blindness

MEDICAL MANAGEMENT

- alpha-adrenergic blocking agents for hypertensive crises

SURGICAL MANAGEMENT

Surgical management is the treatment of choice.
- unilateral or bilateral adrenalectomy (removal of adrenal gland(s))

NURSING MANAGEMENT

MEDICAL

- Administer alpha-adrenergics as prescribed.
- Monitor blood pressure closely.
- Assess neurologic status for changes.
- Promote rest.
- Prohibit beverages or food with caffeine.

SURGICAL

POSTOPERATIVE CARE

In addition to routine postoperative care:
- Assess for signs/symptoms of shock (profound shock can develop as catecholamine levels drop) and hemorrhage (due to high vascularity of the adrenal glands).
- Prevent shock by:
  — administration of IV replacement fluids as prescribed
  — administration of IV pressor agents titrated to blood pressure parameters
  — monitoring of urine output

- Assess for signs of adrenal insufficiency (profound weakness; severe abdominal, back or leg pain; hyperpyrexia followed by hypothermia; and coma).

FOCUSED DISCHARGE CARE

Instruct client regarding:
- importance of daily hormonal replacement
- medication injection technique when client not able to tolerate oral medications
- signs of under- and overdosage
- need to call for dosage adjustment if experiencing emotional or physical stress
- need for Medic Alert bracelet and card

(For more information, see pp. 1243-1246 of Polaski and Tatro, *Luckmann's Core Principles and Practice of Medical-Surgical Nursing.*)

Pituitary Tumors

OVERVIEW

- Pituitary tumors usually occur in the anterior lobe of the pituitary and are benign, small and encapsulated. They usually can be removed successfully via surgery by a procedure called transphenoidal hypophysectomy (see Surgical Management).

CLINICAL MANIFESTATIONS

Pituitary tumors cause hyperpituitarism resulting in:
- visual changes or deficits
- irregular or absent menstrual cycles and infertility in females
- decreased libido or impotence in males
- decreased body hair; elevated blood pressure; warm, moist, coarse skin; coarse facial features; headache
- height and weight changes
- decreased production of other stimulating hormones
- early signs of increasing intracranial pressure

SURGICAL MANAGEMENT

- transphenoidal hypophysectomy — removal of the tumor via an incision made inside the mouth, at the junction between the upper lip and gum

NURSING MANAGEMENT

Transphenoidal Hypophysectomy

Postoperative Care

Nursing care following transphenoidal hypophysectomy is similar to care following craniotomy (see "Intracranial Tumors", p. 397).

In addition to routine postoperative care:

- Monitor for diabetes insipidus [dilute urine output of from 2 to 15 liters/day — due to a lack of antidiuretic hormone (ADH)].
    - Accurate intake and output, assessing for polyuria and polydipsia.
    - Obtain urine specific gravity every 2 hours, assessing for dilute urine (specific gravity 1.000 to 1.005).
    - Assess for electrolyte imbalance.
    - Weigh daily.
- Assist with frequent oral hygiene with saline rinses and use of foam toothettes (toothbrushes are not used at first as this may disrupt the suture line).
- Advance diet and instruct client to avoid rough foods.
- Administer replacement hormones, as prescribed.
- Administer intravenous or inhalation vasopressin (Pitressin) or desmopressin (DDAVP) for treatment of diabetes insipidus, as prescribed.
- Maintain nasal packing to control bleeding.
- Instruct client to avoid all activities (bending, straining, coughing, sneezing) that may increase intracranial pressure.

FOCUSED DISCHARGE CARE

Instruct client/significant other regarding:

- replacement hormone therapy and signs/symptoms of under- or overdose
- correct use of vasopressin (Pitressin), if prescribed

- diabetes insipidus, importance of adequate fluids and how to assess adequate fluid balance
- signs/symptoms of infection
- oral wound care
- importance of follow-up laboratory tests and visits to physician

See also "Syndrome of Inappropriate Antidiuretic Hormone", p. 599.

(For more information, see p. 341 of Polaski and Tatro, *Luckmann's Core Principles and Practice of Medical-Surgical Nursing*.)

Plastic Surgery

OVERVIEW

- Plastic surgery is the surgical subspecialty concentrating on the restoration of function and form to body structures damaged by trauma, the aging process, disease processes such as skin cancer and congenital defects.
- Plastic surgery is divided into two major areas:
  (1) aesthetic (cosmetic) surgery — alteration of any physical feature that is already within the "normal" range
  (2) reconstructive surgery — attempt to restore an abnormal body part to normal. The abnormality may be due to injured tissue, disease or missing tissues.
- Deformities can be actual (that is, objectively measured by others) or perceived (the client is aware of the deformity, but it may not be noticeable to others).
- Plastic surgeons strive for minimal scarring by:
  — making incisions parallel to natural skin lines
  — use of elliptical incisions (the incision lines are longer than the lesion)

— use of precise suturing techniques.
- Types of surgical modalities:
  — microvascular surgery:
    — implants — different types of materials are used to augment or replace tissue
    — skin expansion — technique used to increase the amount of local tissue available to reconstruct a defect. An inflatable silicone balloon is implanted under the skin or muscle adjacent to the defect. The expander is inflated over a period of time to stretch the overlying tissue.
    — lasers — use of a precise beam of light to cause cell destruction with the advantages of reduced bleeding and swelling
  — grafts — tissue that is harvested without a blood supply from a donor site. It is transferred to a recipient site, where it develops a new blood supply. A *split-thickness skin graft* is a very thin graft containing epidermis and a very thin layer of dermis. A *full-thickness graft* contains all of the epidermis and dermis.
  — flaps — tissue that is elevated with its blood supply intact. It may be rotated to reconstruct an adjacent defect or detached from its blood supply at the donor site and reattached to veins and arteries at the recipient site by microvascular anastomosis.

NURSING MANAGEMENT

In addition to routine preoperative care:
- Assist to develop realistic postoperative expectations — report unrealistic expectations to the surgeon.
- Reinforce the fact that the body is naturally asymmetric.
- Instruct client to avoid aspirin and aspirin-containing compounds (interfere with platelet agglutination and promote bleeding and hematoma formation); nicotine (potent vasoconstrictor); and smoking (can result in flap necrosis).

In addition to routine postoperative care:
- Assess and document skin color, temperature, sensation; the blanching time of the surgical site; presence of blisters; the presence or absence of edema or

seroma (accumulation of serosanguinous drainage); and any pain, pressure or bleeding.

— Report cool, pale or cyanotic skin; prolonged blanching time; and changes in sensation.

— Report any sign of decreased vascularity (blue color, change in temperature, change in size or tightness). Be aware that venous stasis and edema can impair tissue perfusion.

— Report to the physician any blisters (these indicate decreased circulation and impaired tissue viability).

- Assess the client's coping mechanisms.
- Assist client to explore and express feelings.
- Gently assist client to look at and touch surgical site (help client to incorporate it into self-concept and body image).
- Encourage client to take measures (such as taking walks in the halls or accepting visitors) to begin desensitization to reactions of others.
- Encourage client to discuss reaction of others. Support grief reactions.
- Remind client that achieving the desired results takes time, and not to be discouraged if progress seems slow.

In addition:

Postoperative Flaps:
- Position client so that the flap is relaxed and elevated.
- Prevent tension on the flap.
- Report pallor or hematoma immediately.

Implants:
- Monitor for and instruct client on signs/symptoms of infection or rejection: change in temperature, drainage, increasing edema, redness of skin and increasing skin temperature.
- Instruct on percutaneous saline injections into the expander which will be performed to stretch the skin.
- Instruct to keep incision and injection site clean and free of infection.
- Discuss how to camouflage the expander with clothing.
- Discuss sleeping positions that protect the expander from pressure.

Laser Surgery:
- Discuss use of ointment to area for two to four weeks.
- Discuss protection from sun exposure to treated area.

FOCUSED DISCHARGE CARE

Discharge teaching depends upon the specific operation and the surgeon's preferences.

(For more information, see pp. 1390-1396 of Polaski and Tatro, *Luckmann's Core Principles and Practice of Medical-Surgical Nursing*.)

Pleural Effusion

- Pleural effusion is an accumulation of fluid in the pleural space between the visceral and parietal pleura.
- Causes include congestive heart failure; liver or renal failure; infections or tumors in the pleura or pleural spaces; and lymphatic obstruction.
- Clinical manifestations depend upon the amount of fluid present. Dyspnea on exertion, decreased or absent tactile fremitus and dull or flat percussion notes may be seen or there may be no symptoms at all.
- Thoracentesis is used to remove the fluid. The fluid is analyzed by the laboratory to aid in diagnosis.
- For recurrent pleural effusion with respiratory compromise or persistent pleural pain, obliteration of the pleural space may be performed:
  (1) Pleurectomy — surgically stripping the parietal pleura away from the visceral pleura. This produces an intense inflammatory reaction that promotes adhesion formation between the two layers during healing.
  (2) Pleurodesis — instillation of a sclerosing substance (e.g., unbuffered tetracycline, nitrogen mustard, talc) into the pleural space via a thoracotomy tube. This creates an inflammatory response that

scleroses tissue together. The tube will remain clamped for a specified period of time with special positioning changes prescribed.

- Nursing care includes:
  — monitoring respiratory status, especially for dyspnea
  — administering analgesics and assessing effectiveness
  — documenting alleviation or persistence of pleural pain
  — encouraging pulmonary hygiene
  — maintaining closed chest tube drainage system (if appropriate)
  — monitoring for signs/symptoms indicating return of pleural effusion

(For more information, see pp. 624-625 of Polaski and Tatro, *Luckmann's Core Principles and Practice of Medical-Surgical Nursing.*)

Pneumonia

OVERVIEW

- Pneumonia (pneumonitis) is an inflammatory process of lung parenchyma usually associated with a marked increase in interstitial and alveolar fluid.
- Pneumonia may occur as a result of bacteria, viruses, mycoplasmas, fungal agents and protozoa. It also may result from (1) inhalation of toxic or caustic chemicals, smoke, dusts or gases or (2) aspiration of food, fluids or vomitus.
- Pseudomonas aeruginosa is the most common cause of hospital-acquired gram-negative pneumonia.
- Streptococcus pneumoniae is the most common cause of community-acquired pneumonia.
- Risk factors include: smoking, air pollution, upper respiratory infection, prolonged immobility, malnutrition, prolonged debilitating disease, advanced age and chronic illness.

CLINICAL MANIFESTATIONS

- fever, chills, sweats, pleuritic chest pain
- cough, sputum production, hemoptysis, dyspnea
- headache or fatigue
- crackling breath sounds
- increased tactile fremitus over areas of pneumonia

MEDICAL MANAGEMENT

- antibiotic therapy

NURSING MANAGEMENT

- Encourage fluid intake.
- Assess lung sounds and monitor for changes.
- Monitor arterial blood gases and observe for signs/symptoms of hypoxia or hypercapnia.
- Assist with turning, coughing and deep breathing every 2 hours.
- Instruct on splinting the chest wall for comfort during coughing.
- Position to facilitate breathing, i.e., 45 degrees.
- Encourage use of incentive spirometer while awake.
- Assess the baseline level of activity and monitor tolerance of activity.
- Schedule activity after treatments or medications.
- Provide adequate rest.
- Instruct on pursed-lip and diaphragmatic breathing. (See p. 158.)

FOCUSED DISCHARGE CARE

- Instruct client/significant other regarding:
  — coughing and deep breathing
  — importance of completing prescribed antibiotics
  — need for adequate rest and gradual resumption of activity
  — avoidance of conditions that increase oxygen demand: temperature extremes, weight gain, stress and smoking
  — need for adequate nutrition
  — complications to report to physician: return of fever, chest pain, hemoptysis, chills

- Encourage immunization for the next winter.

(For more information, see pp. 585-589 of Polaski and Tatro, *Luckmann's Core Principles and Practice of Medical-Surgical Nursing.*)

Pneumothorax

- Pneumothorax is the presence of air in the pleural space that prevents complete lung expansion.
- An open pneumothorax is air in the pleural space from a hole in the chest wall or diaphragm. This almost always occurs due to a penetrating chest injury.
- A closed (or spontaneous) pneumothorax is air in the pleural space from a puncture or tear in an internal respiratory structure (bronchus, bronchioles or alveoli). This may occur spontaneously or be due to a fractured rib, chest surgery, chest trauma or may be the result of underlying pulmonary disease, such as emphysema, pulmonary neoplasms or pneumonia.
- Clinical manifestations:
  — moderate pneumothorax—tachypnea; dyspnea; sudden sharp pain on the affected side with chest movement, breathing or coughing; asymmetric chest expansion; diminished or absent breath sounds on the affected side; restlessness; anxiety and tachycardia
  — severe pneumothorax — all of the preceding along with distended neck veins; PMI (point of maximal impulse of heartbeat) shift; subcutaneous emphysema; decreased tactile and vocal fremitus; tracheal deviation toward the unaffected side; and progressive cyanosis
- Management
  — x-ray confirmation if time permits
  — emergency thoracentesis (if respiratory distress is too severe to wait for x-ray confirmation)
  — insertion of a chest tube into the pleural space and connection to closed-chest drainage (see "Closed Chest Drainage", p. 167)

— thoracotomy — surgical opening into the chest cavity. May be done to explore the chest and repair the site of origin of the pneumothorax.

(For more information, see p. 1575 of Polaski and Tatro, *Luckmann's Core Principles and Practice of Medical-Surgical Nursing.*)

Pneumothorax, Open

- An open pneumothorax occurs with "sucking" chest wounds. A traumatic opening in the chest wall is large enough for air to move freely in and out of the chest cavity during ventilation. This abnormal movement of air through the chest wound produces a "slurping" or "sucking" noise.
- Open sucking chest wounds may occur from accidental injuries or surgical trauma.
- Treatment
  - The wound must be immediately covered with anything available, e.g., a towel. Ask someone to bring a sterile petroleum gauze dressing. Apply this to replace the temporary covering, as soon as possible.
  - When covering the wound, ask the client to take a deep breath and attempt to blow it out while keeping the mouth and nose closed. When the client does this, apply the dressing before the client can inhale. This forces air out the wound.
- After the dressing is applied, stay with the client. Assess closely for signs/symptoms of tension pneumothorax and mediastinal shift. This may develop if the air leak is in the lung or bronchus which permits air to escape into the pleural space. In such a situation, closing the chest wound prevents the outflow of escaping air. Thus, an open pneumothorax has been converted into a tension pneumothorax, which is a more dangerous situation. If it appears that a tension pneumothorax is developing after sealing the wound, immediately remove the seal.

- Closed chest drainage will be necessary to remove air from the pleural space to allow lung re-expansion (see "Closed Chest Drainage", p. 167).

Also see "Pneumothorax, Tension and Mediastinal Shift", p. 522.

(For more information, see pp. 1576-1577 of Polaski and Tatro, *Luckmann's Core Principles and Practice of Medical-Surgical Nursing.*)

Pneumothorax, Tension and Mediastinal Shift

- Tension pneumothorax is a serious type of pneumothorax in which air enters the pleural space with each inspiration, becomes trapped there and is not expelled during expiration. Pressure continues to build in the chest and may collapse the lung on the affected side which then may cause a mediastinal shift. A mediastinal shift occurs when the contents of the mediastinum (heart, trachea, esophagus and great vessels) are pushed or "shifted" toward the unaffected side of the chest.
- Mediastinal shift may cause:
  — compression of the lung opposite the pneumothorax
  — compression, traction, torsion or kinking of the great vessels
  — decreased cardiac output and blood pressure
- Common causes of tension pneumothorax are blunt traumatic injuries and flail chest injuries.
- Tension pneumothorax produces serious circulatory and pulmonary impairment that can be rapidly fatal and is an emergency requiring prompt assessment and intervention.
- Clinical manifestations include:
  — marked, severe dyspnea
  — tachypnea, tachycardia
  — crepitus (subcutaneous emphysema in the neck and upper chest)
  — progressive cyanosis

- — chest pain on the affected side
- — asymmetric chest wall movement
- — diminished or absent breath sounds on the affected side
- — neck vein distention
- — PMI (point of maximal impulse) shift laterally or medially
- — muffled heart sounds
- — laryngeal and tracheal deviation/shift to the unaffected side
- Management

    The goal is to convert the tension pneumothorax into an open pneumothorax (a less serious disorder).

    - — insertion of an 18-gauge needle into the pleural space at the level of the second intercostal space at the midclavicular line to remove air
    - — insertion of a chest catheter and connection to a waterseal drainage system after emergency treatment

    Also see, "Closed Chest Drainage", p. 167.

(For more information, see pp. 1575-1576 of Polaski and Tatro, *Luckmann's Core Principles and Practice of Medical-Surgical Nursing.*)

Poisoning and Overdose

- Accidental or intentional poisonings (overdoses) requiring emergency care occur frequently.
- Poison Control Centers, the Poison Index and toxicology texts may be consulted for full information about various toxins.
- Emergency nursing care:
    - — Obtain an accurate history.
    - — Assess and stabilize airway, breathing and circulation.
    - — Start intravenous lines, insert a urinary catheter, initiate an ECG monitor and obtain appropriate laboratory studies.
    - — Induce emesis *if appropriate*.

- — Client must have an intact gag reflex and be able to cooperate with emetic therapy.
- — Syrup of ipecac is the safest and most effective way to induce emesis (home remedies are often unsafe and ineffective).
- — Syrup of ipecac must be preceded or followed by several hundred milliliters of water or other solution (juice).
- — Emesis should occur within fifteen to twenty minutes. A second dose may be given, but do not exceed two doses. It is important that enough oral fluid be given to prevent retching and possible esophageal tears.
- — Emesis is saved for toxicologic analysis; note the presence of any pill particles.
- — Syrup of ipecac in large doses may be cardiotoxic. If the client does not vomit, lavage may be necessary.
- — Reassess the client frequently. If the client becomes more obtunded, gastric lavage may need to be performed because of the risk of aspiration with emesis.
- Gastric lavage may be indicated for clients with a diminished or absent gag reflex; central nervous system depression; or those unable to cooperate with emetic therapy.
- Absorptives, such as activated charcoal, may be used.
- Antidotes/antagonists may be used in selected cases for management or diagnosis of the toxic substance. Remember that the half-life of the substance may be longer than the antidote.
- Diuresis, fluid loading, cooling or warming, anticonvulsive therapy, antidysrhythmic therapy, hemodialysis or exchange transfusions also may be necessary.
- If the overdose was intentional:
  - — Facilitate psychiatric consult.
  - — Provide empathy and understanding and foster communication.
  - — Implement suicide precautions.
  - — Arrange for someone to stay with the client for the first several days after discharge.
  - — Provide a telephone number for crisis intervention, if the client does not wish to have them contacted while hospitalized.

— Provide written instructions for follow-up.
- For accidental overdoses, provide clear instructions for needed follow-up and signs/symptoms to report to physician.

(For more information, see pp. 1589-1591 of Polaski and Tatro, *Luckmann's Core Principles and Practice of Medical-Surgical Nursing.*)

Poliomyelitis, Acute Anterior (Polio)

- Acute anterior poliomyelitis (polio) is characterized by destruction of motor cells (particularly of the anterior horn cells in the spinal cord and brain stem) and flaccid paralysis of muscles innervated by affected neurons. Poliomyelitis spreads from the gastrointestinal tract to the nervous system.
- Associated paralysis may or may not occur. Paralysis may be spinal or bulbar. Spinal paralysis is flaccid, asymmetric and scattered in distribution. Bulbar paralysis involves the muscles supplied by the cranial nerves because bulbar nuclei are affected. These muscles may be paralyzed alone or in combination with spinal musculature. Bulbar paralysis is often unilateral. Respiratory muscle paralysis also can occur. Clients may need mechanical ventilation.
- Clinical manifestations include headache, stiff neck, fever and asymmetric flaccid paralysis without sensory loss.
- Immunization with the trivalent oral poliomyelitis vaccine in infancy is the best means of prevention.
- There is a recently recognized disorder affecting victims of polio called "post-polio syndrome." It is characterized by new onset of progressive muscle weakness, fatigue, decreased endurance, pain in the joints and muscles and respiratory problems beginning thirty or more years after the original attack. The etiology and pathophysiology are not well understood. Clients with post-polio syndrome need much support.

(For more information, see p. 363 of Polaski and Tatro, *Luckmann's Core Principles and Practice of Medical-Surgical Nursing.*)

Polycythemia

OVERVIEW

- Polycythemia is defined as an increase in both the numbers of circulating erythrocytes and the concentration of hemoglobin within the blood. Red blood cells may number as high as 8 to 12 million/mm³, and the hemoglobin concentration rises to 18 to 25 g/100 ml.
- Polycythemia vera is classified as a myeloproliferative disorder (meaning overgrowth of bone marrow). The precise cause remains unknown. The three major hallmarks are (1) relentless, unrestrained production of erythrocytes, (2) excessive production of myelocytes (in the bone marrow), and (3) overproduction of platelets. This inordinate mass production results in (1) an increase in blood viscosity, (2) an increase in total blood volume, and (3) severe blood congestion of all tissues and organs.
- Polycythemia vera usually develops during middle age, particularly among Jewish men.
- Secondary polycythemia occurs when the body's demand for oxygen increases, and the bone marrow must produce more red cells in order to prevent hypoxia. Polycythemia may be precipitated by conditions that cause prolonged hypoxia, such as:
  — chronic lung disease
  — congenital heart disease
  — prolonged exposure to altitudes of 10,000 feet or more.

CLINICAL MANIFESTATIONS

Polycythemia Vera

- asymptomatic — early stage
- feeling of fullness in the head
- epistaxis
- dizziness, headache, tinnitus, visual disturbances
- ruddy complexion
- dusky red mucosa
- hypertension

- shortness of breath, orthopnea (due to congestive heart failure)
- evidence of thrombotic event (due to cerebral vascular accident, myocardial infarction, peripheral gangrene)
- bleeding tendencies and ecchymosis
- enlargement of liver and spleen
- painful, swollen joints (gout) — secondary to increased uric acid
- distended superficial blood vessels

SECONDARY POLYCYTHEMIA

- same as polycythemia vera except white blood cell and platelet counts are normal and splenic enlargement is absent

MEDICAL MANAGEMENT

POLYCYTHEMIA VERA

- phlebotomy — removal of 500 to 2000 ml of blood until hematocrit reaches 45 per cent
- myelosuppressive agents — radioactive phosphorus, chlorambucil, busulfan, hydroxyurea
- anticoagulant therapy
- radiation therapy — to decrease the production of red blood cells in the marrow

SECONDARY POLYCYTHEMIA

- treatment of underlying disease or condition causing hypoxia

NURSING MANAGEMENT

- Assist with phlebotomy and monitor hemodynamic status post procedure.
- Administer prescribed medications.
- Monitor vital signs and breath sounds.
- Assess for signs/symptoms of a thrombotic event.
- Encourage oral intake (to reduce blood viscosity).
- Monitor for signs of bleeding (if on anticoagulant therapy).
- Monitor laboratory findings — CBC, platelet count, prothrombin time.

- Prevent thrombi secondary to circulatory stasis:
  — encourage client to ambulate
  — elevate feet when possible
  — instruct to wear support hose
  — turn bedridden client frequently and exercise extremities
- Initiate appropriate safety measures.
- See "Radiation Therapy", p. 543.
- See "Chemotherapy", p. 145.

FOCUSED DISCHARGE CARE

Instruct the client regarding:
- importance of medication regime
- signs/symptoms to report to physician
- safety measures to prevent bleeding if on anticoagulant therapy (soft toothbrush, electric razor, fall prevention, etc.)
- increased fluid intake unless otherwise contraindicated
- importance of regular exercise
- importance of follow-up appointments

(For more information, see pp. 852-854 of Polaski and Tatro, *Luckmann's Core Principles and Practice of Medical-Surgical Nursing.*)

Polyps (Uterine or Cervical)

- Polyps are pedunculated tumors arising from the mucosa and extending into the opening of a body cavity. They occasionally may undergo malignant changes.
- Cervical polyps may bleed following vaginal intercourse and are prone to infection.
- Uterine polyps may cause hypermenorrhea, intermenstrual bleeding and postmenopausal bleeding.
- Cervical polyps may be removed in the physician's office.
- Uterine polyps are not easily removed because of their location within the uterus.

(For more information, see p. 1489 of Polaski and Tatro, *Luckmann's Core Principles and Practice of Medical-Surgical Nursing.*)

Portal Hypertension

OVERVIEW

- Portal hypertension is a persistent increase in blood pressure within the portal venous system of the liver as a result of increased resistance or obstruction of the blood flow through the portal venous system.
- The normal flow to and from the liver depends on proper functioning of the portal vein (inflow), hepatic artery (inflow) and the hepatic veins (outflow).
- Disease processes that damage or alter the flow of blood through the liver or its major vessels are responsible for the development of portal hypertension.
- Cirrhosis is the leading cause of portal hypertension. Hepatic tumors or obstruction of the portal vein by a thrombus are other common causes.
- Complications arising from portal hypertension include:
  - (1) hemorrhage — portal pressure causes swollen dilated veins (varices) of the superior rectal veins, abdominal wall veins and esophagogastric veins. These varices may rupture and bleed. Portal pressure also causes damage to the spleen. As the spleen enlarges, it tends to destroy blood cells, especially platelets, which increases the risk of hemorrhage and anemia.
  - (2) hepatic encephalopathy — this may follow a period of bleeding into the gastrointestinal tract. Digestion of this blood takes place in the intestines. Because blood is a protein substance, this process increases ammonia in the gut and bloodstream. Excessive ammonia disturbs brain function.

CLINICAL MANIFESTATIONS

- tortuous epigastric vessels visible through the skin that branch off the umbilicus and lead toward the sternum and ribs
- enlarged palpable spleen
- hemorrhoids
- ascites
- bruits

MEDICAL MANAGEMENT

- propranolol (Inderal) to reduce portal pressure
- vasopressin (Pitressin) — directly infused into the superior mesenteric artery to lower portal pressure
- sclerotherapy — passing an endoscope into the esophagus and injecting a sclerosing agent that flows to the varices
  - causes inflammation of the vein wall; this results in fibrosis

To treat hemorrhage:
- direct ligation of bleeding varices
- transhepatic embolization of the left gastric vein
- insertion of a Sengstaken-Blakemore or Minnesota tube
  - the tube is passed into the stomach and then the esophageal and gastric balloons are inflated
  - the pressure of the balloon against the varices may stop the bleeding

SURGICAL MANAGEMENT

- creation of a portosystemic shunt — sends portal blood directly into the inferior vena cava bypassing the liver, thus reducing portal hypertension. However, this process increases the incidence of hepatic encephalopathy because the shunted blood is not cleansed of toxic substances.

NURSING MANAGEMENT

MEDICAL

- Monitor daily weights.
- Measure abdominal girth daily.
- Monitor fluid balance.

- Monitor for signs/symptoms of bleeding or hemorrhage.
- Monitor hemoglobin, hematocrit and blood ammonia levels.
- Monitor for signs/symptoms of hepatic encephalopathy:
  — mental confusion
  — impaired memory or attention span
  — decreased concentration or rate of response
  — change in level of consciousness
  — drowsiness with sleep pattern reversal (awake at night, sleepy during the day)
  — change in handwriting or speech
  — asterixis (rapid extension and flexion of the fingers and wrists when the arms are extended and the hands are dorsiflexed — also called "liver flap")
- If hemorrhage occurs, monitor blood pressure, pulse, respirations and urine output continually and assist with interventions to restore blood volume.
- Monitor for side effects of vasopressin: hyponatremia, myocardial ischemia, stimulation of uterine and gastrointestinal contraction (cramping and diarrhea).
- Maintain Sengstaken-Blakemore/Minnesota tube:
  — Periodically deflate esophageal balloon as ordered to prevent esophageal necrosis.
  — Provide suction to remove secretions and saliva that accumulate above the balloon level to prevent aspiration. (The Minnesota tube has a fourth port for this; if no suction port is present, a nasogastric tube may be passed to the balloon level to allow for suctioning.)
  — Label each port of the balloon.
  — Cleanse and lubricate the nares to prevent erosion of the nares.
  — Keep emergency scissors at the bedside — if airway obstruction occurs, the tube must be cut and pulled out immediately. (Airway obstruction can occur if the gastric balloon deflates or breaks and the esophageal balloon migrates up to the oropharynx.)
- Instruct client on factors that may cause rupture of varices and must be avoided:
  — coughing, straining at stools or any other activities that increase intra-abdominal or intrathoracic pressure

— spicy or rough foods that may irritate the esophageal mucosa

PORTOSYSTEMIC SHUNT SURGERY

In addition to routine postoperative care:
- Monitor for postoperative hemorrhage.
- Monitor cardiovascular function carefully due to the increased venous return to the heart.
- Monitor for hepatic encephalopathy.

FOCUSED DISCHARGE CARE

- Instruct client/significant other regarding:
  — factors that may rupture varices
  — signs/symptoms of bleeding
  — what to do, who to call if hemorrhage occurs
  — signs/symptoms of hepatic encephalopathy
  — when to contact physician
  — shunt care (if performed)
- Refer to alcoholic treatment program or support groups as needed

See also "Hepatic Encephalopathy", p. 315, and "Cirrhosis", p. 164.

(For more information, see pp. 1026-1029 of Polaski and Tatro, *Luckmann's Core Principles and Practice of Medical-Surgical Nursing*.)

Prostate Cancer

OVERVIEW

- Prostate cancer is the most common cancer among men, and the third leading cause of death among men in the United States.
- Most clients with clinically detectable prostate cancer are over age 50. A man's risk of prostate cancer increases with each decade after age 50.

- Annual digital rectal examination is recommended for all men over the age of 40 because colon and prostate cancer can be screened for at the same time.

CLINICAL MANIFESTATIONS

There may be no symptoms unless benign prostatic hyperplasia is also present because the tumor is usually found in the periphery of the posterior lobe.
- hip or back bone pain — late symptoms caused by metastases
- rectal pressure or obstruction from local tumor growth
- painful ejaculation
- hard nodule in the prostate

MEDICAL MANAGEMENT

- radiation therapy:
  — external
  — interstitial — using iodine (^{125}I) seed implants
  — combination of the above two methods
- androgen blockers — block the action or secretion of androgens which stimulate tumor growth — Eulexin, Zoladex
- estrogen preparations — suppress the release of pituitary gonadotropin and reduce serum testosterone levels — Diethylstilbestrol (DES)
- chemotherapy - Cytoxan, 5-FU, Adriamycin

SURGICAL MANAGEMENT

- transurethral resection for small, well defined tumors or to relieve obstruction
- radical prostatectomy — via a perineal or retropubic approach
- cryosurgery — an experimental surgery using liquid nitrogen at subzero temperatures inserted via tiny punctures into the prostate gland

NURSING MANAGEMENT

MEDICAL

- See "Chemotherapy", p. 145.

- See "Radiation Therapy", p. 543.

SURGICAL

- See "Benign Prostatic Hyperplasia", p. 77.

(For more information, see pp. 1458-1460 of Polaski and Tatro, *Luckmann's Core Principles and Practice of Medical-Surgical Nursing.*)

Prostatitis

OVERVIEW

- Prostatitis, inflammation of the prostate gland, may be (1) acute bacterial, (2) chronic bacterial, or (3) non-bacterial.
- Routes of infection include (1) urethral ascent, (2) descent from the urinary bladder or kidneys, (3) direct extension or lymphatogenous spread from the rectum, and (4) hematogenous spread (via blood).
- Bacterial prostatitis usually is caused by gram-negative rods, especially E. coli and Pseudomonas.

CLINICAL MANIFESTATIONS

- Bacterial
  — Acute:
    – chills and fever
    – low back and perineal pain
    – urinary frequency, urgency, nocturia, and dysuria
    – tender, swollen prostate
    – positive urine cultures identifying the infecting organism
  — Chronic — less severe inflammation:
    – may be asymptomatic but organisms found on routine urinalysis
    – urgency, frequency, nocturia, and dysuria
    – low back or perineal pain
    – myalgia and arthralgia

- Non-bacterial — most common form of prostatitis:
  - same symptoms as bacterial, but no causative organism is identified
  - prostate massage yields abnormal numbers of inflammatory cells

MEDICAL MANAGEMENT

- antimicrobial medications
- anti-inflammatory agents

SURGICAL MANAGEMENT

- rarely required

NURSING MANAGEMENT

MEDICAL

- Administer antibiotics as prescribed.
- Monitor intake and output.
- Encourage oral intake.
- Promote rest.
- Administer PRN analgesics.
- Offer sitz baths.
- Administer stool softeners, as constipation increases the pain of prostatitis.

FOCUSED DISCHARGE CARE

Instruct the client regarding:
- importance of completing antibiotic therapy
- need to maintain oral intake of 2000-3000 ml/day (unless otherwise contraindicated)

(For more information, see pp. 1460-1461 of Polaski and Tatro, *Luckmann's Core Principles and Practice of Medical-Surgical Nursing.*)

Psoriasis Vulgaris

OVERVIEW

- Psoriasis vulgaris is a chronic, recurrent, erythematous, inflammatory skin disorder. The term "vulgaris" means common.
- Rapidly proliferating epidermal cells form small, scaly patches of skin that develop into erythematous, dry scaling patches of various sizes. Psoriatic patches are covered with silvery white scales.
- The eruptions are usually symmetric and occur on the scalp, elbows, knees and sacral regions.
- The course of psoriasis is prolonged and unpredictable. Exacerbations and remissions are common, and anxiety and stress often precede flare-ups. Spontaneous clearing is uncommon.
- The cause is unknown.

MEDICAL MANAGEMENT

- natural sunlight or topical therapy including tar preparations and topical corticosteroids — for mild psoriasis
- injection of small diluted amounts of corticosteroids into or just below the lesion
- topical anthralin to lesions
- tar shampoos with keratolytic agents, followed by topical corticosteroid lotions
- whole body irradiation with ultraviolet light for widespread involvement
- etretinate (Tegison) — a vitamin A derivative used for pustular and erythrodermic psoriasis
- antimetabolites (e.g., Methotrexate) in small doses

NURSING MANAGEMENT

- Instruct client regarding:
  - use of medications — application and possible side effects
  - treatment regimen
  - use of anthralin
    - must not be used in women of childbearing age

- avoid contact with normal skin surrounding lesions
- may stain fabric, hair, skin, nails, furniture and bathroom fixtures
- importance of birth control for clients on antimetabolites
- prevention of infection in open lesions
- Provide psychological support and encourage ventilation of feelings about change in body image (smell of tar preparations or staining of skin may compound feelings).

(For more information, see pp. 1350-1351 of Polaski and Tatro, *Luckmann's Core Principles and Practice of Medical-Surgical Nursing.*)

Pulmonary Embolism

OVERVIEW

- Pulmonary embolism (PE) is an occlusion of a portion of the pulmonary blood vessels by an embolus. An embolus is a detached intravascular solid, liquid or gaseous mass that is carried by the bloodstream from its point of origin to a distant site.
- Emboli travel to the lungs and lodge in the pulmonary vasculature. Blood flow is obstructed, resulting in decreased perfusion of that section of the lung. The lung is still ventilated. A ventilation-perfusion mismatch occurs and hypoxemia results.
- Nearly 99 per cent of all emboli develop from thrombi (clots). Other sources include tumors, air, fat, bone marrow, amniotic fluid, septic thrombi and vegetations on heart valves that develop with endocarditis.
- The most common source of pulmonary emboli is venous thrombosis in the thigh and pelvis.
- Pulmonary embolism is one of the four most common causes of sudden death in the United States. The mortality rate for untreated PE is between 20 and 35 per cent.

- Risk factors include: surgery on or trauma to the lower legs or pelvis, immobility, obesity, estrogen replacement therapy and clotting abnormalities.
- Measures to reduce the risk of pulmonary embolism include early ambulation of clients, leg exercises for bedridden clients, avoidance of smoking and use of prophylactic heparin.

CLINICAL MANIFESTATIONS

- chest pain (usually pleuritic)
- dyspnea, tachypnea, apprehension
- cough, hemoptysis, crackles
- split second heart sound, tachycardia
- fever, diaphoresis, syncope

MEDICAL MANAGEMENT

- anticoagulation with heparin to raise the partial thromboplastin time (PTT) to 2 to 2.5 times normal
- initiation of coumadin about 3 days before heparin is stopped
- oxygen therapy
- inotropic agents and/or fluids for hypotension
- analgesics
- fibrinolytic therapy (controversial, may dissolve the clot but does not improve the mortality rate)

SURGICAL MANAGEMENT

- vein ligation to prevent the embolus from traveling to the heart
- vena cava plication (insertion of an umbrella filter to allow blood flow, but trap emboli)
- embolectomy—surgical removal of emboli from the pulmonary arteries. This is a very high risk surgery.

NURSING MANAGEMENT

- Monitor vital signs every 15 minutes until stable.
- Auscultate lung sounds every 2 to 4 hours.
- Auscultate heart sounds every 4 hours (assess for murmurs or extra heart sounds).
- Monitor for hypoxemia, respiratory compromise and hypotension.

- Monitor blood gas values.
- Place in semi-Fowler's position.
- Provide oxygen as ordered.
- Monitor for right-sided heart failure:
  — peripheral edema
  — distended neck veins
  — liver engorgement
- Monitor partial thromboplastin time (PTT) (goal is 2 to 2.5 times the normal value).
- Monitor for excessive anticoagulation: blood in urine or stool, petechiae, bruising, bleeding of gums, change in level of consciousness, flank pain, and coffee ground emesis.
- Avoid intramuscular and subcutaneous injections; no rectal temperatures or probes.
- Use soft toothbrush or foam toothettes for oral care.
- Provide emotional support.

FOCUSED DISCHARGE CARE

Instruct client regarding:
- signs/symptoms of change in respiratory status and to report to physician
- coumadin therapy:
  — measures to prevent bleeding/injury
  — avoidance of medications/foods that potentiate or interfere with coumadin
  — notification of all physicians/dentists that client is on anticoagulant therapy
  — signs/symptoms of overcoagulation or bleeding
  — importance of follow-up laboratory tests

(For more information, see pp. 620-623 of Polaski and Tatro, *Luckmann's Core Principles and Practice of Medical-Surgical Nursing.*)

Pyelonephritis, Acute

OVERVIEW

- Acute pyelonephritis is an inflammation of the renal pelvis caused by a bacterial infection.

- It often occurs after bacterial contamination of the urethra or after instrumentation, such as catheterization or cystoscopy.
- Risk factors include diabetes, hypertension, chronic renal calculi, or chronic cystitis.

CLINICAL MANIFESTATIONS

- high fever, chills, nausea, headaches and muscular pain
- flank pain on the affected side, often radiating down the ureter or toward the epigastrium
- dysuria, frequency, urgency
- cloudy, bloody, or foul smelling urine
- costovertebral angle tenderness

MEDICAL MANAGEMENT

- parenteral antibiotics (specific to the causative organism) for 3-5 days until the client is afebrile for 24-48 hours. Oral administration follows for 2-4 weeks.
- elimination of any contributing factors (such as calculi)

SURGICAL MANAGEMENT

- Surgery is done only to correct any underlying defects that caused the pyelonephritis.

NURSING MANAGEMENT

MEDICAL

- Administer antibiotic therapy as prescribed.
- Monitor results of culture and sensitivity tests.
- Monitor intake and output.
- Assess for adequate hydration without overhydrating, as this may dilute the effectiveness of antimicrobials.
- Administer analgesics, anti-emetics, and antipyretics as prescribed.
- Also see, "Urinary Tract Infection", p. 641.

FOCUSED DISCHARGE CARE

Instruct client regarding:

- completing the full course of antibiotic therapy
- need for compliance with follow-up urine cultures, since bacteriuria may be asymptomatic
- ways to prevent further urinary tract infection (see, "Urinary Tract Infection", p. 641)
- signs/symptoms of urinary tract infections and to report these to physician immediately.

(For more information, see pp. 951-952 of Polaski and Tatro, *Luckmann's Core Principles and Practice of Medical-Surgical Nursing.*)

Pyelonephritis, Chronic

OVERVIEW

- Chronic pyelonephritis is an inflammation of the renal pelvis caused by a bacterial infection. It usually occurs with chronic disorders or after chronic obstruction with reflux. Fibrosis and scar tissue develop, altering tubular reabsorption and secretion which lead to decreased renal function. It is a slowly progressive disease associated with acute attacks.
- Risk factors include diabetes, hypertension, chronic renal calculi, or chronic cystitis.

CLINICAL MANIFESTATIONS

- no specific symptoms except hypertension

MEDICAL MANAGEMENT

- antibiotics
- antihypertensive medications
- prevention of further renal damage

SURGICAL MANAGEMENT

- Surgery is done only to correct any underlying defects that caused the pyelonephritis.

NURSING MANAGEMENT

- See "Pyelonephritis, Acute", p. 539.

FOCUSED DISCHARGE CARE

- See "Pyelonephritis, Acute", p. 539.

(For more information, see pp. 951-952 of Polaski and Tatro, *Luckmann's Core Principles and Practice of Medical-Surgical Nursing.*)

R

Radiation Therapy

OVERVIEW

- One-half of all clients with cancer receive radiation therapy (RT) at some point during their disease course.
- Radiation therapy is the use of high-energy, ionizing rays that destroy the cell's ability to reproduce by damaging the cell's DNA. Rapidly dividing cells, such as some cancer cells, are more vulnerable to radiation than are slower dividing cells.
- Three treatment modalities for radiation therapy are:
  — primary treatment modality
    — radiation therapy is the only treatment used and provides local cure of the cancer
  — adjuvant treatment modality
    — in conjunction with surgery, either preoperatively or postoperatively
    — in conjunction with chemotherapy to treat disease in sites not readily accessible to systemic chemotherapy, such as the brain
  — palliative treatment modality
    — to relieve pain due to obstruction, pathologic fracture, or spinal cord compression
- Types of radiation therapy:
  — external radiation therapy
    — administered by high energy x-ray or radioisotope machines
    — the maximum effect of radiation occurs within the tumor, not on the skin surface
  — internal radiation therapy
    — placement of radioisotopes directly into or near the tumor itself (sealed source) or into the systemic circulation (unsealed source) by injection or oral route

- Factors that determine side effects are:
  — size of the treatment area
  — the area of the body being irradiated
  — total dose of radiation
- Interventions to limit side effects:
  — fractionating the total dose into small frequent doses
    — increases the probability that tumor cells will be in a vulnerable phase of the cell cycle
    — allows normal cells time to repair themselves
  — alternating the sites of entry (ports) of radiation
  — customized shielding blocks
- Radiation safety — consists of three principles to protect caregivers from excessive radiation:
  — distance – greater the distance from the radiation source, the less exposure
  — time – the less time spent close to source, the less exposure
  — use of shields – provides a block between radiation source and caregiver

NURSING MANAGEMENT

EXTERNAL RADIATION

- Monitor for skin changes over area of radiation.
- Monitor for side effects of radiation therapy (are dependent upon the specific area being irradiated):
  — nausea, vomiting, diarrhea
  — cystitis
  — diminished blood counts
  — edema or inflammation of the brain or spinal cord
  — pneumonitis
- Schedule activities to allow for rest periods.
- Encourage a well balanced diet.

INTERNAL RADIATION

Sealed source differs from unsealed sources in that the radioisotope is completely enclosed by nonradioactive material. Consequently, the client's excretions (urine, sweat, blood or vomitus) are not radioactive.

Sealed Source:
- Place client in a private room.

- Plan care so minimal time is spent in direct contact with the client.
- Use a lead apron or lead shield while in the room.
- Mark the room with appropriate signage.
- Check all linen for presence of foreign bodies.
- Keep long-handled forceps and lead-lined container in client's room.
- Minimize exposure by not exceeding the specified time limitation for the shift.
- Maintain time exposure limitations for visitors and other personnel.
- Maintain bedrest and utilize pressure-relieving devices.
- Check that the applicator is properly placed.
  — if dislodged, use forceps to place in a lead container

Unsealed Source:
- Place client in a private room.
- Maintain and enforce time and distance restrictions and wearing of protective gown, gloves and shoe covers for yourself, visitors and other personnel.
- Instruct client to flush toilet several times after use (isotope may be excreted in body fluid).
- Use disposable dishes and utensils.
- Use telephone or intercom to communicate with patient to decrease time of exposure.

FOCUSED DISCHARGE CARE

Instruct client regarding:
External Radiation
- skin care
- management of side effects
- importance of follow-up appointments

Internal Radiation
Sealed Source:
- perineal care
- importance of follow-up visits

Unsealed Source:
- avoidance of crowds initially
- importance of clinic and laboratory follow-up

(For more information, see pp. 6-9 of Polaski and Tatro, *Luckmann's Core Principles and Practice of Medical-Surgical Nursing.*)

Raynaud's Disease

OVERVIEW

- Raynaud's phenomenon is characterized by intermittent episodes during which small arteries or arterioles in the extremities constrict, causing temporary pallor and cyanosis of the digits and changes in skin temperature. These episodes occur in response to cold temperature or strong emotion.
- Raynaud's disease is a primary vasospastic disorder. If the disorder is secondary to another disease or underlying cause, the term "Raynaud's phenomenon" is used.
- Criteria for diagnosing primary Raynaud's disease include:
  — intermittent attacks of pallor or cyanosis of the digits with exposure to cold or emotional stimuli.
  — bilateral or symmetric involvement
  — no evidence of occlusive disease or systemic disease that may be causing the changes
  — gangrene which (when it occurs) is limited to the skin of the tips of digits
  — history of manifestations for at least 2 years
- Raynaud's disease appears to be caused by (1) a hypersensitivity of digital arteries to cold, (2) release of serotonin, and (3) congenital predisposition.
- Eighty per cent of clients with Raynaud's disease are women between twenty and forty-nine years of age.

CLINICAL MANIFESTATIONS

- feelings of cold, numbness and pain and finally intense redness accompanied by tingling and throbbing of the digits
- color changes of the digits from pallor to cyanosis
- gangrene which is limited to the skin of the tips of the digits

MEDICAL MANAGEMENT

- smoking cessation
- vasodilator therapy

SURGICAL MANAGEMENT

- sympathetic ganglionectomy — excision of a ganglion in the sympathetic nervous pathway to produce vasodilation

NURSING MANAGEMENT

- Administer vasodilator therapy.
- Provide warm environment.
- Instruct on relaxation techniques.

FOCUSED DISCHARGE CARE

Instruct client regarding:
- disease process and treatment regime
- importance of managing stress
- measures to avoid cold exposure
- smoking cessation programs
- limitation of caffeine and chocolate in diet
- safety measures related to orthostatic hypotension (vasodilator therapy)

(For more information, see pp. 808-809 of Polaski and Tatro, *Luckmann's Core Principles and Practice of Medical-Surgical Nursing.*)

Renal Calculi

OVERVIEW

- Renal calculi are stones formed in the kidney.
- Stones may be of one crystalline type or a combination of types. Types include:
  — calcium (due to hypercalciuria)
  — oxalate (may be closely related to diet)
  — struvite (composed of calcium, magnesium and ammonium phosphate)
    — cause is bacteria, usually proteus

— uric acid stones (cause is increased urine excretion, fluid depletion and a low urinary pH)
- Risk factors include urinary stasis or supersaturation (increased concentration) of the urine. Stasis may be caused by immobility; supersaturation may be caused by dehydration or an increase in calcium or other ions. Alteration in purine metabolism (e.g., gout) is a risk factor for uric acid stones.

CLINICAL MANIFESTATIONS

- severe, sharp pain of sudden onset
- renal colic — lumbar pain radiating to bladder (female) or testicles (male)
- ureteral colic — pain radiates to genitalia and thigh
- pain may last minutes to days or be intermittent
- nausea, vomiting, pallor, diaphoresis
- pain also may be dull, aching or heavy

MEDICAL MANAGEMENT

- cystoscopy with placement of ureteral catheters to drain urine proximal to the stone and dilate the ureter to prompt passage of the stone
- cystoscopy with use of ureteral catheters to mechanically guide stones downward for removal
- chemical irrigation to dissolve the stone
- use of special catheters with loops and expanding baskets through a cystoscope to snare the stone
- extracorporeal lithotripsy - administration of electrically generated shock waves to the area of the stone in order to fracture it
- medications to lower uric acid for uric acid stones (such as allopurinol)

SURGICAL MANAGEMENT

- percutaneous lithotripsy — involves insertion of tubes into the area of stone formation. A contrast dye is injected, and forceps are used to remove the stones. Ultrasonic waves are used to break up stones for easier removal.
- nephroscope — may be used for small stones. The stone is removed by alligator forceps or a stone basket through a nephroscope inserted percutaneously.

- an open surgical procedure is needed, if the above measures fail

NURSING MANAGEMENT

- Administer antispasmodics and narcotics to control pain and assess effectiveness.
- Strain all urine through a strainer or gauze pad. (Stones may be as small as sand. Rubbing the material of the strainer between 2 gloved fingers may help detect small stones.)
- Force fluids.
- Monitor intake and output.
- Instruct client to void every two hours.

FOCUSED DISCHARGE CARE

Instruct client regarding:
- prevention of recurrence:
  — maintain fluid intake to ensure 2500 to 3000 ml of urine output daily
  — dietary restrictions based on stone analysis:
    — calcium stones — limit calcium and phosphate intake
    — oxalate stones — avoid tea, instant coffee, chocolate, cola drinks, beer, rhubarb, beans, cabbage, apples, grapes, peanuts, peanut butter
    — uric acid stones — low purine diet and avoid wine, cheese, organ meats
  — medications to prevent recurrence based on stone analysis
  — need to void every two hours
  — maintaining acidic urine
- signs/symptoms of recurrence and to report to physician
- need for follow-up urinalysis and laboratory tests

(For more information, see pp. 975-980 of Polaski and Tatro, *Luckmann's Core Principles and Practice of Medical-Surgical Nursing.*)

Renal Cancer

OVERVIEW

- Renal cell carcinoma (adenocarcinoma) accounts for 90% of all kidney neoplasms.
- Benign kidney tumors are rare; at least 85% of all renal tumors are malignant.
- Common sites of metastasis include: lungs, mediastinum, liver, bone, skin, spleen, and brain.
- The exact cause is unknown. There have been links established to tobacco, lead, cadmium and phosphate.

CLINICAL MANIFESTATIONS

Tumor growth may be advanced before the disease is discovered. Signs/symptoms may seem unrelated to the disease (e.g., abdominal mass).

- Hematuria (gross and intermittent), flank pain, and a palpable abdominal or flank mass.
- Less frequent signs/symptoms are fever, weight loss, fatigue, hypertension, anemia, abnormal serum liver profile, hypercalcemia, elevated sedimentation rate.

MEDICAL MANAGEMENT

- radiation therapy may be used in conjunction with chemotherapy and surgery.
- irradiation may be used for preoperative preparation of the tumor or postoperatively to destroy residual tumor or to treat lymphatic involvement or metastatic sites.
- chemotherapy
  — vinblastine is the most effective single agent

SURGICAL MANAGEMENT

- nephrectomy (removal of the kidney) is the conventional and principal intervention for renal cancer, although radiation and chemotherapy may be used as adjuncts to surgical removal.
- radical nephrectomy (removal of the kidney, adrenal gland, and perinephric fat with the retroperitoneal lymphatics) is the surgical procedure of choice for renal cell carcinoma.

NURSING MANAGEMENT

MEDICAL

- For general care during irradiation or chemotherapy, see "Radiation Therapy", p. 543 and "Chemotherapy", p. 145.

SURGICAL

POSTOPERATIVE CARE

In addition to routine postoperative care:
- Assist with coughing and deep breathing (this is painful for the client due to the close proximity of the incision to the diaphragm).
- Administer analgesics and position comfortably to control pain and facilitate coughing and deep breathing.
- Monitor closely for pneumothorax and paralytic ileus which may occur postoperatively.
- Monitor intake and output hourly, to ensure the remaining kidney is functioning adequately. Monitor closely for renal failure.
- Provide routine wound care.

FOCUSED DISCHARGE CARE

- depends upon the stage of cancer and the need for further treatment

(For more information, see pp. 980-982 of Polaski and Tatro, *Luckmann's Core Principles and Practice of Medical-Surgical Nursing.*)

Renal Failure, Acute (ARF)

OVERVIEW

- Acute renal failure (ARF) refers to the abrupt loss of kidney function. Over a period of hours to a few days the glomerular filtration rate falls, and serum creatinine and urea nitrogen levels rise.
- Causes are divided into 3 major categories:
  — Pre-renal — interferes with renal perfusion

- includes hypotension, fluid volume shifts, circulatory volume depletion, decreased cardiac output, increased vascular resistance and vascular obstruction
- Renal — parenchymal changes from disease or nephrotoxic substances
  - includes acute tubular necrosis, infectious disease, diabetes, hypokalemia, phosphatemia and glomerulonephritis
- Post renal — obstruction in the urinary tract
  - includes prostatic hypertrophy, calculi, and tumors
- Risk factors include hypovolemia, hypotension and nephrotoxic agents.
- ARF has several phases:
  - Onset phase — from precipitating event to development of renal symptoms
  - Oliguric-anuric or nonoliguric phase — this second phase lasts 1 to 8 weeks and is either oliguric (urine production falls below 400 ml/day) or nonoliguric (urine production may be as much as 2 L/day)
  - Diuretic phase — urine output may be 1,000 to 2,000 ml/day; glomerular filtration returns and leveling of the blood urea nitrogen (BUN) occurs
  - Recovery phase — lasts 3-12 months; return to pre-renal failure level

CLINICAL MANIFESTATIONS

- Nonoliguric Renal Failure:
  - urine output up to 2,000 ml/day
  - dilute urine
  - hypertension
  - tachypnea
  - fluid overload
- Oliguric Renal Failure — urine production below 400 ml/day
  The signs and symptoms vary depending upon whether the cause of renal failure is pre-renal, renal, or post-renal.
  - Pre-renal:
    - high specific gravity of urine
    - little or no proteinuria
    - elevated BUN:CR ratio
  - Intrinsic-renal:
    - fixed specific gravity
    - high sodium concentration of urine

- proteinuria
- weight gain
- edema
- hemoptysis
- weakness
- hypertension
— Post-renal:
  - fixed specific gravity
  - elevated sodium concentration of urine
  - little or no proteinuria

MEDICAL MANAGEMENT

- dialysis
- fluid replacement
- electrolyte replacement
- diuretic therapy may be used, but is controversial
- early identification and treatment of infection
- high calorie, low protein diet, which also may be low in sodium and potassium

NURSING MANAGEMENT

- Strict intake and output.
- Monitor fluid status every 4 hours by assessing mucous membranes, skin turgor, apical pulses, vital signs with postural blood pressures, lung sounds, heart sounds and mental status.
- Daily or twice per day weights.
- Maintain fluid restriction as ordered and decrease thirst by providing frequent oral hygiene and lip ointment.
- Provide meticulous skin care, frequent turning, and protective mattress as needed.
- Protect from secondary infections and assess for early signs/symptoms of infection.
- Monitor for electrolyte imbalances, especially hyperkalemia.
- Monitor for pericarditis (occurs in 18% of renal failure clients).
- Monitor for anemia; administer packed red blood cells as ordered.
- Monitor for seizures (the seizure threshold is lowered due to the rising BUN).
- Discuss importance of prescribed diet, when appropriate.

FOCUSED DISCHARGE CARE

Instruct client/significant others regarding:
- renal function, signs/symptoms of renal failure and the need for ongoing treatment
- signs/symptoms of further renal damage or that client has progressed to chronic renal failure
- dietary modifications
- obtaining weights and intake and output
- need for follow-up appointments with nephrologist

(For more information, see pp. 958-962 of Polaski and Tatro, *Luckmann's Core Principles and Practice of Medical-Surgical Nursing.*)

Renal Failure, Chronic (CRF)

OVERVIEW

- Chronic renal failure (CRF) is a progressive reduction of functioning renal tissue such that the remaining kidney mass no longer can maintain the body's internal environment.
- Destruction of nephrons occurs with progressive loss of renal function. It may develop insidiously over many years or can occur as a result of acute renal failure (ARF) from which the client fails to recover.
- The most common causes of chronic renal failure are diabetic and hypertensive nephropathy, glomerulonephritis and chronic pyelonephritis.

CLINICAL MANIFESTATIONS

- Electrolyte Imbalances
  - hyponatremia is seen initially with hypernatremia in end stage disease
  - serum potassium remains normal until late in the disease when hyperkalemia may occur
  - hypocalcemia, hyperphosphatemia and elevated magnesium
- Metabolic Changes
  - rising serum BUN/creatinine

- proteinuria and serum hypoproteinemia
- carbohydrate intolerance
- elevated triglycerides
- metabolic acidosis
- impaired insulin production and metabolism
- Hematologic Changes
  - normocytic, normochromic anemia
- Gastrointestinal Changes
  - anorexia, nausea, vomiting
  - metallic, bitter or salty taste in the mouth
  - stomatitis, gingivitis, parotitis
- Immunologic Changes
  - increased susceptibility to infection
- Changes in Medication Metabolism
  - high risk for medication toxicity
- Cardiopulmonary Changes
  - hypertension
  - volume overload
  - pulmonary edema
- Musculoskeletal Changes:
  - bone demineralization
  - joint pain
- Integumentary Changes:
  - severe pruritus, dry skin, brittle hair and nails
  - peripheral neuropathy
- Reproductive Changes:
  - decreased libido
  - impotence in males
  - menstrual irregularities in females
- Psychosocial:
  - personality changes
  - labile emotions
  - withdrawal
  - depression

MEDICAL MANAGEMENT

- conservative interventions include: correction of contributing factors, controlling blood pressure, and adjusting the fluids and diet
- dialysis or renal transplantation eventually is needed by most clients. See "Dialysis", p. 215.
- electrolyte replacement
- diuretics in the early phase
- regulation of fluids and sodium
- sodium bicarbonate to correct acidosis

- erythropoietin — the primary treatment to correct anemia
- antihypertensive therapy
- dietary management depends upon the results of blood chemistries
- topical lotions, antihistamines and ultraviolet B light for pruritus

SURGICAL MANAGEMENT

- See "Renal Transplantation", p. 557.

NURSING MANAGEMENT

- Monitor for fluid volume deficit or overload.
  - obtain daily or twice daily weights.
  - assess skin turgor, mucous membranes.
  - monitor vital signs and orthostatic blood pressure.
  - strict intake and output.
- Monitor for electrolyte imbalances, especially hyperkalemia.
- Monitor for pericarditis and seizures.
- Maintain fluid restriction and instruct on methods to reduce thirst:
  - frequent oral hygiene
  - lip balms
  - ice chips or water in a spray bottle with judicious use.
- Arrange for dietary consultation to discuss dietary modifications.
- Implement measures to alleviate nausea, vomiting and stomatitis to improve appetite.
- Instruct on use of bran and stool softeners to relieve constipation.
- Discuss importance of balancing rest and activity.
- Provide and instruct client on meticulous skin care and measures to reduce dry skin and pruritus.
- Encourage client and significant other to discuss feelings regarding coping with long-term illness, changes in body image and uncertain future.
- Maintain safety precautions if changes in mentation are present.
- Protect from infection.
- See also "Dialysis", p. 215 and "Renal Transplantation", p. 557.

FOCUSED DISCHARGE CARE

- Instruct the client/significant other regarding:
  — how to monitor fluid status and signs/symptoms to report to physician
  — how to do daily weights and how to interpret relationship of weight loss/gain to need for sodium and water
  — how to take blood pressure
  — prevention of infection
  — need for meticulous skin and oral care
  — safety precautions if change in mentation present
  — medications and changes in medication metabolism
  — dietary regimen
  — importance of follow-up laboratory and physician appointments
  — also see information in "Nursing Management" on the previous page
- Provide referrals for patient and significant other for support and assistance in coping.

(For more information, see pp. 962-975 of Polaski and Tatro, *Luckmann's Core Principles and Practice of Medical-Surgical Nursing*.)

Renal Transplantation

OVERVIEW

- Renal transplantation is the surgical implantation of a human kidney as an intervention for irreversible kidney failure.
- Complications of transplantation may include graft rejection, infection, and urinary tract complications. Additional systems that may be affected include cardiovascular, respiratory, gastrointestinal, integumentary, and musculoskeletal.

NURSING MANAGEMENT

PREOPERATIVE CARE

In addition to routine preoperative care:
- Provide preoperative teaching and prepare donor and recipient for psychological reactions that may occur post-surgically. (The donor may feel anger over need to protect the remaining kidney or abandonment when the focus shifts to the recipient.)
- Instruct that dialysis will be performed, and immunosuppressive therapy started.

POSTOPERATIVE CARE

In addition to routine postoperative care:
- Monitor fluid status and maintain circulatory function.
  - Obtain weights as ordered.
  - Strict intake and output, hourly or half-hourly.
  - Monitor laboratory results, particularly electrolytes, BUN, creatinine, hemoglobin/hematocrit, WBC, and platelets.
  - Monitor vital signs, watch closely for hypertension.
- Monitor for signs/symptoms of graft rejection (fever, graft tenderness, anemia and malaise).
- Monitor for urinary tract complications, cardiac dysrhythmias and congestive heart failure.
- Protect from infection:
  - cough, turn and deep breathe every 2 hours
  - strict aseptic technique for wound or line care
  - meticulous oral care and antifungal mouthwashes as prescribed.
- Administer immunosuppressants as prescribed.
- Provide emotional support to assist client to incorporate new kidney as part of whole being.
- Provide education and counseling to client/significant other to assist with lifestyle and role changes. Make referrals as needed.

FOCUSED DISCHARGE CARE

- Instruct client/significant other regarding:
  - medications—purpose, dosage, administration, side effects and toxic effects

      — signs/symptoms of infection and rejection —report to physician if they occur
      — information about the transplant to give to dentists and other physicians
      — prevention of infection
      — signs/symptoms of other complications to report to physician
      — importance of compliance with follow-up appointments/laboratory tests
- Provide referrals as needed for psychosocial support.
- See also "Renal Failure, Chronic", p. 554.

(For more information, see pp. 970-971 of Polaski and Tatro, *Luckmann's Core Principles and Practice of Medical-Surgical Nursing.*)

Retinal Detachment

OVERVIEW

- Retinal detachment is the separation of the retina from the choroid layer, which is its blood supply. It may take the form of small holes or tears or the actual peeling of the retina from the choroid.
- The retina may become increasingly detached over a period of hours to years.
- The risk of detachment increases after the fourth decade and most often occurs between the ages of fifty and seventy.
- Predisposing factors to retinal detachment include:
  — cataract extraction
  — trauma
  — degeneration of the retina

CLINICAL MANIFESTATIONS

- sudden onset that may be accompanied by a burst of black spots or floaters (indicates bleeding has occurred)
- description of a shadow falling across the field of vision

- experiences flashes of light
- no pain

MEDICAL MANAGEMENT

None

SURGICAL MANAGEMENT

- cryopexy (use of a freezing probe) or photocoagulation (a laser light is focused on the epithelium which absorbs the light and converts it to heat) — used to seal hole if has not progressed to detachment
- scleral buckling — procedure used to place the retina back in contact with choroid
  - prior to the buckling, an intraocular injection of air and/or a sulfahexafluoride (SF6) gas bubble may be used to apply pressure on the retina from the inside of the eye. The air/gas bubble is slowly absorbed.

NURSING MANAGEMENT

PREOPERATIVE CARE

In addition to routine preoperative care:
- Maintain activity restrictions dependent upon size and location of detachment.
- Administer preoperative eye drops to dilate the pupil.
- Administer preoperative sedatives.

POSTOPERATIVE CARE

In addition to routine postoperative care:
- Maintain eye patch in place.
- Position as ordered if air/gas bubble injected (so that bubble can apply maximal pressure on the retina by the force of gravity).
- Administer PRN analgesics.
- Monitor for signs/symptoms of increased intraocular pressure (pain, nausea).
- Apply either warm or cold compresses for comfort.
- Administer postoperative medications:
  - IV Diamox to reduce increased intraocular pressure

— antibiotic-steroid combination eye drops to prevent infection and reduce inflammation
— cycloplegic agents to dilate the pupil and relax ciliary muscles
- Assist with ambulation and activities of daily living.

FOCUSED DISCHARGE CARE

Instruct client regarding:
- eye care
- measures to avoid increasing intraocular pressure:
  — no lifting of heavy objects
  — no bending at the waist
  — no straining with stool
  — avoidance of coughing and vomiting
- technique for instilling eye drops
- signs/symptoms of increased intraocular pressure (pain, nausea, decreased vision)
- signs/symptoms of infection (redness, swelling, drainage, blurred vision or pain)
- need to wear eye protection (shield or glasses)
- need to avoid air travel initially (if air/gas bubble injected) because air or gas will expand at high altitudes
- safety in the home environment
- need for follow-up appointments

(For more information, see pp.443-445 of Polaski and Tatro, *Luckmann's Core Principles and Practice of Medical-Surgical Nursing.*)

Rheumatoid Arthritis

OVERVIEW

- Arthritis is defined as joint inflammation. Rheumatoid arthritis (RA) is a progressive, chronic, systemic, inflammatory connective tissue disorder (collagen disease) affecting mainly the small peripheral joints in a pattern of symmetric distribution. RA, as a connective tissue disorder, may involve the collagen in lungs, heart, muscles, blood vessels, pleurae, or tendons.

- The pathologic processes involved in rheumatoid arthritis are Type III (immune complex) and Type IV (cell-mediated) reactions. If unarrested, pathologic changes progress through four stages: (1) synovitis — proliferative inflammation localized in the joint capsule, primarily in the synovial membrane, (2) pannus formation — inflammatory granulation tissue derived from synovial membrane extends over the articular surface into the joint interior, (3) fibrous ankylosis — subluxation and distortion of the affected joints, and (4) bony ankylosis — firm bony union develops as the fibrous tissue calcifies and changes into osseous tissue.
- Women are affected with rheumatoid arthritis 2 to 3 times more often than are men. Although it may occur at any age, rheumatoid arthritis is most common in people between the ages of 20 and 40.
- There are no specific risk factors for the development of RA. There are risk factors, however, for exacerbation of the disease, including the presence of physical and emotional stress.
- RA is a disease of remissions and exacerbations. Each exacerbation seems more difficult to treat than the previous one, with more residual damage occurring. Although permanent remission can occur, though rarely, rheumatoid arthritis is usually progressive and deformity producing.

CLINICAL MANIFESTATIONS

- red, warm, swollen, stiff and tender joints
- red palms, enlarged dorsal veins of the hand
- low-grade temperature
- guarded movement, limited range of motion and strength
- malaise and weight loss
- paresthesias of the hands and feet
- symptoms are worse in the morning and subside during the day with moderate activity
- painless subcutaneous nodules over bony prominences, especially near the elbow
- chronic deformities of the hands and feet

- depression and early afternoon fatigue

MEDICAL MANAGEMENT

- analgesics and anti-inflammatory agents
  — salicylates
  — non-steroidal anti-inflammatory medications—
  ibuprofen (Motrin), naproxen (Naprosyn),
  sulindac (Clinoril)
  — corticosteroids
  — gold salts
- immunosuppressive (cytotoxic) agents — methotrexate (blocks inflammatory process)
- prescribed rest
- physical therapy
- heat/cold compresses to inflamed joints

SURGICAL MANAGEMENT

- tendon transfer — prevents progressive deformity
  caused by muscle spasms
- osteotomy — excising or cutting through the bone in
  a joint or limb to relieve pressure
- joint replacement—implants composed of Vitallium,
  stainless steel, and polyurethene to replace affected
  joints in the hip, knee, shoulder, fingers, or toes

NURSING MANAGEMENT

MEDICAL

- Administer analgesics and anti-inflammants as pre-
  scribed.
- Maintain bedrest during acute episodes.
- Position client to prevent contractures.
- Perform activities and exercises as outlined by physi-
  cal therapy.
- Consult physical and occupational therapy for adap-
  tive devices.
- Encourage warm shower in A.M. to decrease stiff-
  ness.
- Monitor response to activity.
- Provide adequate rest periods.
- Apply cold/heat to inflamed joints. Never massage
  acutely inflamed joints, because this may aggravate
  the inflammation.

563

PREOPERATIVE CARE

In addition to routine preoperative care:
- Teach the client how to use crutches and/or walker and encourage practice.
- Assist to practice transfer technique from bed to chair.
- Instruct and assist to practice postoperative exercises.

POSTOPERATIVE CARE

In addition to routine postoperative care:
Total Hip Replacement
- Maintain affected leg in abducted position and straight alignment while recumbent.
- Encourage and supervise prescribed exercises.
- Prevent hip flexion greater than 90 degrees when positioning or transferring.
- Assess nerve function and circulation in affected leg every 1 to 2 hours.
- Institute measures to prevent thrombophlebitis:
    — support stockings
    — low-dose Heparin
    — sequential compression devices
    — in-bed exercises.
- Monitor white blood count, temperature, and incision site for signs of infection.
- Administer prophylactic antibiotics as prescribed (steroid therapy, cytotoxic therapy, and implantation of a foreign object put the client at risk for infection).
- Monitor for signs/symptoms of a pulmonary embolism or fat embolism:
    — respiratory distress
    — tachycardia
    — hypertension
    — tachypnea
    — fever
    — petechiae (fat embolism)
- Initiate weight-bearing and ambulation as ordered.

Total Knee Replacement
- Maintain knee in maximum extension.
- Encourage and supervise prescribed exercises.

564

- Maintain continuous passive motion machine as prescribed.
- Institute weight bearing and ambulation as ordered.
- Monitor for possible complications: thrombophlebitis, pulmonary embolism, fat embolism, infection, and adrenal insufficiency.

FOCUSED DISCHARGE CARE

Instruct the client regarding:
- techniques to reduce stress to joints, tendons, and ligaments:
  — monitor response to activity - if pain lasts more than one hour after activity, avoid that activity for awhile
  — alternate between light and heavy tasks
  — plan rest periods
  — assess the joints — if warm or swollen, use as little as possible
- importance of controlling emotional and physical stress
- importance of medication regime
  — advise to take salicylates and non-steroidal anti-inflammants with food or antacids
- prescribed exercises
- application of heat/cold compresses to inflamed joints

SURGICAL MANAGEMENT

- importance of not flexing hip greater than 90 degrees and avoiding extremes of internal rotation for six months to one year
- importance of prescribed exercises
- avoidance of actions that place a strain on the hip joint — excessive bending, heavy lifting, jogging, and jumping
- use of adaptive devices (crutches/walker) until full weight bearing is allowed
- driving restrictions
- importance of prophylactic antibiotics if undergoing procedures that may cause bacteremia, such as tooth extraction

(For more information, see pp. 219-230 of Polaski and Tatro, *Luckmann's Core Principles and Practice of Medical-Surgical Nursing.*)

Rhinoplasty

- Rhinoplasty is the surgical correction of external nose deformities. The incisions are made inside the nose.
- Types of procedures performed may include reshaping the bony dorsum of the nose, the tip of the nose and/or cartilage along the nares.
- Rhinoplasty usually is performed as day surgery under local anesthesia and sedation or general anesthesia.
- Postoperatively, assess for excessive swallowing which may be the only symptom of bleeding in a client sleepy from anesthetic.
- Discharge teaching - instruct the client on the following:
  — sleep with the head of bed elevated for one week
  — do not remove the external splint or nasal packing
  — do not blow the nose
  — sneeze only with the mouth open
  — remain on a soft diet for two days
  — avoid decongestant nasal sprays
  — it will take approximately three months before the client will be able to tell the final results of the surgery

(For more information, see pp. 1398-1399 of Polaski and Tatro, *Luckmann's Core Principles and Practice of Medical-Surgical Nursing.*)

S

Sciatic Nerve Injury

- Sciatica is severe, usually constant, pain in a lower extremity that occurs along the course of the sciatic nerve and its branches.
- There are many causes of sciatica, but in about 90 per cent of clients, the causes are ruptured intervertebral disc or osteoarthritis of the lumbosacral spine, producing mechanical pressure on the nerve or its spinal roots. Sciatic nerve injury can also result from incorrect medication injection technique.

CLINICAL MANIFESTATIONS

- pain begins in the buttocks and extends down the back of the thigh and leg to the ankle
- limited straight-leg raising on the affected side
- complete extension of leg not possible when thigh flexed on abdomen (Lasegue's sign)

TREATMENT

- treatment of the underlying cause

(For more information, see p. 414 of Polaski and Tatro, *Luckmann's Core Principles and Practice of Medical-Surgical Nursing.*)

Scleroderma

OVERVIEW

- Scleroderma is a connective tissue disorder characterized by fibrosis and degenerative changes of the

skin, synovium, digital arteries and small arteries of the internal organs.
- It is 2 to 3 times more common in women than men and occurs between the ages of 30 to 50 years.
- The cause is unknown, although abnormal serologic features suggest an altered immune status.
- Scleroderma typically progresses slowly. Death is usually from infection, renal failure or cardiac failure.

CLINICAL MANIFESTATIONS

- subcutaneous edema
- fever
- malaise
- thick, hide-like skin with loss of normal skin folds
- ulcerations around the fingertips
- polyarthritis and polyarthralgias
- dysphagia (secondary to esophageal dysfunction)
- hypermotility and malabsorption (secondary to fibrosis and atrophy of the gastrointestinal tract)
- low oxygen diffusing capacity (secondary to pulmonary fibrosis and decreased lung compliance)
- hypertension (secondary to renal involvement)
- vasospasms of small peripheral arteries (Raynaud's phenomenon)
- mild anemia

MEDICAL MANAGEMENT

- steroid therapy
- immunosuppressants

NURSING MANAGEMENT

- Provide measures to prevent skin breakdown.
- Administer analgesics.
- Initiate progressive activity program and monitor client response.
- Implement dietary modifications for dysphagia.
- Monitor laboratory results — renal profile, nutritional panel, blood counts, arterial blood gases.
- Provide restful environment.
- Apply heat/cold compresses to affected joints.

FOCUSED DISCHARGE CARE

Instruct client regarding:
- importance of medication regime
- skin breakdown prevention measures
- avoidance of activities that trigger pain associated with Raynaud's phenomenon, polyarthralgia, and polyarthritis:
  - respond to pain that lasts for more than one hour or two by stopping that particular activity
  - alternate light and heavy tasks
  - plan for rest
  - if joints are red or swollen, use them as little as possible
  - avoid extreme cold, wear gloves when hands are exposed to cold
  - eliminate smoking
- dietary modification
- importance of follow-up visits

(For more information, see p. 234 of Polaski and Tatro, *Luckmann's Core Principles and Practice of Medical-Surgical Nursing.*)

Scoliosis

OVERVIEW

- Scoliosis is defined as a lateral curvature of the spine when viewing from the posteroanterior view. Adult scoliosis is a spinal curvature existing after skeletal maturity.
- A curve may be present in any area of the spine — cervical, thoracic, thoracolumbar and lumbar. There is usually a second compensatory curve in the opposite direction.
- Adult scoliosis occurs in individuals aged forty years or older.
- Curves of less than 40 degrees, without symptoms, generally remain stable and do not require intervention.

CLINICAL MANIFESTATIONS

- shortness of breath and fatigue (thoracic spine curve)
- back pain
- decreased height
- cosmetic deformity

MEDICAL MANAGEMENT

- pain management

SURGICAL MANAGEMENT

- application of spinal instrumentation either through an anterior or posterior approach.
- bone grafted fusions
- The client may or may not have a partial body cast postoperatively and may or may not be placed on a Stryker or Foster frame.

NURSING MANAGEMENT

MEDICAL

- Administer analgesics as prescribed.

SURGICAL

POSTOPERATIVE CARE

In addition to routine postoperative care:
- Nursing care will depend on the type of surgical procedure.
- Consult physical therapy for activity/exercise instructions.

FOCUSED DISCHARGE CARE

Instruct client regarding:
- pain management
- management of postoperative immobilization device

(For more information, see p. 1298 of Polaski and Tatro, *Luckmann's Core Principles and Practice of Medical-Surgical Nursing.*)

Sexual Assault, Alleged

OVERVIEW

- "Alleged sexual assault" is the term health care providers are required to use when caring for clients who may be victims of rape. The client should be advised of this, to avoid the perception that the health care provider is insensitive.
- The goal of emergency care for these clients is to provide sensitive, thorough physical care, coupled with empathetic psychosocial support, and to carefully gather vital information and evidence that is usually legally evaluated.
- Sexual assault victims often experience both acute and long-term physical and psychological trauma. The psychological trauma, known as rape-trauma syndrome, may last only a few days to weeks or may last many years.

NURSING MANAGEMENT

- Assess and maintain airway, breathing and circulation. Assess for trauma to the larynx or mandible.
- Ensure privacy and explain to the client not to wash, gargle or douche until all necessary specimens are obtained.
- Obtain a detailed history and physical examination after explaining the need for detail.
- Perform thorough assessment, recording extent, location and treatment of all injuries. Pictures may be included.
- Provide emotional support throughout gynecological examination.
- Obtain specimens for laboratory studies, including cultures for gonorrhea; hanging drop analysis and smears for the presence of sperm and their motility; acid phosphatase of vaginal secretions; analysis of foreign pubic hairs by the police laboratory and serologic fluorescent treponemal antibody studies.
- Ask the client's permission to contact a sexual assault counselor. Be aware that relative calmness or seeming unconcern does not mean that the client is handling it well.

- Note the condition of the client's clothing and document tears, stains or dishevelment. Make arrangements for clean clothes to be brought to the client and place torn clothes in a bag for the police.
- Administer penicillin, 4.8 million units intramuscularly, 30 minutes after one gram of oral probenecid for venereal disease prophylaxis, as prescribed.
- A short course of contraceptive pills may be used if pregnancy is suspected.
- Suggest that someone stay with the client after the event for support.
- Document carefully the history, assessment, interventions and discharge teaching.

FOCUSED DISCHARGE CARE

Instruct client regarding:
- follow-up care in four to six weeks for test results, pregnancy test and psychosocial support
- the name and number of rape counseling resources if the client is unable or unwilling to use counseling resources at the time of emergency treatment (the client may later desire this information)
- possible emotional responses to this type of trauma
- importance of taking prescribed course of contraceptive pills
- reinforcement of information on referral services and information provided by sexual assault counselor

(For more information, see pp. 1584-1585 of Polaski and Tatro, *Luckmann's Core Principles and Practice of Medical-Surgical Nursing*.)

Shock

OVERVIEW

- Shock is defined as inadequate tissue perfusion. Inadequate tissue perfusion can be caused by various disorders that result in decreased oxygenation at the cellular level.

- Inadequate oxygenation leads to an abnormal physiologic state in which there is altered cellular metabolism and accumulated waste products in cells. If the condition is untreated, cell and organ death occurs.
- For adequate blood circulation to occur, three factors must function effectively together:
  — circulating blood volume
  — vascular tone or the resistance of the blood vessels
  — cardiac pump or pumping action of the heart
    When these three components are functioning properly, mean arterial pressure (MAP) is maintained at normal levels.
- Shock is commonly discussed in three major categories:
  (1) hypovolemic shock—due to inadequate circulating blood volume
  — common causes:
    — hemorrhage
    — burns — shift of plasma from the vascular space to the interstitial space or loss of plasma through the surface of the burn
    — dehydration
  (2) cardiogenic shock — results from direct pump failure
  — clients with hypovolemic shock may develop cardiogenic shock. This happens because the rapid heart rate initiated to compensate for decreased volume and to increase cardiac output does not allow time for the coronary arteries to fill with blood, decreasing the oxygen supply to the myocardium.
  — common causes:
    — myocardial infarction
    — valvular insufficiency
    — dysrhythmias
    — obstructive conditions — pulmonary embolism, pericardial tamponade, tension pneumothorax
  (3) distributive shock (vasogenic shock) — results from inadequate vascular tone. The blood volume remains normal, but the size of the vascular space increases dramatically because of massive vasodilation.

573

- — common causes:
  - — allergic reaction (anaphylactic shock)
  - — loss of innervation to blood vessels (neurogenic shock)
  - — massive sepsis (septic shock)
- Risk factors include:
  - — major trauma
  - — previous myocardial damage
  - — immunosuppressive therapy
  - — exposure to allergen
- Stages of shock:
  - (1) compensated stage — cardiac output is slightly decreased but the body's compensatory mechanisms are able to maintain BP and tissue perfusion to the vital organs
    - (a) blood moves from tissues into the vascular system
    - (b) sympathetic nervous system stimulation causes vasoconstriction and tachycardia
  - (2) decompensated stage
    - (a) persistent vasoconstriction causes capillary dilation, decreased venous return, and decreased circulation of reoxygenated blood
    - (b) lactic acidosis occurs as a result of anaerobic metabolism
    - (c) acidosis causes increased capillary permeability, which allows fluid to move back into the tissues, decreasing venous return
    - (d) mean arterial pressure and cardiac output decrease
    - (e) decrease in circulating volume and capillary flow does not allow adequate perfusion and oxygenation of vital organs and tissues
  - (3) progressive stage — occurs if the cycle of inadequate tissue perfusion is not interrupted. Cellular ischemia and necrosis lead to organ failure and death of the client.

CLINICAL MANIFESTATIONS

Early recognition of shock is vitally important.
- rapid, shallow breathing
- cyanosis
- rapid, weak, thready pulse
- hypotension

- narrowing pulse pressure (the difference between systolic and diastolic pressure readings) — during shock, the pulse pressure is more significant than the blood pressure because it tends to parallel cardiac stroke volume.
- restlessness, anxiety and irritability during early stages
- decreased level of consciousness
- weakness
- dizziness or faintness when sitting up from horizontal position
- decreased urinary output
- diaphoresis
- ashen pallor progressing to cyanosis in decompensated shock
- flat neck veins
- slow capillary refill and collapse of superficial veins in extremities
- dilated pupils
- thirst, dry mucous membranes
- cold, clammy skin, goosebumps
- nausea, vomiting
- decreased bowel sounds
- hypothermia

Specific clinical manifestations for each type of shock:

HYPOVOLEMIC

- cool, clammy skin
- cyanosis
- increased urine osmolality and specific gravity initially (due to sodium and water reabsorption)

CARDIOGENIC

- cold, clammy skin
- tachycardia
- decreased urinary output
- jugular venous distention

DISTRIBUTIVE

- anaphylactic
  — initially, feeling of uneasiness or doom
  — complaint of headache

- — feeling of a "lump in the throat"
- — coughing, dyspnea, stridor
- — wheezing and prolonged expiratory phase
- — pruritus and urticaria
- — edema of the eyelids, lips or tongue (angioedema)
- neurogenic
  - — bradycardia and hypotension (loss of ability to vasoconstrict)
  - — below level of injury, skin temperature takes on same temperature as room (poikilothermia)
  - — dry skin (inability to sweat)
- septic
  - — peripheral edema (increased permeability of the vasculature)
  - — fever (caused by the release of cytotoxins) is one of the earliest signs of septic shock
  - — systemic vascular resistance and blood pressure are lowered (due to generalized vasodilation)

MEDICAL MANAGEMENT

- respiratory support
  - — supplemental oxygen
  - — hyperventilation (to restore acid-base balance)
  - — mechanical ventilation
  - — endotracheal intubation
- circulatory support
  - — MAST (medical antishock trouser suit) — encases the body in a one piece, three-chambered (two leg and one abdominal chamber) suit from the lower costal margin to the ankles. The suit is inflated causing increased vascular resistance which decreases the diameter of the blood vessels in the abdomen and legs. This results in impedance of blood flow and decreases leakage into the tissues. Cardiac output increases and arterial blood pressure improves (most often used in trauma settings).
  - — IABP (intra-aortic balloon pump) — (used primarily in cardiogenic shock) — a balloon-tipped catheter is placed in the descending thoracic aorta. It inflates during diastole and deflates just before systole. This counterpulsation displaces blood back into the aorta and improves coronary artery circulation.

- external counterpulsation device — device uses the same general principles as an IABP but is applied externally to the legs. Pressure is applied to the legs during diastole and released in systole.
- positioning — to promote venous return without compressing the abdominal organs against the diaphragm
  - modified shock position with lower extremities elevated about 45 degrees, knees straight, trunk horizontal or slightly raised, and neck comfortably positioned with head level to chest or slightly higher
    - not used in cardiogenic shock when there is already circulatory overload
- fluid therapy — all forms of shock involve a decreased effective circulating blood volume
  - crystalloid or balanced salt solutions — normal saline, Ringer's lactate, half-normal saline, or 5 per cent dextrose in water
  - colloid solutions — contain molecules large enough to remain in general circulation:
    - plasma
    - dextran (can interfere with blood type and crossmatch procedures and with clotting factors; therefore, it should be used only after type and crossmatch have been done and until blood is available to transfuse)
    - hetastarch
    - albumin
  - blood transfusion — when hemorrhage is the primary cause of shock
- pharmacologic management
  - vasoconstrictors — elevate systemic blood pressure and increase blood flow to the brain and heart
    - high dose dopamine (Inotropin)
    - norepinephrine (Levophed)
    - phenylephrine (Neo-Synephrine)
  - vasodilators — induce vasodilation of blood vessels or inhibit vasoconstriction
    - amrinone (Inocor)
    - dobutamine (Dobutrex)
    - epinephrine (Adrenalin)
    - isoproterenol (Isuprel)
    - nitroprusside (Nipride)

- — low-dose dopamine (Inotropin)
- — vasoconstrictor/vasodilator combination — to offset profound effects of some vasoconstrictors or to provide the benefit of both types of drugs
- — antibiotics — when shock is due to infection
- — steroids — precise mechanism in shock is unknown
- — Heparin therapy — to prevent or treat some complications of shock (disseminated intravascular coagulation) and in myocardial infarction to prevent thrombi formation near area of infarction
- — calcium replacement — needed for normal functioning of nervous and cardiovascular systems and for blood clotting
- — stress ulcer prophylaxis — histamine hydrogen-receptor antagonists
    - — cimetidine
    - — famotidine
    - — ranitidine
- — antihistamine therapy — anaphylactic shock
    - — diphenhydramine hydrochloride (Benadryl)
- — narcotics — do not administer narcotics to a client suffering from multiple trauma without first knowing that the blood volume is adequate. Narcotic administration causes vasodilation, which results in severe hypotension and shock
- — cardiotonic medications
    - — digitalis – used if there is evidence of cardiac failure, to strengthen inotropic action of the heart
    - — antidysrhythmics – to improve cardiac efficiency
    - — atropine – to treat bradycardia which predisposes to cardiogenic shock
- renal support
    - — diuretics for low urine output
    - — fluid replacement
    - — correction of metabolic acidosis
- thermoregulation — even though client feels cold and clammy, do not apply heat to the skin (will dilate vessels and draw blood away from vital organs and will increase metabolism and oxygen demand). The environment is kept warm to prevent chilling, which also increases energy demands.
- nasogastric suction — early response in shock is decreased splanchnic circulation, causing inadequate

tissue perfusion and delayed gastric emptying; thus, increasing vomiting and aspiration potential.

- Summary of the Management of Hypovolemic Shock:
  — stop external bleeding
  — decrease intra-abdominal or retroperitoneal bleeding by applying MAST suit
  — administer crystalloids
  — transfuse with fresh whole blood, packed cells, plasma
  — administer plasma expanders (albumin, heta-starch, dextran)
- Summary of the Management of Cardiogenic Shock:
  — fluid challenge to rule out hypovolemia (unless congestive heart failure or pulmonary edema is present)
  — insert central venous pressure or pulmonary artery catheter
  — administer fluids to maintain left ventricular filling pressure
  — administer dopamine or dobutamine
  — administer vasodilators
  — administer diuretics
  — administer cardiotonics
  — IABP or external counterpulsation device if unresponsive to therapies
  — pericardiocentesis, if tamponade present
  — thrombolytic or anticoagulant therapy
  — treat dysrhythmias
- Summary of Management of Distributive Shock
  — anaphylactic shock
    — airway management
    — epinephrine administration
    — fluid therapy replacement
    — steroid administration
    — vasopressor administration
    — Benadryl administration
    — aminophylline administration
    — gastric lavage to remove ingested antigen
    — ice pack to injection or sting site
  — septic shock
    — identify origin of sepsis
    — apply MAST suit
    — IV fluid resuscitation
    — antibiotic therapy
    — dopamine or dobutamine therapy
    — vasoconstrictor administration

- steroid therapy
- temperature control
- neurogenic (spinal) shock
  - treat bradycardia with atropine
  - vasopressor administration
- vaso-vagal shock
  - place client in head-down or recumbent position
  - administer atropine if bradycardic
  - eliminate pain

NURSING MANAGEMENT

- Provide emergency measures as indicated:
  - apply MAST suit
  - control bleeding — direct pressure or pressure dressings to wound, nasogastric lavage, etc.
- Assess cardiac, respiratory and neurologic status.
- Administer and monitor fluid therapy replacement to prevent fluid overload.
- Provide respiratory support:
  - supplemental oxygen
  - mechanical ventilation
- Monitor vital signs and hemodynamic values.
- Monitor urinary output.
- Continuous cardiac monitoring.
- Place patient in modified shock position (unless in cardiogenic shock).
- Administer and monitor prescribed vasoactive drug therapy:
  - Vasoconstrictors
    - Monitor arterial blood pressure; watch for undesirable blood pressure elevation.
    - Titrate IV medications to obtain desirable blood pressure.
    - Assess for major adverse effects:
      - increased myocardial oxygen consumption
      - ventricular dysrhythmias
      - decreased blood flow to kidneys and splanchnic area
      - pulmonary edema or left ventricular failure
    - Monitor IV administration sites closely to detect infiltration early.
  - Vasodilators
    - Monitor blood pressure and central venous pressure for severe hypotension.

> — Keep clients lying relatively flat to prevent orthostatic hypotension.

- Administer epinephrine (to stop the release of histamine) and Benadryl (to relieve symptoms) in anaphylactic shock.
- Administer electrolyte replacement therapy.
- Monitor laboratory values — arterial blood gases, electrolytes, hemoglobin, oxygen saturations.
- Maintain nasogastric tube to suction.
- Monitor nasogastric aspirant for blood and pH value to assess for development of a stress ulcer.
- Administer histamine hydrogen-receptor antagonists and antacids.
- Administer antibiotics as prescribed (septic shock).
- Administer cardiotonic medications as prescribed (to improve contractility).
- Monitor for complications of immobility (pulmonary embolism, deep vein thrombosis, pressure sores, etc.).

(For more information, see pp. 1540-1560 of Polaski and Tatro, *Luckmann's Core Principles and Practice of Medical-Surgical Nursing.*)

Sinusitis

OVERVIEW

- Sinusitis is an infection of one of the paranasal sinuses. It occurs when ostia in the nose are obstructed or ciliary action is impaired, causing mucous accumulation and infection.

CLINICAL MANIFESTATIONS

- pain in the sinus area, worsened with bending
- pain or numbness in the upper teeth
- purulent or discolored nasal discharge

MEDICAL MANAGEMENT

- antibiotics to treat infection
- decongestants to reduce edema
- steroid nasal sprays to reduce mucosal inflammation
- humidification to prevent nasal crusting and to moisten secretions
- antral or sinus lavage if the above measures are not effective

SURGICAL MANAGEMENT

- Functional endoscopic sinus surgery (FESS) is often the first surgical technique performed to reestablish sinus ventilation and mucociliary clearance. Small sinus endoscopes are passed through the nasal cavity and into the sinuses. Diseased tissue is removed, and sinus ostia enlarged.
- Caldwell-Luc is another surgical procedure for maxillary sinusitis. The diseased mucous membrane is removed through an incision into the gingival buccal sulcus above the lateral incisor teeth. An opening also may be created between the maxillary sinus and lateral nasal wall (nasal antral window) to increase aeration of the sinus and permit drainage into the nasal cavity.

NURSING MANAGEMENT

SURGICAL

FUNCTIONAL ENDOSCOPIC SINUS SURGERY (FESS)

Postoperative Care
In addition to routine postoperative care:
- Monitor placement of nasal packing (usually removed within several hours of procedure).
- Apply ice compresses to the nose and cheek to minimize edema and control bleeding.
- Monitor amount of nasal bleeding; change drip pad as needed.
- Monitor for increased bleeding, respiratory distress and edema for the first 24 hours after surgery.
- Monitor for visual changes; blindness can occur rarely from intraorbital hematoma formation or direct injury to the optic nerve.

- Maintain semi-Fowler's to high-Fowler's position for 24 to 48 hours after surgery to minimize edema.

CALDWELL-LUC

Postoperative Care

In addition to routine postoperative care:
- Monitor placement of nasal and maxillary sinus packing. Nasal packing generally is removed the morning after surgery; antral packing remains in place for 36-72 hours. Assess oral cavity for blood or dislodged packing that may obstruct the pharynx.
- Assess for increased bleeding, respiratory distress, and edema for the first 24 hours after surgery.
- Assess for any numbness of the upper teeth due to interruption of the sensory nerves from the incision (this may last several weeks).
- Apply ice compresses to the nose and cheek to minimize edema and control bleeding.
- Maintain semi-Fowler's to high-Fowler's position for 24-48 hours after surgery to minimize edema.
- Administer mild analgesics as prescribed.

FOCUSED DISCHARGE TEACHING

FUNCTIONAL ENDOSCOPIC SINUS SURGERY (FESS)

Instruct client regarding:
- increasing fluids to moisten secretions
- avoidance of blowing the nose for 7-10 days
- using nasal saline sprays as recommended (usually started 3-5 days postoperatively)
- avoidance of strenuous activity, lifting or straining for 2 weeks
- importance of follow-up to physician's office for removal of crusts and debris

CALDWELL-LUC

- Same as for FESS procedure above.

(For more information, see pp. 563-565 of Polaski and Tatro, *Luckmann's Core Principles and Practice of Medical-Surgical Nursing.*)

Skin Cancer

OVERVIEW

- Skin cancer is a malignant condition caused by uncontrolled growth and spread of abnormal cells in a specific layer of skin.
- There are several kinds of skin cancer:
  - Basal cell cancer — malignant epithelial tumor of the skin that arises from basal cells in the dermis; almost never metastasizes.
  - Squamous cell cancer — tumor of the epidermal keratinocytes; usually found on rim of the ear, the face, the lips and mouth, and the dorsa of the hands. It may metastasize to the lymph nodes and be subsequently fatal. It rarely occurs in dark-skinned clients.
  - Malignant melanoma — deadliest form of skin cancer. The incidence and mortality have risen by 7 to 15 per cent per year in countries populated with fair-skinned whites. The tumor can metastasize, usually to the brain, lungs, bones, liver and skin. It is universally fatal.
- More than 90 per cent of skin cancers are either basal cell or squamous cell cancer. Both have an excellent cure rate of 95 per cent or greater with treatment.
- The cause of skin cancer is prolonged or intermittent exposure to ultraviolet radiation from the sun, especially when it results in sunburn and blistering.
- Clients with red, blonde or light-brown hair with light complexions or freckles, many of Celtic or Scandinavian origin are most susceptible.
- Danger signals suggesting malignant changes in pigmented nevi are:
  - changes in color (especially red, white and blue)
  - change in diameter
  - change in outline
  - change in surface characteristics
  - change in consistency
  - change in symptoms
  - change in shape
  - change in surrounding skin.

CLINICAL MANIFESTATIONS

Basal Cell Carcinoma
- painless and slow-growing lesions appearing on sun-exposed skin, face, ears, head, neck or hands
- lesions with "pearly" texture

Squamous Cell Carcinoma
May present in any of the forms below. These tumors are poorly marginated with the edge blending into the skin.
- ulcer
- flat red area
- cutaneous horn
- indurated plaque
- hyperkeratotic papule or nodule

Malignant Melanoma
- lesion with shades of brown and black plus red, white or blue coloration
- bleeding of a mole or change in color, size or thickness
- notching or indentation of the border of a lesion

SURGICAL MANAGEMENT

Treatment of skin cancer requires removal of the lesion. The tumor removed needs to have a specified margin free of tumor to guarantee full removal of the tumor.
- Moh's surgery for basal cell and squamous cell carcinoma — a special surgical technique used for the removal of skin malignancies. The technique is based upon a series of excisions. Careful microscopic tissue assessment "maps" the presence or absence of malignant cells within each specimen.
- excision of basal cell or squamous cell carcinoma and closure of the area with a skin flap
- wide local excision with a 1 to 3 cm margin of normal skin is the initial treatment for malignant melanoma
- possible radiation therapy, surgical removal of metastatic lesions, chemotherapy and local hyperthermia for metastatic melanoma

NURSING MANAGEMENT

- Instruct client/significant other regarding:
  — wound care after surgical removal

- need for regular self inspection
- signs/symptoms of recurrent skin cancer
- avoidance of ionizing radiation
- avoidance of excessive exposure to the sun
- use of sunscreen and other sun protection
- importance of follow-up
- Malignant melanoma:
  - signs/symptoms to report to physician
- See "Chemotherapy", p. 145.
- See "Radiation Therapy", p. 543.
- Provide emotional support to client and significant other.
- Make referrals to cancer support groups, home health care agencies and community resources as appropriate.

(For more information, see pp. 1357-1359 of Polaski and Tatro, *Luckmann's Core Principles and Practice of Medical-Surgical Nursing.*)

Spinal Cord Injury

OVERVIEW

- Injury to the spinal cord can range in severity from mild flexion-extension "whiplash" injuries to complete transection of the cord with quadriplegia. Trauma to the cord can occur at any level but most commonly occurs in the cervical and lower thoracic-upper lumbar vertebrae.
- Each year approximately 10,000 individuals sustain a spinal cord injury. Most of these individuals are males under the age of 40.
- Trauma is the most common cause of spinal injury. Traumatic spinal injury may be due to automobile or motorcycle accidents, gunshot or knife wounds, falls, or sporting mishaps. Disorders that may result in spinal cord injury include:
  - cervical spondylosis – producing spinal canal narrowing, causing injury to the cord and roots
  - myelitis – infective or inflammatory process

- — osteoporosis – causing compression fractures of the vertebrae
- — syringomyelia – cavitation of the cord
- — tumors – both infiltrative and compressive
- — vascular disease – infarction or hemorrhage
- Pathophysiology:

Mechanism of injury

(1) flexion-rotation, dislocation, or fracture dislocation
  - — occurs in cervical spine (C_5 and C_6)
  - — ruptures supporting ligaments, fractures the vertebrae, damages blood vessels and leads to ischemia of the spinal cord

(2) hypoextension
  - — seen in elderly clients with degenerative vertebral changes and in clients involved in automobile and diving accidents
  - — injury stretches the spinal cord against the ligamenta flava and can lead to dorsal column contusion and posterior dislocation of the vertebrae
  - — complete transection of the cord can occur

(3) compression
  - — caused by falls or jumps in which the individual lands on the feet or buttocks
  - — force of impact fractures the vertebrae compressing the cord
  - — lumbar and lower thoracic vertebrae are most commonly injured

Level of injury

- — injury to the cervical spine and cord produces quadriplegia
- — injuries above C_4 may be fatal due to loss of innervation to the diaphragm and intercostal muscles
- — injuries to the thoracic or lumbar spine produce paraplegia

- Syndromes causing partial paralysis

(1) central cord syndrome
  - — produces more weakness in upper extremities than lower
  - — weakness is caused by edema and hemorrhage

(2) anterior cord syndrome
  - — complete motor function loss and decreased pain sensation

587

— touch, position and vibration sensation remain intact
(3) Brown-Sequard syndrome
    — lateral hemisection of the cord
    — ipsilateral motor paralysis, loss of vibratory and position sense
    — contralateral loss of pain and temperature sensation
- Complete transection
    — results in immediate loss of all sensation and voluntary movement in areas below the transection
    — initially, all reflex activity is lost, but recovery does occur, although reflexes may be hyperactive.
    The immediate response is spinal shock (post traumatic areflexia)
        — is the immediate response to cord transection
        — complete loss of skeletal muscle function, touch and bladder tone, sexual function and autonomic reflexes
        — loss of venous return and hypotension
        — hypothalamus cannot control temperature, and client assumes temperature of surrounding air
        — may last 7 days to 3 months
        — return of reflexes, the development of hyperreflexia rather than flaccidity, and the return of reflex emptying of the bladder and bowel indicate shock is resolving
- Autonomic dysreflexia
    — exaggerated sympathetic response to noxious stimulus (this is a medical emergency)
    — occurs in clients with injury above T_7 and can occur up to 6 years after injury
    — stimuli include bladder and bowel distention, pressure ulcers, spasms, pain
    — symptoms include extreme hypertension, pounding headache, flushing, diaphoresis, blurred vision, bradycardia, restlessness
    — treatment — removal of noxious stimulant, administration of anti-hypertensives

CLINICAL MANIFESTATIONS

- Initial clinical manifestations of acute spinal cord injury depend upon the level and extent of injury. Below the level of injury or lesion there is loss of (1) voluntary movement, (2) sensation of pain, temperature, pressure and proprioception, (3) bowel and bladder function, and (4) spinal and automatic reflexes.

MEDICAL MANAGEMENT

- spinal cord immobilization (anyone who has sustained multiple trauma should be handled as if there are spinal injuries until proven otherwise)
- respiratory support
- hemodynamic monitoring — heart rate, blood pressure, respirations, temperature, fluid balance
- shock therapy — vasopressors, fluid replacement
- skeletal traction (cervical injuries)
- steroid therapy — to decrease inflammation
- antispasmodic therapy — dantrolene (Dantrium)

SURGICAL MANAGEMENT

- decompressive laminectomy — lamina of vertebrae are removed to minimize pressure on the spinal cord — controversial
- fusion — insertion of metal plates and screws for stabilization — controversial
- immobilization in a brace or halo jacket — a ring is fixed to the skull with pins and then attached to a jacket by rods for cervical fracture stabilization

NURSING MANAGEMENT

- Monitor respiratory status.
- Maintain traction as ordered.
- Encourage to cough, deep breathe and to use incentive spirometer.
- Monitor arterial blood gas results and oxygen saturations.
- Suction PRN.
- Initiate aspiration precautions.
- Provide frequent oral care.

- Provide measures to maintain skin integrity:
  — reposition as ordered
  — assessment of skin and pressure points
  — pressure reducing beds or mattresses
  — Roto Rest bed — keeps body aligned while oscillating from side to side
- Provide nutritional support — dietary supplements, tube feedings, etc.
- Monitor the client for indications of autonomic dysreflexia:
  — severe hypertension
  — throbbing headache
  — profuse diaphoresis
  — flushing of the skin above the lesion
  — nasal stuffiness
  — blurred vision
  — nausea
  — bradycardia
- Intervene if autonomic dysreflexia occurs:
  — Monitor blood pressure closely.
  — Elevate head of bed to sitting position.
  — Notify physician.
  — Check for possible sources of irritation (kinked or clogged catheter, distended bowel or bladder, and pain).
  — Remove stimulus.
  — Administer antihypertensives as prescribed.
- Initiate safety measures to prevent injury secondary to muscle spasms.
- Avoid unnecessary stimulation of areas that elicit reflex spinal automatisms — flexion and contraction of muscles by the limbs and abdomen, evacuation of bladder and bowel, sweating and flushing below the lesion.
- Accurate intake and output.
- Encourage up to 3000 ml/day unless otherwise contraindicated.
- Assess bladder control.
- Implement measures to preserve bladder capacity and muscle tone.
- Establish and maintain a routine pattern of bowel elimination.
- Assure urinary catheter patency (obstruction may cause autonomic dysreflexia).
- Observe for signs of urinary infection.

- Assess for indications of constipation or paralytic ileus.
- Maintain nasogastric tube and NPO status, if paralytic ileus present.
- Institute measures to prevent constipation and impaction:
  — forced fluids
  — diet high in bulk and roughage
  — stool softeners
  — routine daily pattern of elimination
- Administer PRN analgesics and antispasmodics; evaluate effectiveness.
- Monitor for complications of decreased venous return (secondary to loss of muscle contractions in lower extremities) — pulmonary embolus, deep vein thrombosis.
- Institute measures to decrease venous pooling and clot formation:
  — passive/active range of motion exercises
  — antiembolic stockings
  — sequential compression devices
  — subcutaneous Heparin as prescribed
- Injections should be given above the level of the cord lesion whenever possible (absorption may not be adequate below the level of the lesion).
- Institute measures to prevent complications from immobility:
  — frequent position changes
  — proper positioning of joints
  — use of splints and removable casts
  — intermittent turning to a prone position
  — positioning of upper extremities away from the body
  — draping bed linens
  — keeping knees flexed at 15° when supine
  — use of active and passive conditioning exercises
- Collaborate with physical therapy for exercise program, transfer techniques, use of brace or corset, and weight-bearing activities.
- Monitor for orthostatic hypotension when changing position (secondary to venous pooling).
- Encourage independence in activities of daily living within physical limitations.
- Collaborate with occupational/physical therapy for adaptive devices.

- Assist the client/family in working through the grief process and to develop adaptive coping strategies.

FOCUSED DISCHARGE CARE

Most spinal cord injured clients are transferred from an acute care hospital to a rehabilitation facility. After functional capabilities are maximized, the client is discharged home.

Instruct the client regarding:
- measures to prevent skin breakdown in desensitized and paralyzed areas:
  — repositioning techniques
  — daily inspection of pressure areas
  — pressure relieving devices for bed/chair
  — meticulous skin care
- exercise regime
- safety measures related to sensory loss:
  — avoid wearing ill-fitting shoes
  — avoid use of heating pads or hot water bottles
  — tepid bath water
  — shifting of body weight while sitting
  — regular foot and nail care
- bladder training program:
  — intermittent catheterization (by client or caregiver)
  — methods to empty bladder without catheterization:
    — Credé Maneuver — client makes a fist and presses directly over bladder and down towards pubic area with a kneading motion
    — Valsalva Maneuver — client inhales deeply, holds breath and bears down as if for a bowel movement
    — rectal stretch — client inserts finger into rectum; when sphincter relaxes, the client gently pulls on the sphincter to relax the perineal floor
    — reflex stimulation — tapping the suprapubic area, stroking the glans penis, thigh or vulva, etc.
  — maintain an established elimination schedule
  — fluids to 3000 ml/day
- bowel training program:
  — maintain an established elimination schedule

- — fluids to 3000 ml/day
- — dietary modification—high bulk, increased roughage
- use of adaptive devices and ambulation aids
- factors that may precipitate muscle spasms:
  - — cold temperature
  - — prolonged sitting
  - — emotional upset
  - — cutaneous stimulation (tickling, stroking or pinching)
- pulmonary hygiene
  - — cough, deep breathe
  - — incentive spirometry
- factors that may precipitate autonomic dysreflexia and necessary interventions
- measures to prevent deep vein thrombosis:
  - — antiembolic stockings
  - — passive range of motion exercises
  - — assess for signs of deep vein thrombosis
- Refer to community resources.

(For more information, see pp. 390–406 of Polaski and Tatro, *Luckmann's Core Principles and Practice of Medical-Surgical Nursing.*)

Spinal Tumors

OVERVIEW

- Spinal tumors are most common in young or middle-aged adults and most often involve the thoracic region.
- Spinal tumors may occur outside the spinal cord (extramedullary) or within the substance of the spinal cord (intramedullary). Neurofibromas and meningiomas are the most common spinal tumors. Both are benign and operable and may not produce permanent damage if removed early enough. Spinal cord compression is the most common pathologic feature of all tumors within the spinal canal, because there is little room for expansion.

CLINICAL MANIFESTATIONS

Early
- pain
- sensory loss
- muscle weakness and wasting

Progressive
- spastic weakness below level of lesion
- decreased sensation
- hyper-reactive reflexes

Severe
- paraplegia and quadriplegia

SURGICAL MANAGEMENT

Treatment of Choice
- tumor removal
- partial resection of the tumor followed by radiation therapy (complete surgical removal of an intramedullary tumor is rare)

NURSING MANAGEMENT

See "Herniated Intervertebral Disc", p. 323.

(For more information, see p. 412 of Polaski and Tatro, *Luckmann's Core Principles and Practice of Medical-Surgical Nursing.*)

Splenectomy

OVERVIEW

- The spleen is a lymphoid organ located in the left upper quadrant of the abdomen beneath the diaphragm. It is a storage organ for red corpuscles and a blood filter for foreign materials and cellular debris.
- Despite the important functions of the spleen, it can be removed (splenectomy) without harm in adults.

Its role can be taken over by other organs (e.g., liver, lymph nodes, bone marrow).
- Indications for splenectomy include:
  — splenic rupture
  — hypersplenism — the spleen destroys excessive numbers of one of the blood cell types (erythrocytes, platelets, leukocytes).

NURSING MANAGEMENT

SURGICAL

POSTOPERATIVE CARE

In addition to routine postoperative care:
- Monitor for the development of hemorrhage:
  — vital signs
  — increased abdominal girth
  — abdominal pain

See page 500, "Perioperative Nursing Care."

FOCUSED DISCHARGE CARE

Instruct client regarding:
- care of the incision
- activity limitations
- need for prophylactic antibiotics
- early signs/symptoms of infection (fever, chills, productive cough) and when to report to physician
- routine immunization against influenza and pneumonia
- avoidance of people with infections

(For more information, see pp. 866-867 of Polaski and Tatro, *Luckmann's Core Principles and Practice of Medical-Surgical Nursing.*)

Squamous Cell Carcinoma of the Oral Cavity

OVERVIEW

- Squamous cell carcinoma is the leading type of oral cancer. It is a malignant growth arising from tiny flat squamous cells that line mucous membranes. It most often is seen on the lower lip and tongue.
- The primary cause is chronic irritation of the mucous lining of the mouth and oral cavity.
- Squamous cell cancer of the tongue has a poor prognosis due to the extensive vascular and lymphatic supply of the tongue.
- Cancer of the lip has a high cure rate.
- Risk factors include alcohol and tobacco overuse, poor oral hygiene, or chronic chemical or thermal trauma.

CLINICAL MANIFESTATIONS

- sore or lesion in the oral cavity
- irritation of the tongue
- sore throat, tongue or ear pain
- trouble wearing dentures

MEDICAL MANAGEMENT

Treatment depends upon the site and staging of the tumor.
- chemotherapy
- radiation therapy

SURGICAL MANAGEMENT

- local excision or laser therapy of small tumors
- extensive surgical excision and possible removal of associated lymph nodes for invasive tumors:
  — glossectomy — removal of the tongue
  — hemiglossectomy—removal of part of the tongue
  — mandibulectomy — removal of the mandible
  — radical neck dissection — removal of all tissue under the skin, from the jaw down to the clavicle,

and from the anterior border of the trapezius muscle to the midline

NURSING MANAGEMENT

MEDICAL

- Discuss prevention of further oral lesions:
  — Avoid chemical, physical and thermal oral trauma
  — Perform oral hygiene at least 3 times a day.
  — See a dentist for ill-fitting dentures.
  — See a physician for any mouth lesions that do not heal in 2-3 weeks.
  — Maintain a well-balanced diet
- Discuss "Radiation Therapy", see p. 543.
- Discuss "Chemotherapy", see p. 145.
- Promote and encourage adequate nutrition:
  — Provide analgesics 30 to 45 minutes before meals.
  — Encourage small frequent meals.
  — Provide/encourage oral care before and after meals.
  — Provide artificial saliva and administer pilocarpine, as prescribed for xerostomia (dryness of the mouth) due to radiation therapy. Sugarless gum or candy and frequent oral rinses also will provide moisture.

SURGICAL

PREOPERATIVE CARE

In addition to routine preoperative care:
- Discuss purpose and care of tracheostomy (temporary/permanent) and feeding tube as appropriate.
- Make referrals to assist with coping with changes in appearance.

POSTOPERATIVE CARE

Nursing care required depends upon the extent of the surgery.
In addition to routine postoperative care:
Local Excisions
- Monitor the amount of drainage.
- Monitor intactness of dressing and packing.

- Instruct the client on gentle oral care.
- Instruct on oral rinses every 4 hours of half strength hydrogen peroxide and water or saline (after removal of dressings and packing).

Extensive Surgery
- Maintain a patent airway.
  - Maintain semi- to high Fowler's position.
- Monitor for hemorrhage.
- Protect suture lines from trauma.
- No oral hygiene or suctioning until approved by the physician.
- Monitor condition of donor and graft sites if a skin graft was performed.
- Provide tracheostomy care, see "Tracheostomy",p. 616.
- Maintain adequate hydration by IV. Begin tube feedings as prescribed when bowel sounds return.
- Provide means of communication if tracheostomy present.
- Resume oral feedings as prescribed when adequate healing has occurred.
  - Assess swallowing ability.
  - Instruct that there is decreased sensation in the oral cavity.
  - Instruct to avoid putting food directly on surgical site.
  - Instruct to perform oral hygiene after meals.

If a radical neck dissection was performed, also see "Laryngeal Cancer", p. 411.

FOCUSED DISCHARGE CARE

- Instruct client regarding:
  - diet
  - signs/symptoms of complications and to report these to physician
  - oral care
  - wound care
  - tracheostomy care (as appropriate)
  - tube feedings (as appropriate)
- Provide referrals to home health care agency for assistance with respiratory support, nutritional support and wound care.
- Provide referrals to support groups for coping with cancer or change in body image.

(For more information, see pp. 1013-1016 of Polaski and Tatro, *Luckmann's Core Principles and Practice of Medical-Surgical Nursing.*)

Syndrome of Inappropriate Antidiuretic Hormone (SIADH)

OVERVIEW

- SIADH is a disorder associated with excessive amounts of antidiuretic hormone (ADH), resulting in a water imbalance.
- SIADH is the opposite of diabetes insipidus. Instead of large fluid losses, clients with SIADH retain fluids and may develop water intoxication (a condition where all body fluid compartments experience expansion with effects related to circulatory overload, interstitial edema, cerebral edema, and electrolyte dilution). Under normal circumstances, ADH regulates serum osmolality. When serum osmolality falls, a feedback mechanism inhibits ADH. This promotes increased water excretion by the kidneys to raise serum osmolality. When the feedback mechanism fails, ADH levels are sustained and fluid retention results. Ultimately serum sodium falls, resulting in hyponatremia and water intoxication.
- There are a wide variety of causes, including the stress of surgery, certain disorders and medications.
- Risk factors include:
  — treatment of diabetes insipidus with vasopressin
  — a variety of malignancies

CLINICAL MANIFESTATIONS

- hyponatremia
- central nervous system dysfunction (secondary to hyponatremia):
  — alterations in level of consciousness
  — seizures
  — coma

MEDICAL MANAGEMENT

- fluid restriction
- replacement of sodium chloride
- administration of diuretics and demeclocycline (a tetracycline that increases free-water clearance)

NURSING MANAGEMENT

- Maintain fluid restriction.
- Monitor intake and output.
- Assess cardiovascular status for signs of overload.
- Daily weights.
- Assess neurologic status.
- Keep head of bed flat or at no more than a 5 degree elevation (helps prevent possible development or worsening of cerebral edema and avoids stimulation of receptors in the atrium of the heart that are sensitive to volume changes that can increase ADH secretion).
- Maintain dietary modifications (low sodium).

FOCUSED DISCHARGE CARE

Instruct the client regarding:
- need for fluid and sodium restrictions
- daily weights — report gain of 2 pounds or more per day
- need to avoid aspirin and nonsteroidal anti-inflammatory agents (can increase hyponatremia)

(For more information, see pp. 1251-1253 of Polaski and Tatro, *Luckmann's Core Principles and Practice of Medical-Surgical Nursing.*)

Syphilis

OVERVIEW

- This systemic, infectious disease is caused by the spirochete, Treponema pallidum, and is highly infectious.

- The organism enters the body through intact mucous membranes or abraded skin almost exclusively by direct sexual contact (acquired syphilis). Sexual transmission requires exposure to the moist mucosal or cutaneous syphilitic lesion. After entry, the organisms multiply locally and disseminate through the lymphatics and the bloodstream.
- Syphilis has become dramatically less prevalent with the advent of antibiotics but has not been eradicated. It is the third most commonly reported communicable disease in the United States.
- Adolescents, young adults, and homosexual males are at the greatest risk.

CLINICAL MANIFESTATIONS

Syphilis is characterized by well-defined stages that occur over a period of of years: primary, secondary, latent, and late.
- Primary Stage:
  — appearance of chancre — an oval ulcer with a raised border that does not bleed readily and is painless unless infected. The chancre is at the site of inoculation, usually the genitalia, anus, or mouth. If untreated, a chancre disappears after 4-6 weeks.
  — lymphadenopathy — local lymph glands at the chancre swell painlessly
- Secondary Stage (begins 2 weeks to 6 months after chancre disappears):
  — generalized skin rash — a maculopapular rash appears on the palms and soles of the feet
  — generalized lymphadenopathy
  — mucous patches — gray, superficial patches on mucous membranes in the mouth
  — Condylomata lata — broad-based, flat papules develop in warm, moist body areas, most commonly the labia, anus, or at the corners of the mouth. Condylomata are highly contagious.
  — generalized flu-like symptoms
  — patchy hair loss from eyebrows and scalp
  — secondary stage symptoms usually disappear after 2-6 weeks, and the latency period begins
- Latent Stage (begins 2 or more years after primary lesion):
  — typically no symptoms

- disease is not transmitted by sexual contact during this phase. However, transmission through the bloodstream by blood donation can occur.
- about two-thirds of infected clients remain in this phase without further problems. Some clients relapse into the primary or secondary stage during the first 2 years of latency.
- Late Stage:
  - chronic bone and joint inflammation
  - cardiovascular problems (e.g., valve involvement, aneurysms)
  - granulomatous lesions on any part of the body
  - central nervous system problems (including mental illness, slurred speech, ataxic gait, paralysis, judgment loss, and senility)
  - not infectious during this stage

MEDICAL MANAGEMENT

All sexual contacts should be evaluated and treated.
- penicillin
  - early stages: benzathine penicillin G IM, single dose
  - late stage: benzathine penicillin G IM, weekly for 3 weeks (cardiovascular syphilis) or aqueous penicillin IV every 4 hours for 10-14 days (neurosyphilis)
- follow-up cultures

All stages respond to antibiotic therapy, but the structural changes are irreversible.

NURSING MANAGEMENT

- Administer antibiotics as prescribed.
- Monitor cardiac and neurological changes in late stages.

FOCUSED DISCHARGE CARE

Instruct the client regarding:
- the importance of completing the antibiotic regime and follow-up
- the importance of abstaining from sexual contact for at least one month after treatment for primary or secondary syphilis

- the importance of treating all sexual contacts
- information about transmission, reinfection (infection does not confer lasting immunity), early detection, treatment and follow-up

(For more information, see pp. 1509-1510 of Polaski and Tatro, *Luckmann's Core Principles and Practice of Medical-Surgical Nursing.*)

Systemic Lupus Erythematosus (SLE)

OVERVIEW

- Systemic lupus erythematosus (SLE) is a chronic, inflammatory connective tissue disease. It produces inflammatory, biochemical, and structural changes in vascular and connective tissue as well as in the viscera, joints, fascia, tendons, and bursae. SLE has an insidious onset and is characterized by remissions and exacerbations.
- Abnormal serum protein factors and ANA (antinuclear antibodies) found with SLE suggest an autoimmune mechanism. These mainly affect the DNA within the cell nuclei, leading to inflammation of vessels (vasculitis) and organs. The leading cause of death in clients with SLE is renal failure.
- SLE is 10 times more common in women than men and occurs between the ages of 15 and 40 years.
- Causes of exacerbations include exposure to sunlight or other forms of ultraviolet light, physical and emotional stress, and pregnancy.
- There is a form of drug-induced SLE associated with adverse reactions to some drugs including procainamide (Pronestyl) and hydralazine (Apresoline). Some drugs, phenytoin (Dilantin) and phenobarbital are known to produce an SLE-like syndrome. The drug-induced problems resolve when the drugs are discontinued.

CLINICAL MANIFESTATIONS

Chronic SLE
- fever
- malaise
- anorexia and weight loss
- erythema of exposed skin
- generalized lymphadenopathy
- severe hemolytic anemia
- thrombocytopenic purpura
- pericarditis
- tachycardia
- gallop rhythm
- peripheral vascular syndrome (e.g., Raynaud's phenomena)
- ulcerative mucous membrane lesions
- hepatic dysfunction
- glomerulonephritis
- psychosis and coma

Acute SLE
- fever
- musculoskeletal aches and pains
- butterfly rash on the face
- pleural effusion
- basilar pneumonia
- pericarditis
- tachycardia, gallop rhythm
- hepatosplenomegaly
- delirium, convulsions
- coma

MEDICAL MANAGEMENT

- non-steroidal anti-inflammatory agents — aspirin, ibuprofen
- antimalarial drugs
- corticosteroids
- cytotoxic agents — cyclophosphamide, methotrexate
- plasmapheresis — removes circulating auto-antibodies and immune complexes

NURSING MANAGEMENT

- Administer anti-inflammatory agents as prescribed and monitor side effects.

- Monitor laboratory findings — renal profile, nutritional panel, blood counts.
- Assess cardiopulmonary status and response to activity.
- Provide physiologic support to prevent skin breakdown.
- Encourage nutritionally balanced diet.
- Minimize the risk of opportunistic infections.
- Maintain quiet, restful environment.
- Provide emotional support to the client facing a chronic, potentially fatal disease.

FOCUSED DISCHARGE CARE

Instruct the client regarding:
- importance of medication regime
  — advise to take anti-inflammants with food or antacids
- measures to decrease exposure to sunlight or ultraviolet light
- importance of avoiding emotional or physical stress that may trigger an exacerbation
- importance of follow-up appointments

(For more information, see pp. 232-234 of Polaski and Tatro, *Luckmann's Core Principles and Practice of Medical-Surgical Nursing.*)

T

Testicular Disorders

HYDROCELE

- Hydrocele is a painless collection of clear, yellow fluid along the spermatic cord.
- Treatment:
  — aspiration or surgical drainage

HEMATOCELE

- Hematocele is a collection of blood in the tunica vaginalis.
- Treatment:
  — aspiration or surgical drainage

SPERMATOCELE

- Spermatocele is a collection of milky fluid and spermatozoa originating in the epididymis.
- Treatment:
  — aspiration or surgical drainage

VARICOCELE

- Varicocele is dilation and varicosity of the network of veins supplying the testicles.
- Clinical Manifestations:
  — pulling sensation
  — dull ache or scrotal pain
- Treatment:
  — scrotal support
  — surgery if varicocele is thought to contribute to infertility

(For more information, see pp. 1462-1463 of Polaski and Tatro, *Luckmann's Core Principles and Practice of Medical-Surgical Nursing*.)

Testicular Tumors

OVERVIEW

- Testicular cancer is the most common and serious solid tumor cancer in males between the ages of 15 and 35.
- The major risk factor is cryptorchidism (undescended testicles). It is now recommended that any child born with an undescended testicle have an orchiopexy as soon as possible after birth.

CLINICAL MANIFESTATIONS

- painless enlargement, noted as heaviness in the testicles
- findings suggesting metastasis include back pain, vague abdominal pain, nausea and vomiting, anorexia, and weight loss

MEDICAL MANAGEMENT

- radiation therapy
- chemotherapy - Cisplatin, Vinblastine, Bleomycin

SURGICAL MANAGEMENT

Primary treatment for testicular cancer:
- radical orchiectomy — the amputated testicle can be replaced with a testicular prosthesis
- radical orchiectomy with retroperitoneal lymph node dissection — major complication is impotence
- radical orchiectomy followed by a course of chemotherapy for known lymph node involvement or as prophylaxis

NURSING MANAGEMENT

MEDICAL

- Administer prescribed chemotherapy. See "Chemotherapy", p. 145.
- Monitor for and intervene if side effects develop.
- Provide emotional support.

607

- Provide routine postoperative care.

FOCUSED DISCHARGE CARE

Instruct the client regarding:
- management of side effects if receiving chemotherapy
- wound care for postoperative client

(For more information, see pp. 1461-1462 of Polaski and Tatro, *Luckmann's Core Principles and Practice of Medical-Surgical Nursing.*)

Tetanus

- Tetanus is caused by the anaerobic spore-forming rod Clostridium tetani. The spores produce a toxin when introduced into a wound. The toxin suppresses spinal and brain stem inhibitory neurons and may act on skeletal muscle at the point of entry.
- Clinical manifestations include:
  — painful muscular spasms and contractions in the affected extremity
  — spasms of the jaw muscles
  — spasms of muscles of the neck, trunk, limbs and the respiratory and pharyngeal muscles
  — seizures
  — impaired respiration
- Interventions:
  — surgery to debride wound
  — single dose of antitoxin (hyperimmune serum)
  — ten day course of penicillin G or alternate agents
  — respiratory support (possible mechanical ventilation)
  — chlorpromazine, meprobamate or diazepam to control muscle spasms
  — nasogastric feeding, if the client has dysphagia
  — prophylactic anticoagulation to prevent thrombus formation
- The mortality rate is 25 to 50 per cent.

- The best prevention is immunization with regular booster doses of toxoid.

(For more information, see pp. 361-362 of Polaski and Tatro, *Luckmann's Core Principles and Practice of Medical-Surgical Nursing.*)

Thalassemias

OVERVIEW

- The thalassemias are a group of inherited, chronic, hemolytic anemias.
- The production of extremely thin, fragile erythrocytes called target cells characterizes the thalassemias. The severity of the anemia depends upon whether the afflicted client is homozygous or heterozygous for the trait. Thalassemia major and intermedia, both characterized by profound anemia, appear in homozygotes. Thalassemia minor, characterized by a mild anemia, develops in heterozygotes.
- The outlook for clients with thalassemia major is poor. Many fail to live through puberty. Thalassemia minor, on the other hand, does not affect life expectancy.
- Clients from Mediterranean, central African, African American, southern Chinese or southern Asian backgrounds are at risk.

CLINICAL MANIFESTATIONS

THALASSEMIA MAJOR

- jaundice (accumulation of bilirubin)
- cholelithiasis (excess bilirubin from red blood cell breakdown causes gallstones)
- enlarged spleen
- chronic fatigue
- pallor
- mongoloid faces and thickening of the cranium (bone hyperactivity)

- asymptomatic except for mild anemia
- diagnosis made on blood smear

MEDICAL MANAGEMENT

THALASSEMIA MAJOR

- transfusion therapy on a monthly or bimonthly basis

SURGICAL MANAGEMENT

- splenectomy if the transfused cells are being rapidly destroyed by the spleen

THALASSEMIA MINOR

Treatment usually not required; however, clients who carry the trait should have genetic counseling.

NURSING MANAGEMENT

- Administer transfusion therapy as ordered. See "Blood Component Transfusion", p. 88.
- Monitor laboratory findings — CBC.
- Monitor response to activity and provide rest periods.

FOCUSED DISCHARGE CARE

Instruct client regarding:
- importance of treatment regime
- need for follow-up appointments

(For more information, see pp. 849-850 of Polaski and Tatro, *Luckmann's Core Principles and Practice of Medical-Surgical Nursing.*)

Thoracic Outlet Syndromes

OVERVIEW

- Thoracic outlet syndromes produce symptoms affecting the neck, shoulder, and upper extremities. They are caused by compression or mechanical irritation of the brachial plexus, subclavian artery or subclavian vein as these structures pass through the thoracic outlet.

CLINICAL MANIFESTATIONS

NEUROLOGIC TYPE

Fifty per cent occur following hyperextension injury of the neck or upper spine
- aching or throbbing pain of the neck or upper limb
- paresthesias

ARTERIAL TYPE

Chronic compression of subclavian artery
- embolization leads to severe ischemia of the upper extremity

VENOUS TYPE

External compression of the axillosubclavian vein
- sudden swelling
- pain
- cyanosis

MEDICAL MANAGEMENT

VENOUS TYPE

- anticoagulation or thrombolytic therapy

SURGICAL MANAGEMENT

ARTERIAL TYPE

- embolectomy

(For more information, see p. 809 of Polaski and Tatro, *Luckmann's Core Principles and Practice of Medical-Surgical Nursing.*)

Thromboangiitis Obliterans (Buerger's Disease)

OVERVIEW

- Thromboangiitis obliterans is a vasculitis of small and medium-size veins and arteries in the extremities.
- The cause remains unknown. Almost all clients are moderate to heavy smokers.
- The disease process starts distally and progresses upward, involving both upper and lower extremities.
- The disease occurs in the second to fourth decade and is seen predominantly in men.

CLINICAL MANIFESTATIONS

- intermittent claudication — occurs in the arch of the foot or calf of the leg
- rest pain with persistent ischemia of one or more digits
- cold sensitivity
- paresthesias
- weak or absent peripheral pulses
- abnormally red or cyanotic extremity (advanced cases), particularly when dependent
- color or temperature changes involving only one extremity, certain digits or portions of digits (advanced cases)
- ulceration and gangrene
- edema of the leg
- changes in skin and nails

MEDICAL MANAGEMENT

- smoking cessation

- pain control
- vasodilators - calcium channel blockers, prazosin

SURGICAL MANAGEMENT

- amputation if conservative measures fail

NURSING MANAGEMENT

MEDICAL

- Administer analgesics.
- Administer vasodilators.
- Discuss safety measures related to postural hypotension (vasodilator therapy).
- Provide measures to increase body warmth.

SURGICAL

- See "Amputation", p. 30.

FOCUSED DISCHARGE CARE

Instruct client regarding:

MEDICAL

- disease process and treatment regime
- importance of avoiding exposure to cold
- signs/symptoms of advancing disease
- smoking cessation program
- pain control

SURGICAL

- See "Amputation", p. 30.

(For more information, see p. 808 of Polaski and Tatro, *Luckmann's Core Principles and Practice of Medical-Surgical Nursing.*)

Thyroid Cancer

OVERVIEW

- Malignant tumors of the thyroid are rare. They account for three or four new cases per 100,000 population per year. Thyroid cancer develops mainly in women between the ages of 40 and 60 years.
- Clients receiving large doses of radiation to the head and neck are at the greatest risk of developing thyroid cancer.

CLINICAL MANIFESTATIONS

- hard, painless nodule in an enlarged thyroid gland
- palpable lymph glands
- respiratory difficulty and dysphagia

MEDICAL MANAGEMENT

- chemotherapy
- radioiodine treatment with ^{131}I.

SURGICAL MANAGEMENT

- thyroidectomy—removal of all or part of the thyroid
- neck resection may be done for metastases

NURSING MANAGEMENT

MEDICAL

- Administer chemotherapy as ordered; monitor for side effects. See "Chemotherapy", p. 145.
- Maintain radiation precautions for patients receiving ^{131}I. See "Radiation Therapy", p. 543.
- Encourage nutritionally balanced diet.
- Monitor activity tolerance, promote rest periods.

SURGICAL

- For care of client undergoing thyroidectomy, see "Hyperthyroidism", p. 365.

FOCUSED DISCHARGE CARE

Instruct client regarding:
- postoperative home care:
  - importance of taking thyroid replacement hormone (total thyroidectomy)
  - wound care
  - symptoms of thyroid deficiency and excess
- chemotherapy -
  - management of side effects
- radioiodine treatment -
  - necessary radiation precautions

(For more information, see pp. 1220-1221 of Polaski and Tatro, *Luckmann's Core Principles and Practice of Medical-Surgical Nursing.*)

Total Parenteral Nutrition

OVERVIEW

- Total parenteral nutrition (TPN) is the intravenous administration of amino acid-dextrose solutions (usually in conjunction with fat emulsions) in order to provide sufficient nutrients in clients who are unable to ingest, digest or absorb sufficient nutrients to maintain themselves in a state of positive nitrogen balance. TPN may also be used to rest the gastrointestinal tract when there is a fistula or inflammatory bowel disease or after an intestinal obstruction is removed.
- TPN is usually administered through an indwelling subclavian catheter into the superior vena cava.

NURSING MANAGEMENT

- Initiate TPN via an infusion pump at a slow rate. Gradually increase rate as prescribed.
- Never administer any medications in the same line in which TPN is infusing; only intralipids may be infused in the same line.

- Monitor catheter insertion site for redness, tenderness, drainage or edema.
- Never abruptly discontinue TPN as hypoglycemia can occur.
  — If the next TPN bag is unavailable, administer a 10 per cent dextrose solution until the TPN is available.
  — When TPN is to be discontinued, the rate is gradually decreased over a period of time.
- Monitor blood sugars every six hours.
- Monitor for signs/symptoms of hypoglycemia and hyperglycemia.
- Monitor for signs/symptoms of infection and increased temperature.
- Monitor intake and output.
- Obtain daily weights.
- Monitor laboratory values — BUN/Creatinine, electrolytes, minerals, nutritional panel.
- Monitor for venous thrombosis: neck vein distention (unilateral); unilateral edema of the arm, neck or face; shoulder pain.
- Maintain strict aseptic technique when changing TPN solutions or performing dressing changes.
- Change the TPN solution every 24 hours.
- Perform dressing and tubing changes as outlined by healthcare facility policy.

(For more information, see pp. 1033-1034 of Polaski and Tatro, *Luckmann's Core Principles and Practice of Medical-Surgical Nursing.*)

Tracheostomy

OVERVIEW

- A tracheostomy is the surgical creation of a stoma from the trachea to the overlying skin for airway management.
- Indications for a tracheostomy are:
  — need for long-term artificial airway
  — upper airway obstruction
  — upper airway bleeding

— inability to clear lower airway secretions
— altered level of consciousness with inability to protect the lower airway
— need for continuous mechanical ventilation
— prolonged endotracheal tube insertion
— sleep apnea
- Types of tracheostomy tubes:
  — universal or standard tracheostomy tube (e.g., Shiley)—consists of three parts: an outer cannula, an inner cannula and an obturator. The outer cannula fits in the client's tracheostomy stoma to keep it open. The inner cannula is locked inside the outer cannula and maintains airway patency. The obturator is used for insertion and is immediately replaced by the inner cannula after insertion.
  — single-cannula tracheostomy tube — has only one cannula. Not appropriate for clients producing secretions.
  — fenestrated tracheostomy tube — similar to a universal tracheostomy tube, except it has an opening on the curvature of the posterior wall of the outer cannula. When the inner cannula is in place, the tube functions as a universal tracheostomy tube. If the inner cannula is removed, air flows through the upper airway and allows speech and more effective coughing. When the inner cannula is replaced with a short decannulation stopper (tracheostomy plug), all airflow passes through the upper airway. When plugged, the person can speak, cough and breathe deeply. If the tube is cuffed, the cuff must be deflated before plugging the tracheostomy, so that air can pass to the lungs. If this is not done, asphyxiation results.
  — talking tracheostomy — this is a one way valve in a plastic T-piece attached to the 15 mm end of the inner cannula of a universal tracheostomy tube. It permits talking without the need to plug the tracheostomy tube. The cuff of the tracheostomy tube must always be deflated before using a talking tracheostomy adapter. Otherwise, suffocation (from inability to exhale) can result.
  — Communitrach — this tube allows speech but involves coordination on the client's part to oc-

617

clude a distal end of an airflow tube. Speech will not sound normal.

— metal tracheostomy (e.g., Jackson) — most often used following a permanent tracheostomy or laryngectomy. The inner and outer cannulas lock together and are made of sterling silver or stainless steel.

— permanent tracheostomy — this is usually an uncuffed tracheostomy with a low-profile inner cannula that lies flush with the neck. This minimizes the tracheostomy's appearance and allows clothing to be arranged to conceal the tracheostomy.

— tracheostomy button — a short, straight tracheostomy tube that fits into a tracheostomy's stoma, but is not deep enough to enter the tracheal lumen. May be used during weaning as an intermediate device between the standard tracheostomy tube and complete extubation.

• Tracheostomy cuffs — a tracheostomy tube may be cuffed or uncuffed. Inflated cuffs protect the lower airway by creating a seal between the upper and lower airways. When inflated, they seal the area between the outer cannula and tracheal wall. They do not hold the tube in place. A pilot balloon reflects the absence or presence of air in the cuff, but cannot be an absolute indicator of cuff inflation. Most tracheostomy cuffs are designed to exert a low pressure against the tracheal wall, yet accept a high volume of air (high volume — low pressure cuffs). Low cuff pressure is necessary to prevent tracheal mucosal damage. Cuff pressures should not exceed 20 cm H_2O.

• Complications due to prolonged contact between tube cuffs at high pressure and the tracheal wall include: obstruction, cuff inflation problems, tracheoesophageal fistula and malposition of the tube. Other potential problems that may occur with tracheostomy tubes are:

— tube displacement — the tracheostomy tube should lie 1 to 2 cm above the carina. If the tube is not properly placed, it may be in the soft tissues of the neck, or in the right main bronchus (allowing only ventilation of the right lung).

- accidental extubation (tube removal)—dislodgement of the tube from the stoma which may occur if the tube is not properly secured
- airway obstruction—due to: misalignment of the tube (the tube tip is against the tracheal wall); cuff over-inflation; or occlusion of the tube with excessive or dried secretions
- infection—bronchopulmonary infection or stoma site infection may occur

- Weaning from a tracheostomy tube—usually begins by plugging the tracheostomy tube's opening. At first, the plug is inserted for only short times and then the time is gradually lengthened. Ideally, tracheostomy plugging is attempted only when an uncuffed or fenestrated tracheostomy tube is in place.

- Tracheostomy removal (extubation) — performed only after successful tracheostomy plugging and when the client's respiratory status and function are stable.

- Tracheostomy tubes ideally should be changed every six to eight weeks, or more frequently if the client is at risk for tracheobronchial infections. Protocols vary between health care facilities.

- If respiratory arrest occurs, emergency mouth-to-tracheostomy or mouth-to-stoma resuscitation may be necessary.

NURSING MANAGEMENT

Maintain a Patent Airway
- Following a tracheostomy, frequently assess:
  - vital signs
  - mucous membrane color
  - for signs/symptoms of shock, hemorrhage or respiratory insufficiency
- Suction PRN. Provide oxygen and hyperinflate the client's lungs by delivering five or six breaths with a manual resuscitation bag before and after suctioning. Instill artificial saline to thin secretions if necessary.
- Provide adequate hydration and humidification.
- Change the client's position frequently.
- When deflating a tracheostomy cuff, give a deep manual inflation with a resuscitation bag, simultaneously deflating the cuff (this allows secretions trapped at the cuff to be blown up into the mouth,

preventing them from falling into the lower airway).

- Monitor oxygen saturations or arterial blood gas analysis.

Prevent Infection

- Maintain aseptic technique for all care directly involving the tracheostomy.
- Inspect skin around the stoma and the stoma itself for irritation, inflammation, skin breakdown and purulent drainage.
- Assess color, quantity and odor of sputum production.
- Change tracheostomy dressings when damp, and do not use plastic-backed dressings.
- Cleanse the skin around the stoma using hydrogen peroxide and cotton-tipped applicators. Rinse the area with normal saline using cotton-tipped applicators. Use 4x4 gauze sponges to dry.
- For complete tracheostomy care, see Table 20-5, p. 529 of Polaski and Tatro, *Luckmann's Core Principles and Practice of Medical-Surgical Nursing.*

Provide Adequate Nutrition

- Assess for a tracheoesophageal fistula before permitting oral feedings (to assess, give client a "test swallow" of water with blue dye added). If severe coughing occurs, or if blue fluid is suctioned from the tracheostomy, do not give other foods or fluids and call physician.
- Sit client upright to feed.
- Offer foods and fluids with texture (such as pudding), which are easier to swallow.
- Tip the client's chin to the chest to aid in swallowing.
- If the client is receiving nutrition via a G-tube, inflate the tracheostomy cuff one hour before feeding. Suction above the cuff before deflating again.

Provide a Method of Communication

- Ensure that the client has an emergency call system to summon help. Ensure that the staff know the client cannot speak.
- Provide a method agreeable to the client to communicate needs (i.e., picture board, paper and pen, etc.).

Prevent Injury

- Ensure that the tracheostomy tube always is secured and ties knotted (two fingers should be able to slide under the ties to ensure it is not too tight). Do not place the knot over the carotid artery or spine.

- Drain water and condensate in tubing away from the tracheostomy.
- Support ventilator and aerosol tubing to prevent pulling on the tracheostomy tube.
- Do not allow smoking or the use of aerosol cans in the client's room.
- Do not shake bedding or create dust clouds in the room.
- Cover the tracheostomy with a thin cloth during shaving.
- Use only manufactured pre-sewn dressings around the trach (cut dressings may have loose edges that could be aspirated into the tracheostomy).
- Monitor tracheostomy cuff pressure and use the minimal leak technique to inflate the cuff. (See Table 20-4, p. 526 of Polaski and Tatro, *Luckmann's Core Principles and Practice of Medical-Surgical Nursing.*)
- Keep the obturator taped above the head of the bed and keep tracheal dilators (spreaders) in the room.
- Use caution when changing tracheostomy ties to prevent extubation.
  — Hold the tube with two fingers.
  — Use two people, or only change one tie at a time.
  — If accidental extubation occurs and the stoma is less than four days old:
    — call for help immediately
    — maintain ventilation and oxygenation by bag and mask
    — if ventilation is impossible, reinsert the tube
    — if the tracheostomy cannot be reinserted within one minute, call a code for respiratory arrest. An emergency cricothyroidectomy may be necessary.

If accidental extubation occurs greater than four days following a tracheostomy, the same procedure is used, although it is generally easier. If bleeding occurs or the airway is obstructed, emergency measures are indicated.

Maintain Oral Mucosa Integrity
- Provide oral hygiene every two hours.

Prevent Constipation

- Be aware that the client is predisposed to constipation due to inability to perform the Valsalva's maneuver (the glottis and the vocal cords are bypassed with a tracheostomy).
- Use prescribed stool softeners, laxatives as needed.

Reduce Fear and Anxiety

- Provide emotional support and reassurance.
- Frequently check the client.
- Explain all procedures and equipment.

FOCUSED DISCHARGE CARE

- Instruct client/significant other regarding:
  — tracheostomy care and safety measures
  — suctioning, use of a manual resuscitation bag, hyperoxygenating
  — aerosol therapy
  — airway maintenance
  — signs/symptoms of infection
  — clothing to disguise tracheostomy
- Refer to support groups.
- Refer to home health care agency for follow up.
- Involve a pulmonary nurse specialist if appropriate.
- Also see, "Laryngeal Cancer", p. 411.

(For more information, see pp. 525-533 of Polaski and Tatro, *Luckmann's Core Principles and Practice of Medical-Surgical Nursing.*)

Traction

OVERVIEW

- Therapeutic traction is accomplished by exerting a pull in two directions, the pull of traction and the pull of countertraction. Traction (pull) usually is produced by weights. Countertraction is produced by other weights or the weight of the person's own body. Forces also are exerted by the position of the client (e.g., flexion of the knee and hip). It is imperative that the position of the pulleys and the angle of splints not be adjusted without physician order.

- The goal of traction is to return bone fragments to their normal position or to treat muscle sprain, strain and spasm.

- If traction is applied to a long bone, the direction of traction is in line with the bone's long axis. When applied to the head or pelvis, the pull is in line with the person's spinal column.

- Traction techniques include:
  — Running traction (straight traction) — exerts a direct pull on the affected part without a hammock or splint to provide balanced support. It may be applied to the skin or skeleton.
  — Suspension traction (balanced traction) — exerts a pull on the affected part and also supports the extremity in a hammock or splint held in place by balanced weights attached to an overhead bar. It may be either skeletal or skin traction.
  — Continuous versus Intermittent — traction may be continuous (constant pull) or intermittent (pulled periodically by lifting the weights).

- Types of traction include:
  — Skin — traction is applied to the underlying skeletal system and other structures using adhesive backed materials or by encircling a body part with a halter, corset or sling.
  — Skeletal — traction is accomplished by surgically inserting metal wires (Kirschner wires) or pins (Steinmann pins) through bones or by anchoring metal tongs (such as Crutchfield) in the skull. Kirschner wires or Steinmann pins are round stainless steel rods typically inserted with a drill, perpendicular to and completely through bones.
  — Cervical — traction applied via a head halter to treat muscle sprain, strain and spasm.
  — Pelvic — application of a belt above and encircling the iliac crests to apply traction to the lumbar spine.
  — Buck's traction — a form of skin traction exerted by a straight pull in one or both legs. Traction is applied using a prefabricated boot.
  — Russell's traction — a modification of Buck's traction, creating a vertical pull by placing a sling under the leg above the knee.

NURSING MANAGEMENT

- Discuss with client the purpose of traction and contraindicated movements or positions.
- Perform baseline neurovascular assessment before insertion of pins or wires.
- Place corks or adhesive tape over protruding ends of pins or wires to prevent injury or damage to clothing.
- Inspect skin around pin sites for odor, redness or drainage.
- Provide pin site care as prescribed (often a daily dressing change with cleansing using antiseptic solution and application of betadine ointment).
- Cover the affected limb without interfering with traction.
- Ensure that ropes and pulleys hang free.
- Ensure that knots in the rope do not catch in the pulleys.
- Add and remove weights slowly with physician order.
- With pelvic traction, keep hips and knees flexed 30 degrees. Do not excessively elevate the backrest (this creates a shearing force on the sacrum).
- Monitor color, warmth, movement and sensation of extremity distal to traction every shift.
- Assess distal pulses every shift.
- Monitor degree of pain continually — pain should decrease. If pain increases, notify physician.
- Change linen from top to bottom of bed.
- Provide diversional activities—obtain Occupational Therapy consult.
- Provide normal aids to orientation.
- Use a fracture pan for elimination.
- Provide trapeze for assistance with movement.
- Provide analgesics as prescribed (muscle spasms should subside after 48 to 72 hours).
- Assess skin for breakdown.
- Apply therapeutic mattress to bed.
- Perform range of motion exercises every shift to all joints except those immediately proximal and distal to the fracture.
- Assess lung sounds every shift.
- Instruct client on coughing, deep breathing and incentive spirometry.

- Monitor for thrombophlebitis.
- Monitor bowel movements and encourage fluids and high fiber diet.

Following traction removal:
- Assist the client to gradually resume a sitting (and later standing) position (to prevent orthostatic hypotension).
- Prepare client for lack of proprioceptor response (awareness of body position, movement and posture).
- Discuss that joints may be stiff or unstable and client may feel faint or weak for awhile.

(For more information, see pp. 1274-1278 of Polaski and Tatro, *Luckmann's Core Principles and Practice of Medical-Surgical Nursing.*)

Transient Ischemic Attacks

OVERVIEW

- Transient ischemic attacks (TIA's) are brief, reversible episodes of neurologic dysfunction caused by temporary, focal cerebral ischemia.
- During a TIA, a transient decrease occurs in the blood supply to a focal area of the cerebrum or brain stem. Factors that can cause this ischemia include: occlusive disease of the extracranial cerebral vessels; occlusions in the vertebrobasilar system; and emboli.
- Risk factors and preventive measures are essentially the same as those for cerebrovascular accident (CVA) (see "Cerebrovascular Accident", p. 134).

CLINICAL MANIFESTATIONS

Symptoms are transient, lasting usually from two to fifteen minutes up to an hour. They vary, depending upon which area of the brain is affected.
- visual, auditory or vestibular disturbances
- motor and sensory disturbances

- headache
- slowed mental processes
- seizures

MEDICAL MANAGEMENT

(The goal is to prevent the progression of a TIA to a CVA.)
- antihypertensives, antiplatelet drugs or aspirin
- Warfarin (coumadin) to prevent clot development

SURGICAL MANAGEMENT

- carotid endarterectomy — resection of plaque causing occlusion in the common carotid artery. A temporary blood supply to the brain may be created by shunting blood through other vessels during the operation.
- extracranial-intracranial bypass — anastomosis of the superficial temporal artery to the middle cerebral artery, thereby increasing blood flow to the brain. Performed for vascular insufficiency in the distribution of the middle cerebral artery.

NURSING MANAGEMENT

MEDICAL

- Administer antihypertensives, antiplatelet drugs or aspirin as prescribed.
- Administer Coumadin as prescribed; monitor prothrombin time (PT) and for any signs/symptoms of bleeding.
- Monitor blood pressure.
- Monitor neurological status.
- Maintain safety precautions.

SURGICAL - POSTOPERATIVE CARE

In addition to routine postoperative care:

EXTRACRANIAL-INTRACRANIAL BYPASS

Nursing care is the same as for clients undergoing other types of cranial surgery. (See "Intracranial Tumors", p. 403.)
- Monitor vital signs and neurological status closely, reporting any changes immediately to physician.
- Palpate pulse created by surgical anastomosis (lo-

cated just below the curve of the incision) and notify surgeon immediately of any changes in character.

- Keep the head in a straight position.
- Elevate the head of the bed.
- Maintain systolic blood pressure between 120 and 170 mm Hg to ensure cerebral perfusion (blood pressure may be labile due to manipulation of the baroreceptors during surgery).
- Monitor for hematoma formation or excessive neck swelling (can cause airway obstruction).
- Assess neurological status frequently, including pupillary reaction, level of consciousness, motor function and sensory function. Report any changes immediately.
- Assess functioning of the following cranial nerves: facial (VII), vagus (X), spinal accessory (XI) and hypoglossal (XII) (cranial nerve damage usually is temporary but may last for months).

FOCUSED DISCHARGE CARE

MEDICAL MANAGEMENT

Instruct client/significant other regarding:
- Coumadin therapy
  — signs/symptoms of bleeding
  — safety measures
  — importance of follow-up laboratory tests
- antihypertensive or antiplatelet therapy
- signs/symptoms of increasing neurological deficits to report to physician
- safety measures

SURGICAL MANAGEMENT

Instruct client/significant other regarding:
- wound care; signs/symptoms of infection
- no constrictive clothing or jewelry around the neck
- above information under "Medical Management"

(For more information, see pp. 327-329 of Polaski and Tatro, *Luckmann's Core Principles and Practice of Medical-Surgical Nursing.*)

Trichomoniasis

OVERVIEW

- Trichomoniasis is a protozoal infection causing vulvovaginitis.
- Trichomoniasis is caused by the parasite protozoan, Trichomonas vaginalis.
- The organism likes an alkaline environment, and changes in the vaginal flora make a woman susceptible.
- The organism is almost always transmitted sexually, and recurrence is common.

CLINICAL MANIFESTATIONS

- Female:
  — copious, malodorous, yellow-green vaginal discharge
  — itching, burning, excoriation, and maceration of the vulvar tissue
  — cervix may be covered with punctate hemorrhages, "strawberry cervix"
  — vaginal mucosa is reddened and slightly edematous
  — pain with intercourse
  — frequency and burning with urination
- Male:
  — frequency and burning with urination

MEDICAL MANAGEMENT

- single dose of Flagyl (metronidazole) orally for the client and all sexual contacts; for recurrence, a seven day regime.
- for the pregnant client — vaginal clotrimazole cream because Flagyl may adversely affect fetal development.

Single-dose therapy is usually curative but recurrence is common.

NURSING MANAGEMENT

- Administer Flagyl as prescribed.
- Administer PRN medications for pain and itching.

- Instruct regarding perineal care.

FOCUSED DISCHARGE CARE

Instruct the client regarding:
- importance of completing medication regime
- information regarding disease, transmission, treatment, and follow-up
- need to treat all sexual partners
- medication administration
  — no alcoholic intake (including mouthwash and some cold preparations) during and 3 days after Flagyl administration to prevent the side effects of nausea, vomiting, and headaches
- need for the client to refrain from sexual intercourse or to use a condom while infection is active
- perineal hygiene

(For more information, see pp. 1512-1513 of Polaski and Tatro, *Luckmann's Core Principles and Practice of Medical-Surgical Nursing*.)

Trigeminal Neuralgia

OVERVIEW

- Trigeminal neuralgia is pain in the distribution of the fifth cranial nerve, the trigeminal nerve. The trigeminal nerve has three branches: the ophthalmic, maxillary and mandibular. Trigeminal neuralgia may occur in any one or more of these branches.
- The causative mechanisms can be divided into intrinsic (abnormalities of the axon or myelin) or extrinsic (mechanical compression from a tumor or from vascular anomalies).
- It is most common between the ages of 50 and 70 years. Approximately 60 per cent of clients are women.

CLINICAL MANIFESTATIONS

- intermittent episodes of intense pain with sudden onset

- pain not relieved by analgesics
- attacks are triggered by tactile stimulation (touch, facial hygiene) and talking
- the right side of face is more commonly affected

MEDICAL MANAGEMENT

- anticonvulsant therapy—carbamazepine (Tegretol), phenytoin (Dilantin) — decrease the reactivity of neurons in the trigeminal nerve
- antispasmodic therapy — baclofen (Liorsal)

SURGICAL MANAGEMENT

- nerve blocks
- microvascular decompression — craniotomy is performed and the vessel removed from the posterior trigeminal root
- rhizotomy - resection of the root of the nerve (requires a craniotomy)

NURSING MANAGEMENT

MEDICAL

- Administer medications as ordered and assess effectiveness.
- Instruct client on ways to prevent triggering events.

SURGICAL

- See care of client following craniotomy, Nursing Management, "Increased Intracranial Pressure", p. 392.

(For more information, see pp. 414-416 of Polaski and Tatro, *Luckmann's Core Principles and Practice of Medical-Surgical Nursing.*)

Tuberculosis, Pulmonary

OVERVIEW

- Tuberculosis (TB) is a chronic infectious disease that is characterized by the formation of tubercles or granulomas in the lungs. It is caused when droplet nuclei of mycobacterium tuberculosis are aerosolized through coughing, laughing, sneezing or singing and a susceptible client inhales the droplet nuclei. If it penetrates lung tissue, the infection occurs.
- Tuberculosis is a worldwide health problem with an estimated 3 million new cases diagnosed each year.
- Tuberculosis is a reportable communicable disease. Brief exposure usually does not cause infection, but rather those having repeated close contact.
- High risk groups include: the elderly, clients with reduced immunity, clients who are malnourished, Native Americans, Eskimos and blacks, economically disadvantaged or homeless, and clients dependent upon alcohol.
- TB infection may be primary or secondary:
  — Primary infection refers to the first time a client is infected with tuberculosis. The primary tubercles heal over a period of months through the formation of fibrous scars and, ultimately, calcified lesions. These lesions may contain certain living bacilli that later can reactivate and cause secondary infection.
  — Secondary infection (or reinfection) occurs when primary sites of infection containing TB bacilli (which may have been latent for years), reactivate when the client's resistance is lowered.

CLINICAL MANIFESTATIONS

- fatigue, anorexia, weight loss
- persistent, long-term, low grade fever
- chills and sweats (often at night)
- nonresolving bronchopneumonia
- dyspnea, hemoptysis
- chest pain (pleuritic or dull) or chest tightness
- persistent, progressive and often productive cough

MEDICAL MANAGEMENT

- isoniazid 300 mg daily for 9-12 months for prevention of active TB
- use of three or more medications initially for active TB to destroy large numbers of rapidly multiplying organisms; then maintenance therapy with two medications to eliminate most remaining bacilli. Medications used include: isoniazid, ethambutol, rifampin, streptomycin and pyrazinamide.
- the length of each phase of therapy depends upon the client's compliance and the success of treatment. The course of each treatment phase may be anywhere from 6-24 months.
- TB protocols for non-compliant patients may include medications 2 to 3 times weekly.

NURSING MANAGEMENT

- Discuss need for respiratory isolation, if hospitalized.
- Instruct client that public health officials will talk with the client to develop a contact list (persons with whom client has had contact).
- Discuss mode of transmission and methods of preventing spread of disease.
- Monitor for side effects of medications and drug toxicity.
- Collect sputum specimens for acid-fast bacillus smear and culture.
- Discuss mode of transmission of TB and that it is not a shameful disease.

FOCUSED DISCHARGE CARE

Instruct client regarding:
- importance of follow-up visits to ensure that dormant lesions have not reactivated
- signs/symptoms of reinfection (secondary disease)
- importance of compliance with medication regimen
- side effects to report to physician
- need for isolation until 2 to 4 weeks into treatment
- transmission of TB:

- cover mouth and nose when coughing, laughing or sneezing
- TB is not carried on eating utensils or articles
- client must wash hands after handling body substances, masks or soiled tissues
- sputum is highly contaminated
- need to wear mask and change frequently

(For more information, see pp. 590-595 of Polaski and Tatro, *Luckmann's Core Principles and Practice of Medical-Surgical Nursing.*)

Tympanic Membrane Perforation (Ruptured Eardrum)

- The tympanic membrane is a semi-transparent membrane which may become perforated through sports injuries, cleaning the ear with a sharp instrument, falling in water, a hand slap or middle ear infection.
- A perforation may be acute, as seen with trauma or acute infection, or chronic, as seen in repeated infections.
- Acute perforations usually heal spontaneously. There may be hearing loss associated with the perforation, depending upon the size and location.
- Medical management includes use of systemic and local antibiotics (eardrops).
- Surgical management involves a myringoplasty (closure of the perforation). A tympanoplasty may be performed if the middle ear is also involved.

(For more information, see pp. 462-463 of Polaski and Tatro, *Luckmann's Core Principles and Practice of Medical-Surgical Nursing.*)

Ulcerative Colitis

OVERVIEW

- Ulcerative colitis is a type of inflammatory bowel disease. It is characterized by periods of exacerbation and remission. This disease spans the entire length of the colon and involves the mucosa and submucosa. It starts in the rectum and distal colon and spreads upward to the sigmoid and descending colon.
- Ulcerative colitis causes inflammation, thickening, congestion, edema and minute lacerations that ooze blood and eventually develop into abscesses.
- When the inflammatory lesions heal, scarring and fibrosis with narrowing, thickening and shortening of the colon may occur. Loss of haustral folds also may occur.
- Theories of causation include allergic reaction, altered immunity, bacterial origin, destructive enzymes and a lack of protective substances in the bowel wall.
- Young adults, women and Jewish people have a higher incidence of the disease, and it does have a familial tendency.
- Cancer of the colon is more common in clients with ulcerative colitis.
- There are no preventable risk factors, but controlling stress can help keep the disease in remission.

CLINICAL MANIFESTATIONS

- rectal bleeding
- diarrhea of up to 20 or more stools/day
- urgency, cramping, abdominal pain in lower left quadrant
- nausea, vomiting, dehydration, anorexia, fever, weight loss and decreased serum potassium
- decreased plasma proteins and prothrombin

MEDICAL MANAGEMENT

- anti-inflammatory therapy, including steroids
- fluid, electrolyte and blood replacement
- antidiarrheals
- hydrophilic mucilloids
- antispasmodics
- antibiotics and sulfonamides (such as sulfasala-zine)
- bowel rest
- total parenteral nutrition
- antacids, histamine receptor antagonists
- anticholinergics
- high protein and calorie diet
- correction of nutritional deficiencies

SURGICAL MANAGEMENT

- total proctocolectomy with a permanent ileos-tomy:
  — removal of the colon and rectum and closure of the anus
  — the terminal ileum is brought through the abdominal wall and a permanent ileostomy formed
- ileorectal anastomosis:
  — old procedure performed infrequently
  — resection of the colon, leaving a rectal stump; the terminal ileum is anastomosed to this stump
- ileoanal reservoir (J Pouch):
  — excision of the rectal mucosa and colon removal
  — an ileoanal reservoir is created in the anal canal and a temporary loop ileostomy is formed
  — after healing takes place, the ileostomy is reversed, and stool drains into the reservoir
  — prevents the need for an ostomy and preserves the rectal sphincter muscle
- Kock pouch (continent ileostomy)
  — a reservoir is constructed from a loop of ileum
  — stool is retained in the intra-abdominal pouch until the client drains it with a catheter through a special nipple valve
  — the stoma is flat and flush with the skin on the right side of the abdomen
  — there is no external pouch worn — the internal pouch is drained several times a day

NURSING MANAGEMENT

MEDICAL

- Monitor the number, color and consistency of stools.
- Hemoccult all stools.
- Administer antidiarrheals as prescribed.
- Monitor intake and output; daily weights.
- Provide good perianal skin care — cleanse skin with warm water after each bowel movement and apply protective moisture barrier product.
- Monitor hemoglobin and hematocrit.
- Monitor intake of foods and fluids — encourage small servings of bland and easily digested foods.
- Offer nutritional supplements.
- Assess quality, location, severity and duration of pain — changes in pain may indicate development of complications.
- Administer pain medications as prescribed and assess effectiveness.
- Discuss stress management and relaxation techniques (stress may exacerbate).

SURGICAL

PREOPERATIVE CARE —IF OSTOMY WILL BE PERFORMED

In addition to routine preoperative care:
- Discuss role of enterostomal therapist.
- Arrange for preoperative visit from member of an ostomy association.
- Allow client to wear pouch over selected ostomy site 1 to 2 days before surgery to ensure comfort with site selected.
- Encourage discussion regarding feelings about change in body image and feelings about loss of a major body part.

POSTOPERATIVE CARE

In addition to routine postoperative care:
- Assess stomal color and contact physician immediately if pale, dusky or cyanotic.
- Maintain patent nasogastric, gastrostomy or jejunostomy tube to prevent distention. Measure amount of drainage.

- Clamp tube and start ice chips as ordered when bowel sounds return.
- Assess for signs/symptoms of intestinal obstruction after ileostomy: anorexia, abdominal cramps, absence of visible peristalsis, absence of ileostomy drainage or a foul, brown, watery discharge in the pouch.
- Monitor for fluid and electrolyte imbalance.
- Monitor for hemorrhage.
- After Kock pouch, assess for suture line leakage and local or generalized peritonitis.
- After continent ileostomy or Kock pouch, assess for start of ileal drainage (three to four days postoperatively).
- Assist the client to look at and touch the stoma as soon as possible.
- Encourage the client to verbalize feelings about the stoma and its appearance.

FOCUSED DISCHARGE CARE

MEDICAL AND SURGICAL

- Instruct client regarding:
  — factors that exacerbate: emotional stress, overfatigue, dietary indiscretions, laxatives, antibiotics, physical exertion, respiratory infections
  — signs/symptoms of fluid and electrolyte imbalance
  — keeping a record of number of stools, consistency, color and presence of blood
  — need for follow-up colonoscopies and barium enemas if have had disease 5 or more years (higher incidence of cancer)
  — need to report significant weight loss to physician
  — side effects of steroids
- Refer to Crohn's and Colitis Foundations of America.
- Refer to American Cancer Society.

SURGICAL

ILEOSTOMY

- Instruct client regarding:
  — normal appearance of stoma—instruct that stoma will shrink to permanent size within 3 to 4 months
  — assessing stoma for signs of irritation or cyanosis

- — care of the stoma and surrounding skin
- — signs of fungal skin infection
- — applying, changing and emptying pouch
- — where to purchase ileostomy equipment and supplies (include brand name, order number, size of pouch, skin barrier and pouch deodorants)
- — use of deodorizing solutions and tablets
- — foods that create odor: eggs, fish, onion, cabbage or greens
- — foods that reduce odor: spinach, parsley, yogurt or buttermilk
- — drinking at least 1500 mls per day
- — low residue diet, high in protein, carbohydrates and calories
- — foods that may cause problems: berries, whole grains, raw fruits and vegetables
- — foods to avoid: rice, bran, coconuts, popcorn, peanuts, skinned vegetables, tough fibrous meats, high fiber and high cellulose foods
- — sexual activity, concerns and pregnancy — encourage discussion with partner. Discuss emptying pouch before intercourse or wearing soft flannel pouch over it.
- — need for follow-up with enterostomal therapist
- — clothing options
- — medications — enteric coated tablets may not be absorbed in the small intestine
- Encourage to join the Ileostomy Association (associated with American Cancer Society).
- Refer to United Ostomy Association.
- Refer to enterostomal therapist for follow-up ostomy teaching.

Ileorectal Anastomosis

- Instruct client regarding:
  - — importance of defecating before rectum is overly distended
  - — stool will be pasty in consistency
  - — remaining bowel may become diseased
  - — increased risk of rectal cancer
  - — need for regular proctoscopic examinations
  - — need for adequate fluids

- Instruct client regarding:
  — need to respond to sensation to defecate so spillage does not occur
  — need for adequate fluids
  — stool output — eventually there will be 2 to 4 stools/day

CONTINENT ILEOSTOMY OR KOCK POUCH

- Instruct client regarding:
  — need to empty reservoir every 2 hours for first 2 weeks
  — evacuation catheter will be removed about 2 weeks after surgery
  — how to empty the reservoir
  — need for oral intake of at least eight 8 oz. glasses of water daily
  — need for Medic-Alert identification and to carry drainage instructions in case of emergency
  — need to avoid foods such as mushrooms and nuts that could block valve

(For more information, see pp. 1061-1071 of Polaski and Tatro, *Luckmann's Core Principles and Practice of Medical-Surgical Nursing.*)

Urinary Retention

OVERVIEW

- Urinary retention is urine retained in the bladder. It is most often caused by obstruction at or below the bladder outlet.
- Benign prostatic hypertrophy, anesthesia, and scarring from chronic urinary tract infections are common causes.

CLINICAL MANIFESTATIONS

- distended bladder with inability to void

MEDICAL MANAGEMENT

- catheterization with a straight catheter or retention catheter
- urethral dilation with progressively larger catheters used each day
- cholinergic medications sometimes combined with phenoxybenzamine, prazosin, and terazosin (alpha-adrenergic blockers)

SURGICAL MANAGEMENT

- suprapubic catheter placement
- specific procedures done to relieve obstruction below the bladder

NURSING MANAGEMENT

- Differentiate retention from oliguria and anuria.
- Perform non-invasive methods to stimulate voiding:
  — place client in a normal sitting or standing position
  — run water or flush the toilet within earshot of client
  — pour warm water over perineum or provide warm bath
  — immerse client's hand in water or have client blow bubbles with a straw in a glass of water
  — apply ice to or stroke inner thigh to stimulate trigger points.
- Straight catheterize or place retention catheter as ordered.
- Maintain patent drainage system if catheter in place. Keep drainage bag below level of the bladder.
- Maintain strict aseptic technique when handling catheter or drainage system.
- Monitor intake and output.

FOCUSED DISCHARGE CARE

Instruct client regarding:
- suprapubic catheter care after discharge (if present):

      — care of catheter
      — changing leg bag to conventional drainage bag at night
      — cleaning of bags and odor control
- self catheterization as appropriate
- signs/symptoms of urinary tract infection and when to call physician
- prevention of infection and need to force fluids

(For more information, see pp. 928-931 of Polaski and Tatro, *Luckmann's Core Principles and Practice of Medical-Surgical Nursing.*)

Urinary Tract Infection

OVERVIEW

- Urinary tract infection (UTI) refers to an infection within the lower urinary tract. The infection can affect the bladder (cystitis), the urethra (urethritis) and/or the ureters.
- The most common organisms causing urinary tract infections are: Escherichia coli, Enterobacter, Pseudomonas and Serratia.
- Risk factors include: indwelling catheters, pregnancy, and sexual intercourse.
- Factors that contribute to the development of UTIs include
      — decreased resistance to invading organisms
      — loss of integrity of mucosal lining
      — retention of urine in the bladder
      — undertreated cyctitis

CLINICAL MANIFESTATIONS

- frequency, urgency, burning on urination, hematuria
- inability to void or voiding in small amounts
- incomplete emptying of the bladder
- low back, suprapubic, abdominal or flank pain
- positive urine cultures

- chills, fever, malaise, nausea, vomiting
- incontinence

MEDICAL MANAGEMENT

- 10-14 day course of antibiotic therapy
- use of medications containing azo dyes to anesthetize the urinary tract mucosa
- chronic urinary tract infection — acidifying the urine through an acid-ash diet to decrease the rate of bacterial multiplication — this may or may not be ordered depending on the specific antiseptic or antibiotic used. (An acid-ash diet is considered more effective in acidifying the urine than use of cranberry juice or ascorbic acid.)

SURGICAL MANAGEMENT

- Rare, but surgery may include correction of bladder neck strictures or ureteral pelvic junction abnormalities.

NURSING MANAGEMENT

MEDICAL

- Monitor the client's voiding — note frequency, urgency, retention or dysuria.
- Monitor intake and output.
- Provide warm sitz baths - baking soda may be added for a greater soothing effect.
- Encourage fluids.
- Apply a heating pad to the suprapubic area as ordered to reduce bladder spasms.
- Administer anti-infective agents as prescribed — assess for a decrease in the severity of symptoms within 24 hours after the start of medications.
- Monitor culture and sensitivity reports.
- Obtain residuals as ordered.
- Monitor vital signs, consider blood cultures for temperature of 101° F.
- Assess for sepsis (UTI's are the most common cause of gram negative sepsis).

FOCUSED DISCHARGE CARE

Instruct the client regarding:

- Drinking at least eight 8 ounce glasses of water per day.
- Avoidance of caffeine, alcohol , and carbonated beverages (they irritate the bladder).
- Voiding at the first urge and at least every 2-3 hours during the day.
- Voiding 1-2 times per night.
- Women:
  — avoidance of synthetic underwear, panty hose, tight jeans
  — wearing cotton panties
  — avoidance of bubble baths, perfumed toilet paper or sanitary napkins
  — wiping perineum front to back
  — taking baths versus showers
  — if sexually active:
    — wash well before sexual intercourse
    — void immediately after sexual intercourse
    — drink 2 glasses of water after intercourse.
- Taking the full course of medication, even if symptoms disappear.
- Compliance with the schedule of follow-up urine cultures.
- Following the acid-ash diet as ordered.
- Contacting the physician for signs of persistent infection.

(For more information, see pp. 916-922 of Polaski and Tatro, *Luckmann's Core Principles and Practice of Medical-Surgical Nursing.*)

Uterine Prolapse

OVERVIEW

- Uterine prolapse occurs in 3 stages:
  (1) First Degree— the uterus descends into the vaginal canal and the cervix reaches, but does not go through the entrance to the vagina (introitus).
  (2) Second Degree —the body of the uterus is within the vagina but the cervix protrudes through the introitus.

(3) Third Degree — the entire uterus and cervix protrude through the introitus and the vaginal canal is inverted (turned inside out).

- Prolapse commonly follows multiple childbirths, childbirth trauma, aging and failure to maintain the perineal musculature.
- During the stages of prolapse of the uterus, other structures may be pulled down or out of position:
  — cystocele — protrusion of part of the urinary bladder through the vaginal wall due to weakened pelvic muscles
  — rectocele — protrusion of a portion of the rectum through a weak place in the vaginal wall musculature
  — enterocele — herniation of small bowel and/or omentum into the vaginal canal
- When complete prolapse has occurred and involves a cystocele, rectocele and enterocele, the woman is said to have pelvic relaxation.
- With pelvic relaxation, the cervix protrudes through the vaginal orifice and is constantly irritated, causing inflammation and possible malignant degeneration.

CLINICAL MANIFESTATIONS

- feeling that "something is descending internally"
- dyspareunia (pain with intercourse)
- feelings of pressure, dragging and heaviness
- backaches, bowel and bladder symptoms

Cystocele
- urinary frequency, urgency, urinary tract infections, difficulty emptying the bladder, stress incontinence

Rectocele
- constipation, heaviness, hemorrhoids

MEDICAL MANAGEMENT

- Kegel exercises (see Nursing Management)
- use of a pessary

SURGICAL MANAGEMENT

Cystocele
- anterior repair or anterior colporrhaphy — tightening the pelvic muscles to provide better bladder support

Rectocele
- posterior repair or posterior colporrhaphy — surgical tightening of the weakened muscles (this also may be performed in conjunction with an anterior repair and then is called an anteroposterior colporrhaphy or anterior-posterior repair)

Complete Uterine Prolapse
- vaginal hysterectomy — removal of the uterus through the vagina

NURSING MANAGEMENT

MEDICAL

- Instruct client on Kegel exercises (alternately tightening and relaxing rectal and vaginal muscles). These are tightened as if trying to hold back a bowel movement or stop the urinary stream. They should be performed frequently throughout the day or 50 to 100 times once or twice daily.

SURGICAL

POSTOPERATIVE CARE

In addition to routine postoperative care:
- Keep urinary catheter patent to keep bladder decompressed and pressure off the anterior vaginal muscles until healing has occurred.
- Instruct client to void every 2 hours after catheter is removed to keep bladder decompressed.
- Monitor for excessive vaginal bleeding, rigid and distended abdomen or referred shoulder pain. Notify physician, if any of these occur.
- Maintain vaginal packing or drain (usually removed after 24 to 48 hours).
- Provide sitz baths for comfort.

FOCUSED DISCHARGE CARE

Instruct client regarding:
- catheter care (if applicable)
- signs/symptoms to report to physician:
  — excess bleeding
  — distended abdomen
  — inability to void

- — signs of urinary tract infection
- — signs of infection
- activity/lifting restrictions
- use of sitz baths for comfort
- use of analgesics
- bleeding may occur on the 4th, 9th, 14th and 21st days following surgery, as the sutures dissolve
- low residue diet and stool softeners until healing occurs
- avoidance of constipation which can cause recurrence

(For more information, see pp. 1487-1489 of Polaski and Tatro, *Luckmann's Core Principles and Practice of Medical-Surgical Nursing*.)

Uterine Tumors, Benign (Leiomyomas)

OVERVIEW

- Leiomyomas are benign tumors of the uterine muscles. They are the most common tumors of the female genital tract and also are called myomas or fibroids of the uterus.
- They occur in more than 20 to 30 per cent of all women during their menstrual years. The incidence in black women is 2 to 3 times greater than in white women.
- The cause of leiomyomas is unknown, but seems to be related to estrogen stimulation.

CLINICAL MANIFESTATIONS

- abnormal uterine bleeding (excessive in amount or duration) with associated anemia, tiredness, weakness and lethargy
- urinary frequency
- urinary retention
- constipation
- hydroureter, hydronephrosis, abdominal pain and dyspareunia are less common symptoms

MEDICAL MANAGEMENT

Treatment depends upon symptoms, age, location and size of the tumors, onset of complications and the woman's desire to become pregnant.

SURGICAL MANAGEMENT

- myomectomy (removal of tumor without removal of the uterus) for small tumors
- total hysterectomy — removal of the uterus and cervix (performed vaginally or abdominally)
- total abdominal hysterectomy with bilateral salpingo-oophorectomy (TAH-BSO) — removal of the uterus, cervix, fallopian tubes and ovaries

NURSING MANAGEMENT

MEDICAL

- Discuss ways to reduce pain — sitz baths, application of heat to lower abdomen.
- Discuss ways to reduce pain during intercourse — alternate positions, use of water soluble lubricants.
- Pain medications can be used for severe pain.

SURGICAL — HYSTERECTOMY

PREOPERATIVE CARE

In addition to routine preoperative care:
- Discuss fact that reproductive function will be lost if hysterectomy is performed.
- Instruct that sexual intercourse should be pain-free once healing has occurred, and orgasms are still possible.
- If the ovaries will be removed, discuss that surgical menopause will occur.

POSTOPERATIVE CARE

In addition to routine postoperative care:
- Monitor amount of bleeding, number of pads used and drainage on dressings. Also note color and odor.

- If total abdominal hysterectomy was performed, monitor abdominal incision site for redness, drainage or swelling.
- Encourage turning, coughing and deep breathing and increase activity as prescribed.
- Maintain thigh-high antiembolism stockings.
- Encourage ankle and leg exercises.
- Monitor Homan's sign.
- Maintain urinary catheter to dependent drainage and monitor intake and output.
- Encourage 2 to 4 liters of fluid daily when tolerating fluids well.
- Monitor for pain on voiding, voiding frequently in small amounts, inability to void or hematuria when the catheter is removed and report to physician.
- Assess color, odor and clarity of urine — report any changes.
- Provide analgesics and assess effectiveness.
- Provide good perineal care and catheter care (if present) every shift.
- If abdominal hysterectomy was performed, monitor for return of bowel sounds. Encourage ambulation to stimulate peristalsis.
- Provide open environment for patient to discuss feelings regarding loss of uterus and sexual concerns.
- Encourage client to share thoughts/concerns with partner.

FOCUSED DISCHARGE CARE

Instruct client regarding:
Hysterectomy
- performing prescribed abdominal strengthening exercises
- avoidance of heavy lifting for 2 months
- avoidance of activities that increase pelvic congestion (such as dancing, horseback riding and prolonged standing)
- avoidance of vaginal or rectal sexual activities and douching until permitted by surgeon
- avoidance of constrictive clothing for several months
- symptoms to report to physician — abnormal vagi-

nal discharge, bleeding, signs/symptoms of infection, incision not healing
- possible effects of surgical menopause, and interventions to minimize (if ovaries were removed):
  — vasomotor instability (including hot flashes, night sweats, occasional palpitations and dizziness)
    — dress in layers so that clothing can be removed during hot flashes
    — avoid hot environments and keep the thermostat around 65° F. or lower
    — avoid highly seasoned, spicy foods, coffee, tea and alcohol if they trigger hot flashes
    — keep a record of hot flashes to help determine "triggers"
  — vaginal dryness
    — use water soluble jelly for lubrication; estrogen cream if needed
  — osteoporosis
    — take part in weight bearing exercise
    — increase calcium intake
    — stop smoking
    — decrease caffeine and alcohol intake
  — urinary tract infection
    — drink plenty of fluids
    — void frequently
    — perform good perineal hygiene
- hormone replacement therapy, side effects and precautions (if prescribed)

Myomectomy
- need for routine gynecologic examinations

If surgery was not performed:
- interventions to minimize pain during intercourse (e.g., different positions)
- need for routine gynecologic examinations to monitor the leiomyomas

(For more information, see pp.1481-1484 of Polaski and Tatro, *Luckmann's Core Principles and Practice of Medical-Surgical Nursing.*)

Uveitis

OVERVIEW

- Uveitis is an inflammation of the uveal tract that can affect one or more parts of the eye (iris, ciliary body and choroid).
- Uveitis commonly occurs from a hypersensitivity reaction in its acute form or following microbial infection in its chronic form.

CLINICAL MANIFESTATIONS

- pain (ciliary body muscle spasm)
- blurred vision
- photophobia
- redness of the eye
- constricted pupil

MEDICAL MANAGEMENT

- topical atropine (cycloplegic) — relieves spasm
- topical steroid — to reduce inflammation
- analgesics

NURSING MANAGEMENT

- Administer eye drops.
- Administer PRN analgesics.
- Keep room lights dimmed.
- Implement safety measures.

FOCUSED DISCHARGE CARE

Instruct client regarding:
- technique for instilling eye drops
- measures to relieve photophobia — sunglasses, dimmed lights
- signs/symptoms of increased intraocular pressure (pain, nausea, decreased vision)
- measures for a safe home environment

(For more information, see p.450 of Polaski and Tatro, *Luckmann's Core Principles and Practice of Medical-Surgical Nursing.*)

Vaginal Cancer

OVERVIEW

- Vaginal cancer is rare, but is seen in women whose mothers ingested diethylstilbestrol during pregnancy. It typically occurs between menarche and age 30 years.
- Women exposed to diethylstilbestrol in utero should receive twice yearly careful gynecologic examinations beginning at menarche or age 14 years, whichever comes first.
- The prognosis for vaginal cancer is generally poor. The overall cure rate reported by the American Cancer Society is about 35 per cent. One-half of women with vaginal cancer die within 18 months of diagnosis.
- Risk factors also include repeated pregnancies, syphilis, uterine prolapse, pessary use, leukoplakia and leukorrhea.

CLINICAL MANIFESTATIONS

- foul vaginal discharge
- painless vaginal bleeding
- pruritus
- pain

MEDICAL MANAGEMENT

- external or intravaginal radiation therapy

SURGICAL MANAGEMENT

- radical hysterectomy, lymphadenectomy and vaginectomy for early stages (removal of the uterus, cervix, fallopian tubes, ovaries, lymph nodes, upper third of the vagina and parametrium)

- pelvic exenteration (removal of pelvic organs and formation of an ileostomy and an ileal conduit) for more advanced cancer

NURSING MANAGEMENT

- Discuss the potential impact of the disease process and treatment on sexuality (potential problems include fatigue, pain, dyspareunia, decreased libido and altered body image).
- Discuss use of alternate positioning and need for adequate lubricant if a partial vaginectomy was performed.
- Discuss use of vaginal dilator to prevent vaginal fibrosis and scarring.

Irradiation

- Discuss need for vaginal penetration to minimize vaginal adhesions and stenosis (may be accomplished by client's own fingers, a vaginal dilator or sexual partner's fingers or penis).
- Discuss need for water soluble lubricant for vaginal dryness.

See "Uterine Tumors, Benign", p. 646, for post-hysterectomy care.

See "Radiation Therapy", p. 543.

(For more information, see pp.1494-1495 of Polaski and Tatro, *Luckmann's Core Principles and Practice of Medical-Surgical Nursing.*)

Vaginal Fistulas

OVERVIEW

- Fistulas are abnormal tubelike passages from the vagina to the bladder (vesicovaginal), rectum (rectovaginal) or urethra (urethrovaginal).
- Causes of vaginal fistulas include: (1) an abnormal opening between two adjacent organs; (2) a result of spread of a malignant lesion; (3) irradiation for cancer; (4) venereal and other inflammatory diseases; (5) prolonged, difficult labor and delivery.

CLINICAL MANIFESTATIONS

- leakage of urine or feces into the vagina
- excoriation and irritation of the vaginal and vulvar tissues
- infection
- feeling of wetness
- sensation of feeling dirty
- offensive odor (with rectovaginal fistulas)

SURGICAL MANAGEMENT

Treatment depends upon the location, extent and cause of the fistula.

- vesicovaginal, urethrovaginal or rectovaginal fistulectomy — repair of the fistula, which may be performed following a 6 month waiting period during which edema and inflammation subside
- temporary colostomy — may be needed with a rectovaginal fistula

NURSING MANAGEMENT

Preoperative Care

In addition to routine preoperative care:
- Encourage fluid intake if the client has a urinary fistula (restriction of fluids may increase the incidence of infection).
- Instruct the client on perineal hygiene measures:
  — cleaning the perineum every 4 hours
  — sitz baths
  — douches
  — changing perineal pads frequently
- Instruct the client on deodorizing and comfort measures:
  — vitamin A and D ointment
  — deodorant powders
  — heat lamp
  — pouring weak acid or weak base solutions over the perineum, as prescribed
  — deodorizing douches as prescribed

Postoperative Care

In addition to routine postoperative care:

- Maintain patency of urinary catheter to prevent strain on sutures.
- Encourage fluid intake.
- Do not let urinary catheter become occluded as the pressure could reopen the fistula.

(For more information, see pp. 1493-1494 of Polaski and Tatro, *Luckmann's Core Principles and Practice of Medical-Surgical Nursing.*)

Vaginosis, Bacterial

OVERVIEW

- Bacterial vaginosis is caused by the organism, Gardnerella vaginalis.

CLINICAL MANIFESTATIONS

- mild to moderate amount of malodorous ("fishy"), gray, homogenous, thin vaginal discharge
- vaginal irritation
- vaginal pruritus

MEDICAL MANAGEMENT

- Flagyl (metronidazole) by mouth for 7 days (unless pregnant due to adverse effect Flagyl may have on fetal development).

NURSING MANAGEMENT

- Administer Flagyl as prescribed.
- Instruct regarding perineal care.
- Instruct regarding palliative measures — PRN medication for pain and itching, sitz baths, etc.

FOCUSED DISCHARGE CARE

Instruct client regarding:

- importance of completing medication regime
- information regarding disease, transmission, treatment, and follow-up
- medication administration:
  — no alcohol intake during or 3 days following Flagyl regime to prevent side effects of nausea, vomiting and headaches
- need to treat male partners only if recurrent or resistant infection
- need to avoid sexual intercourse during the treatment and condom use to prevent recurrence
- perineal hygiene

(For more information, see p. 1513 of Polaski and Tatro, *Luckmann's Core Principles and Practice of Medical-Surgical Nursing.*)

Valvular Heart Disease

OVERVIEW

- The four heart valves maintain the one-way flow of blood through the heart and lungs. Dysfunction occurs when the heart valves are unable to fully open or close. A stenosed valve may impede the flow of one chamber to the next. An insufficient valve may allow blood to regurgitate back into the chamber from which the blood is being pumped. Either problem increases the workload of the heart. The aortic and mitral valves on the heart's left side become dysfunctional more often than the pulmonary and tricuspid valves on the right side because the left side is a system of higher pressures. For a time the heart can compensate by dilation and eventually hypertrophy, but if valvular damage worsens, without intervention the heart will fail.
- *Mitral stenosis* is a block in blood flow into the left ventricle resulting from an abnormality of the leaflets which prevents opening of the valve during diastole. Causes include: infective endocarditis, calcification of valve leaflets, and systemic disorders.

- *Mitral regurgitation* occurs when blood from the left ventricle is ejected back into the left atrium during systole because of an incompetent mitral valve. Causes include mitral valve prolapse, coronary artery disease, and infective endocarditis.
- *Mitral valve prolapse* occurs when one or both of the valve leaflets bulge into the left atrium during ventricular systole. It is usually a benign disorder.
- *Aortic stenosis* is an obstruction to flow across the aortic valve during systole, creating resistance to ejection and increased pressure in the left ventricle. Causes include congenital defect, aging process, and infective endocarditis.
- *Aortic regurgitation* — blood ejected into the aorta during systole re-enters the left ventricle due to an incompetent aortic valve. Causes include infectious or systemic disorders.
- Tricuspid and pulmonic valve disease is rare; tricuspid disorders usually develop in combination with other structural disorders and pulmonic valve disorders are commonly genetic in origin. Because the tricuspid valve is on the right side of the heart, the major hemodynamic alterations are a decrease in cardiac output and an increase in right atrial pressure. Pulmonic valve disease affects cardiac output.
- Risk factors include:
  — acute rheumatic fever
  — infective endocarditis.

CLINICAL MANIFESTATIONS

- Mitral stenosis:
  — low-pitched murmur
  — loud snapping S_1
  — dyspnea, orthopnea, paroxysmal nocturnal dyspnea (PND)
  — fatigue
  — palpitations
  — pulmonary crackles
  — hemoptysis, cough
  — peripheral edema
- Mitral regurgitation:
  — high-pitched murmur
  — weakness, fatigue
  — left ventricular failure, dyspnea, orthopnea, PND, crackles, S_3 and S_4

- right ventricular failure, neck vein distention, peripheral edema, hepatomegaly
- Mitral valve prolapse:
  - not uncommon to be asymptomatic with only a regurgitant murmur on physical examination
  - tachycardia, lightheadedness, syncope
  - fatigue, weakness
  - dyspnea, chest discomfort
- Aortic stenosis:
  - systolic, harsh murmur
  - dyspnea, orthopnea, PND
  - S_3 and S_4
  - fatigue
  - vertigo, syncope
  - exertional angina
- Aortic regurgitation:
  - diastolic, blowing murmur
  - dyspnea, orthopnea, PND
  - fatigue, weakness
  - syncope
  - palpitations
  - pulmonary congestion
  - S_3 and S_4
  - neck vein distention, peripheral edema, hepatomegaly
- Tricuspid and pulmonic valve disease:
  - diastolic murmur
  - signs of right ventricular failure: peripheral edema, neck vein distention, hepatomegaly
  - dyspnea, fatigue

MEDICAL MANAGEMENT

- Mitral stenosis
  - oral diuretics
  - sodium restricted diet
  - digitalis preparations and beta-blockers to slow heart rate and improve activity tolerance
- Mitral regurgitation:
  - restriction of physical activities that produce fatigue and dyspnea
  - sodium restricted diet
  - diuretics and nitrates
- Mitral valve prolapse:

— beta-blockers to relieve syncope, palpitations, and chest pain
— prophylactic antibiotics prior to invasive procedures to prevent infective endocarditis
- Aortic stenosis:
  — activity restrictions
  — prophylactic antibiotics prior to invasive procedures to prevent infective endocarditis
  — pharmacologic management of dysrhythmias
- Aortic regurgitation:
  — same as aortic stenosis
- Tricuspid and pulmonic valve disease
  — diuretic and digitalis therapy

SURGICAL MANAGEMENT

- Mitral stenosis:
  — valve replacement
  — valve reconstruction (commissurotomy)
- Mitral regurgitation:
  — valve replacement
  — valve reconstruction
- Mitral valve prolapse:
  — surgical intervention usually is not needed
- Aortic stenosis:
  — valve replacement
  — balloon valvuloplasty to dilate valve orifice
- Aortic regurgitation:
  — valve replacement

NURSING MANAGEMENT

MEDICAL

- Auscultate heart and lung sounds.
- Monitor intake and output.
- Daily weights.
- Monitor activity tolerance.
- Assess for peripheral edema, neck vein distention, and hepatomegaly.

SURGICAL

- See "Cardiac Surgery", p. 119.

FOCUSED DISCHARGE CARE

Valvular Disease

Instruct client regarding:
- disease process and treatment regimen
- activity restrictions
- dietary restrictions
- importance of adequate rest
- prophylactic antibiotics before and after dental or surgical procedures
- need to notify the physician if new onset of chest pain, palpitations, shortness of breath, peripheral edema, or signs and symptoms of pharyngitis (streptococcal infection) occur.
- need for follow-up appointments.

Mitral Valve Prolapse

Instruct client regarding:
- if palpitations occur, exercise moderately; the increased heart rate will override the extra beats
- if becomes short of breath, perform deep inhalation and slow pursed-lip exhalation
- if chest pain occurs, lie down, elevate legs to 90 degree angle and push against wall for 3-5 minutes
- exercise program
- decrease caffeine intake, drink plenty of fluids
- stress management

(For more information, see pp. 748-759 of Polaski and Tatro, *Luckmann's Core Principles and Practice of Medical-Surgical Nursing.*)

Varicose Veins

OVERVIEW

- Varicose veins are caused by the loss of valvular competence and the constant elevation of venous pressure, which results in distention and tortuosity of the superficial veins.

- The greater and lesser saphenous veins and perforator veins in the ankle are common sites of varicosities.
- Varicose veins may be either primary or secondary. Primary varicose veins result from a congenital or familial predisposition that leads to loss of elasticity of the vein wall. Secondary varicosities occur when trauma, obstruction, deep vein thrombosis or inflammation damages valves.
- The prevalence increases with age and peaks between the fifth and sixth decades of life. Varicose veins are more common in women.

CLINICAL MANIFESTATIONS

- complaint of aching, heaviness, itching
- dilated tortuous skin veins

SURGICAL MANAGEMENT

- ligation (tying off) of the greater saphenous vein at the saphenofemoral junction, combined with saphenous vein stripping and ligation of incompetent perforator veins. Removal of the vein is performed through multiple, short incisions.
- sclerotherapy — injection of a sclerosing agent into varicosed veins that damages the vein and endothelium, causing aseptic thrombosis that closes the veins. This treatment is palliative and is performed for cosmetic reasons to close small, residual varicosities after surgery.

NURSING MANAGEMENT

POSTOPERATIVE CARE

In addition to routine postoperative care:
- Maintain firm elastic pressure over the whole limb.
- Elevate foot of bed six to nine inches.
- Ambulate as ordered (usually 24 to 40 hours after surgery).
- Instruct client to walk rather than to stand or sit.
- Assess for possible complications:
  — hemorrhage
  — infection
  — nerve damage
  — deep vein thrombosis

FOCUSED DISCHARGE CARE

Instruct client regarding:
- need to wear elastic bandages for six weeks
- signs/symptoms to report to physician
- measures to prevent venous stasis:
    - no crossing legs
    - no constrictive clothing
    - avoid standing or sitting for prolonged periods of time
    - elevate legs when sitting or lying down
    - elastic stockings

(For more information, see pp. 818-819 of Polaski and Tatro, *Luckmann's Core Principles and Practice of Medical-Surgical Nursing.*)

Venous Stasis Ulcers

- Venous stasis ulcers represent the end stage of chronic venous insufficiency. Over a period of years, the excess venous pressure causes small skin veins and venules to rupture, with creation of stasis ulcers. Stasis ulcers are characteristically located in the malleolar area.
- Once the skin is broken, infection occurs, usually due to staphylococcus or streptococcus.
- Interventions include:
    - antibiotic therapy
    - Unna's boot — bandage impregnated with calamine, zinc oxide and glycerin
    - transparent moisture permeable dressing used to promote epithelization
    - ulcer debridement
    - skin grafting
- Instruct the client regarding:
    - wound care
    - elevation of legs above level of heart whenever possible when sitting or lying down
    - not crossing legs
    - use of elastic stockings after wound is healed
    - avoidance of constrictive clothing

661

— avoidance of standing or sitting for prolonged periods of time
— importance of daily skin inspection
— risk factor modification

(For more information, see p. 818 of Polaski and Tatro, *Luckmann's Core Principles and Practice of Medical-Surgical Nursing.*)

Vulvar Cancer

OVERVIEW

- Cancer of the vulva accounts for about 5 per cent of female genital carcinoma and occurs mainly in women over age 50.
- Vulvar cancer has a slow growth rate and remains localized for a long time.
- The prognosis is poor for vulvar invasive lesions.
- Risk factors include: vulvar leukoplakia, sexually transmitted disease, kraurosis (vulvar and mucous membrane skin atrophy and dryness), diabetic vulvitis and other primary malignancies (such as cervical cancer).
- Early detection of vulvar cancer is very important. Significant changes are detected early by women who practice regular vulvar self-assessment using a mirror.

CLINICAL MANIFESTATIONS

- pruritus
- vulvar soreness
- tissue irritation, bleeding
- vulvar edema
- pelvic lymphadenopathy

MEDICAL MANAGEMENT

- chemotherapy is used less often than surgical intervention

- irradiation generally is not used, as the tissue tolerates it poorly

SURGICAL MANAGEMENT

- simple vulvectomy — removal of the labia majora and minora and possibly the glans clitoris
  — the perineal area also may be removed
- radical vulvectomy — excision of tissue from the anus to a few centimeters from the symphysis pubis (skin, labia majora and minora and clitoris)
  — may also involve bilateral dissection of groin lymph nodes

NURSING MANAGEMENT

In addition to routine preoperative care:
- Discuss fears and concerns of client, such as fear of disfigurement, grief over the loss of a body part, fear of death and sexual concerns.
- Discuss preoperative procedures which will include an enema, douche and insertion of a Foley catheter.

(For more information, see pp. 1495-1496 of Polaski and Tatro, *Luckmann's Core Principles and Practice of Medical-Surgical Nursing*.)

Z

Zollinger-Ellison Syndrome

- Zollinger-Ellison syndrome is a condition characterized by abnormal secretion of gastrin by a rare islet cell tumor in the pancreas.
- Hypergastrinemia, diarrhea and hyperplasia of the gastric mucosa are seen.
- Treatment is aimed at suppression of acid secretion.

(For more information, see pp. 1039-1040 of Polaski and Tatro, *Luckmann's Core Principles and Practice of Medical-Surgical Nursing.*)

APPENDICES

APPENDIX A Reference Laboratory Values

Reference Values in Hematology

Acid hemolysis test (Ham)	No hemolysis		Coombs' test		
Alkaline phosphatase, leukocyte	Total score 14–100		Direct		Negative
			Indirect		Negative
Cell counts			Corpuscular values of erythrocytes		
Erythrocytes			Mean corpuscular hemoglobin (MCH)		26–34 pg
Males	4.8–5.5 million/mm³				
Females	4.0–5.0 million/mm³		Mean corpuscular volume (MCV)		80–96 μm^3
Children (varies with age)	4.5–5.1 million/mm³				
Leukocytes			Mean corpuscular hemoglobin concentration (MCHC)		32–36%
Total	5000–10,000 mm³		Erythrocyte sedimentation rate (ESR)		
Differential	*Percentage*	*Absolute*			
Myelocytes	0	0/mm³	Wintrobe method: Males		0–9 mm/hr
Band neutrophils	3–5	150–400/mm³		Females	0–15 mm/hr
Segmented neutrophils	60–70	3000–5800/mm³	Westergren method: Males		0–15 mm/hr
Lymphocytes	20–40	1500–3000/mm³			
Monocytes	2–6	300–500/mm³			

Appendix continued on following page

666

Eosinophils	1–4	50–250/mm^3
Basophils	0–1	15–50/mm^3
Platelets		150,000–400,000/mm^3
Reticulocytes		0.5–1.5% of erythrocytes

Coagulation tests

Bleeding time (template)	2.75–8.0 min
Coagulation time (glass tubes)	5–15 min
Factor VIII and other coagulation factors	50–150% of normal
Fibrin split products (Thrombo-Welco test)	<10 μg/mL
Fibrinogen	200–400 mg/dL
Partial thromboplastin time (PTT)	30–45 sec
Prothrombin time (PT)	10–12.5 sec

	Females	0–20 mm/hr
Haptoglobin		26–185 mg/dL
Hematocrit		
Males		40–54 mL/dL
Females		37–47 mL/dL
Newborns		49–54 mL/dL
Children (varies with age)		35–49 mL/dL
Hemoglobin		
Males		14.0–18.0 gm/dL
Females		12.0–16.0 gm/dL
Newborns		16.5–19.5 gm/dL
Children (varies with age)		11.2–16.5 gm/dL
Hemoglobin, fetal		<1.0% of total
Hemoglobin A$_{1C}$		3–5% of total
Hemoglobin A$_2$		1.5–3.0% of total
Hemoglobin, plasma		0–5.0 mg/dL
Methemoglobin		30–130 mg/dL

Appendix continued on following page

Reference Values for Blood, Plasma, and Serum*

Acetoacetate plus acetone, serum		Adrenocorticotropin (ACTH), plasma	
Qualitative	Negative	6 AM	10–80 pg/mL
Quantitative	0.3–2.0 mg/dL	6 PM	<50 pg/mL
Acid phosphatase (thymol-phthalein monophosphate substrate), serum	0.11–0.60 mU/mL	Alanine aminotransferase (ALT, SGPT), serum	5–35 U/L
Albumin/globulin (A/G) ratio	1.5:1–2.5:1	Albumin, serum	3.5–5.5 gm/dL
Aldolase, serum	1.3–8.2 U/dL	Folate, serum	1.8–9.0 ng/mL
Aldosterone, plasma		Erythrocytes	150–450 ng/mL
Supine	3–10 ng/dL	Follicle-stimulating hormone (FSH), plasma	
Standing		Males	4–25 mU/mL
Males	6–22 ng/dL	Females	4–30 mU/mL
Females	5–30 ng/dL	Postmenopausal	40–250 mU/mL
Alkaline phosphatase (ALP), serum	20–90 mU/mL	γ-Glutamyltransferase, serum	
		Males	5–38 U/L
		Females	5–29 U/L
Alpha-fetoprotein (AFP)	<10 ng/mL	Gastrin, serum	<200 pg/mL

Appendix continued on following page

668

Ammonia nitrogen, plasma	15–49 µg/dL
Amylase, serum	60–160 Somogyi U/dL
Anion gap	8–16 mEq/L
Ascorbic acid, blood	0.4–1.5 mg/dL
Aspartate aminotransferase (AST, SGOT), serum	10–50 mU/mL
Base excess, blood	0 ± 2 mEq/L
Bicarbonate	
Venous plasma	18–23 mEq/L
Arterial blood	
Bile acids, serum	0.3–3.0 mg/dL
Bilirubin, serum	
Conjugated	0.1–0.3 mg/dL
Unconjugated	0.2–0.8 mg/dL
Total	0.1–1.0 mg/dL
Ca-125	<35 U
Calcitonin	<100 pg/mL
Calcium, serum	9.0–11.0 mg/dL
Calcium, ionized, serum	4.25–5.25 mg/dL
Carbon dioxide, total, serum or plasma	24–30 mEq/L
Carbon dioxide tension (Pco_2), blood	35–45 mmHg
Glucose (fasting), plasma or serum	60–100 mg/dL
Growth hormone (hGH), plasma	3 µg/mL
Haptoglobin, serum	26–185 mg/dL
Hepatitis antigens and antibodies	Negative for antigens; positive or negative for antibodies, depending on history
Human chorionic gonadotropin (HCG)	0–5 IU/L
Immunoglobulins, serum	
IgG	500–1900 mg/dL
IgA	60–333 mg/dL
IgM	45–145 mg/dL
IgD	0.5–3.0 mg/dL
IgE	500 ng/mL
Insulin (fasting), plasma	5–25 µU/mL
Iron, serum	50–150 µg/dL
Iron binding capacity, serum	
Total	250–350 µg/dL
Saturation	20–55%
Lactate	
Venous blood	4.5–19.8 mg/dL

Appendix continued on following page

Reference Values for Blood, Plasma, and Serum* (continued)

Carcinoembryonic antigen		Arterial blood	4.5–14.4 mg/dL
Nonsmokers	0–2.5 ng/mL	Lactate dehydrogenase (LD, LDH), serum	60–150 IU/L
Smokers	<3.0 ng/mL		
β-Carotene, serum	40–200 μg/dL	Lipase, serum	0–110 U/L
Ceruloplasmin, serum	23–44 mg/dL	Lipids, total, serum	450–850 mg/dL
Chloride, serum or plasma	96–106 mEq/L	Luteinizing (LH), serum	
Cholesterol, serum or EDTA plasma		Males	6–18 IU/L
		Females	
Desirable range	<200 mg/dL	Premenopausal	5–22 IU/L
LDL cholesterol	60–180 mg/dL	Mid-cycle	3 times baseline
HDL cholesterol	30–80 mg/dL	Postmenopausal	>30 IU/L
Copper		Lysozyme	2.8–15.8 μg/mL
Males	70–140 μg/dL	Magnesium, serum	1.8–3.0 mg/dL
Females	85–155 μg/dL	Metalbumin	Absent
Cortisol, plasma		Osmolality	286–295 mOsm/kg water
8 AM	6–23 μg/dL	Oxygen, blood	
4 PM	3–15 μg/dL	Capacity (varies with hemoglobin)	16–24 vol%
10 PM	<50% of 8 AM value		
Creatine, serum	0.7–1.4 mg/dL	Content, arterial	15–23 vol %
Creatine kinase (CK, CPK), serum		Saturation, arterial	94–100%
		Oxygen tension (Po_2), blood	75–100 mmHg
Males	55–170 U/L	P_{50}	26–27 mmHg

Appendix continued on following page

Females	30–135 U/L
Creatine kinase MB isozyme, serum	0.0–4.7 ng/mL
Creatinine, serum	0.6–1.2 mg/dL
D-Xylase	Blood levels peak (25–40 mg/dL) 2 hours after ingestion; 80–95% excreted in 5 hours
Estrogen receptors	Positive >10 fmol/mg
Ferritin, serum	20–200 ng/mL
Fibrinogen, plasma	200–400 mg/dL
Albumin	3.5–5.5 gm/dL
α_1-globulin	0.2–0.4 gm/dL
α_2-globulin	0.5–0.9 gm/dL
β-globulin	0.6–1.1 gm/dL
γ-globulin	0.7–1.7 gm/dL
Pyruvate, blood	0.3–0.9 mg/dL
Serotonin	50–200 ng/dL
Serum 5'-nucleotidase	0.3–3.2 Bodansky units
Serum gamma-glutamyl transpeptidase (GGTP)	<65 IU/L
Sodium, serum or plasma	135–145 mEq/L
Parathyroid hormone	430–1860 ng/dL
pH, arterial blood	7.35–7.45
Phenylalanine, serum	<3 mg/dL
Phosphate, inorganic, serum	3.0–4.5 mg/dL
Potassium, serum or plasma	3.5–5.0 mEq/L
Prolactin	
Males	1–20 ng/mL
Females	1–25 ng/mL
Protein, serum	
Total	6.0–8.0 gm/dL
Thyroxine, free (FT), serum	0.8–2.4 ng/dL
Thyroxine (T_4), serum	4.5–11.5 μg/dL
Triglycerides, serum	40–150 mg/dL
Triiodothyronine (T_3), serum	70–220 ng/dL
Triiodothyronine uptake, resin (T_3RU)	25–38% uptake
Urate, serum	
Males	2.5–8.0 mg/dL
Females	1.5–7.0 mg/dL
Urea, serum or plasma	24–49 mg/dL
Urea nitrogen, serum or plasma	10–20 mg/dL

* For some procedures, the reference values may vary depending on the method used.

Appendix continued on following page

Reference Values for Blood, Plasma, and Serum* (continued)

Testosterone, plasma		Uric acid	
Males	275–875 ng/dL	Males	2.5–8.0 mg/dL
Females	23–75 ng/dL	Females	1.4–7.0 ng/dL
Pregnant	38–190 ng/dL	Viscosity, serum	1.4–1.8 times water
Thyroid-stimulating hormone	1–10 μU/mL	Vitamin A, serum	20–80 μg/dL
(TSH), serum		Vitamin B$_{12}$, serum	180–900 pg/mL

Reference Values for Urine*

Acetone and acetoacetate, qualitative	Negative	5-Hydroxyindoleacetic acid	
		Qualitative	Negative
Albumin		Quantitative	< 9 mg/24 hr
Qualitative	Negative	17-Ketosteroids	
Quantitative	10–100 mg/24 hr	Males	6–18 mg/24 hr
Aldosterone	3–20 μg/24 hr	Females	4–13 mg/24 hr
δ-Aminolevulinic acid	1.3–7.0 mg/24 hr	Magnesium	6.0–8.5 mEq/24 hr
Amylase	3–35 IU/hr	Metanephrines (see Catecholamines)	
Amylase/creatinine clearance	1–4%	Osmolality	275–295 mOsm/L
ratio		pH	4.5–8.0
Bilirubin, qualitative	Negative		

Appendix continued on following page

672

Calcium (usual diet)	<250 mg/24 hr
Catecholamines	
Epinephrine	<10 µg/24 hr
Norepinephrine	<100 µg/24 hr
Total free catecholamines	4–126 µg/24 hr
Total metanephrines	0.1–1.6 mg/24 hr
Chloride (varies with intake)	110–250 mEq/24 hr
Copper	0–50 µg/24 hr
Cortisol, free	10–100 µg/24 hr
Creatinine	15–25 mg/kg body weight/24 hr
Creatinine clearance (corrected to 1.73 m² body surface area)	
Males	110–150 mL/min
Females	105–132 mL/min
Dehydroepiandrosterone	
Males	0.2–2.0 mg/24 hr
Females	0.2–1.8 mg/24 hr
Estrogens, total	
Males	4–25 µg/24 hr
Females	5–100 µg/24 hr
Phenylpyruvic acid, qualitative	Negative
Phosphate	0.9–1.3 grams/24 hr
Porphobilinogen	
Qualitative	Negative
Quantitative	<2.0 mg/24 hr
Porphyrins	
Coproporphyrin	50–250 µg/24 hr
Uroporphyrin	10–30 µg/24 hr
Potassium	25–100 mEq/24 hr
Pregnanediol	
Males	0.4–1.4 mg/24 hr
Females	
Proliferative phase	0.5–1.5 mg/24 hr
Luteal phase	2.0–7.0 mg/24 hr
Postmenopausal	0.2–1.0 mg/24 hr
Pregnanetriol	<2.5 mg/24 hr
Protein	
Qualitative	Negative
Quantitative	10–150 mg/24 hr
Sodium	130–260 mEq/24 hr
Specific gravity	1.002–1.035
Urate	200–500 mg/24 hr

Appendix continued on following page

Glucose	
Random specimen	Negative
24-hour specimen	<0.5 g/24 hr
Hemoglobin and myoglobin, qualitative	Negative
17-Hydroxycorticosteroids	
Males	3–9 mg/24 hr
Females	2–8 mg/24 hr
Urobilinogen	0–4 mg/24 hr
Vanillylmandelic acid (VMA, 4-hydroxy-3-methoxymandelic acid)	1–8 mg/24 hr

* For some procedures, the reference values may vary depending on the method used.

Reference Values for Cerebrospinal Fluid

Cells	<5/mm³; all mononuclear
Electrophoresis	Predominantly albumin
Glucose	50–75 mg/dL (20 mg/dL less than serum)
IgG	
Children under 14	<8% of total protein
Adults	<14% of total protein
IgG index $\left(\dfrac{\text{CSF/serum IgG ratio}}{\text{CSF/serum albumin ratio}} \right)$	0.3–0.6
Oligoclonal banding on electrophoresis	Absent
Pressure	70–180 mm water
Protein, total	15–45 mg/dL

APPENDIX B Analysis of Arterial Blood Gas Results

Step 1: Classify the pH

Normal: 7.35–7.45

7.35 – 7.45

Acidemia: below 7.35

< 7.35 acid

Alkalemia: above 7.45

> 7.45 base (alkaline)

Step 2: Assess $PaCO_2$

35 – 45

< 35 – BASE

Normal: 35–45 mm Hg

> 45 – ACID

Respiratory acidosis: above 45 mm Hg

Respiratory alkalosis: below 35 mm Hg

Step 3: Assess HCO_3^-*

22 – 26

< 22 acid

> 26 base

Normal: 22–26 mEq/L

Metabolic acidosis: below 22 mEq/L

Metabolic alkalosis: above 26 mEq/L

Step 4: Determine presence of compensation

Compensation present: $PaCO_2$ and HCO_3^- are abnormal (or nearly so) in *opposite* directions, e.g., one is acidotic and the other alkalotic.†

Compensation absent: One component ($PaCO_2$ or HCO_3^-) is abnormal, the other normal.

Step 5: Identify primary disorder, if possible

If pH is clearly abnormal: Acid-base component most consistent with pH is primary disorder.

If pH is normal or near-normal: The more deviant component is probably primary.‡ To verify, note whether pH is on acidotic or alkalotic side of 7.4. The more deviant value should be consistent with this pH.

Step 6: Classify degree of compensation, if present

Partial compensation: Evidence of compensation, but pH is still abnormal.

Complete compensation: Evidence of compensation, pH is normal.

Appendix continued on following page

675

* Base excess (BE) is also reported with ABGs and is a second index of metabolic status. Normal BE is -2 to $+2$. Because fluctuation in BE exactly parallels that of bicarbonate, it is not necessary to classify both.

† It is possible, but less likely, that two opposing primary imbalances (e.g., a mixed disorder) are present, which results in the *appearance* of compensation. The detection of mixed disorders is facilitated by the use of acid-base maps or nomograms (Fig. 15-3), but a mixed disorder cannot always be differentiated from compensation.

‡ It is unlikely that the more deviant value represents compensation, because the body does not overcompensate for imbalance. When pH approaches the normal range, compensatory mechanisms are no longer triggered.

Appendix C — Blood Components

	Composition/Volume	Use	ABO/Rh Compatability
Whole Blood	RBC, plasma, plasma proteins (globulins, antibodies), 63 ml of anticoagulant-preservative 500 ml/unit	Acute, massive blood loss with hypotension, tachycardia, shortness of breath, pallor, and low hemoglobin/hematocrit	Thge ABO type of the donor should be identical with the recipient's Rh— blood can be given to an Rh+ recipient
Red Blood Cells	RBC with CPDA-1 solution (anticoagulant-preservative only), final hematocrit no higher than 80% (80% RBC, 20% plasma) RBC with 100 ml additive solution, final hematocrit about 55-60% 250-350 ml/unit 350-400 ml/unit	Acute or chronic blood loss with tachycardia, shortness of breath, pallor, low hemoglobin/hematocrit, and fatigue	A can match with A or O; B can match with B or O; O can match only with O; AB can match with A, B, or O Rh— blood can be given to either Rh+ or Rh— recipient

Table continued on following page

Appendix C — Blood Components (continued)

Composition/Volume	Use	ABO/Rh Compatability
Single-unit platelets contain a minimum of 5.5 X 10^{10} (1 unit) platelets in 50-70 ml of plasma obtained by separating platelet-rich plasma from 1 unit of whole fresh blood; 6-10 units may be pooled for 1 transfusion	To control or prevent bleeding associated with deficiencies in platelet number or function	Whereas platelets have no ABO or Rh antigens, they are suspended in 200-400 ml of plasma containing donor antibodies and a small number of RBC
	Used prophylactically for platelet counts < 10,000-20,000/mm^3	There is evidence that platelet survival decreases if donor plasma is incompatible, and large volumes of incompatible plasma may cause a positive direct Coombs' test
Single donor platelets contain a minimum of 3.0 X 10^{11} platelets (6 units) obtained from single donor by use of automated cell separator during apheresis; recipient exposed to fewer donors, which decreases complications	Administered if evidence of bleeding with platelet count < 50,000/mm^3	

50-70 ml/unit
200-400 ml/unit

A can match with A or AB; B can match with B or AB; AB can match only with AB; O can match with A, B, AB, or O
Rh— and Rh+ can be given to either Rh+ or Rh— recipient

Fresh Frozen Plasma	91% water, 7% protein (globulin, antibodies, clotting factors), and 2% carbohydrates Freezing within 8 hr of collection preserves all clotting factors	To increase level of clotting factors in clients with demonstrated deficiency If PT and PTT are < 1.5 times normal, FFP is rarely indicated	200-250 ml/unit

679

Table continued on following page

Appendix C — Blood Components (continued)

	Composition/Volume	Use	ABO/Rh Compatability
Cryoprecipitate	Each unit contains about 80-120 units of factor VIII (antihemophilic factor) that represents 50% of antihemophilic factor originally present in unit, von Willebrand's factor, 250 mg of fibrinogen, and 20-30% of factor XIII present in a unit of whole blood, suspended in 10-20 ml of plasma 5-10 ml/unit	To correct deficiencies of factor VIII (hemophilia A), von Willebrand's factor, factor XIII, and fibrinogen Occasionally used to control bleeding in uremic clients	Cryoprecipitate contains no RBC and a small volume of plasma ABO crossmatching not needed, and plasma compatibility preferred but not required

| **Granulocyte Concentrates** | Unit obtained by granulocytapheresis contains a minimum of 1.0×10^{10} granulocytes, variable amounts of lymphocytes (usually < 10%), 30-50 ml of RBC and 100-400 ml of plasma, and 6-10 units of platelets; the platelets can be separated from the unit if the granulocyte recipient is not thrombycytopenic | To treat clients with acquired neutropenia or congenital WBC dysfunction, who have serious infections unresponsive to conventional antibiotics
Granulocytes are not currently licensed by FDA
Long-term therapeutic benefit of granulocyte transfusion still questionable and continues to be evaluated | Granulocytes contain a significant number of RBC and plasma; therefore, ABO of donor should be identical with recipient's
Rh— components may be transfused to an Rh+ recipient |
| | 200-400 ml with platelets
100-200 ml without platelets | | |

681

Table continued on following page

Appendix C — Blood Components (continued)

	Composition/Volume	Use	ABO/Rh Compatability
Plasma Derivatives	*Albumin:* 96% albumin, 4% globulin and other proteins extracted from plasma; available as a 5% solution, oncotically equivalent to plasma, and also a concentrated 25% solution *Plasma protein fraction:* 83% albumin and 17% globulins extracted from plasma; less pure than albumin and has higher degree of contamination with other plasma proteins; in 5% solution only	To provide volume expansion in situations in which crystalloid solutions are not adequate, such as plasma exchange, shock, and massive hemorrhage Also used for treatment of acute liver failure, burns, and hemolytic disease of the newborn	Antibodies destroyed during processing; therefore, compatibility not a factor

	Albumin: 250 and 500 ml (5%); 50 and 100 ml (25%)	
Coagulation Factor Concentrates	*Factor VIII:* Lyophilized concentrate containing large quantities of factor VIII; prepared from large pools of donor plasma, but heat treatment during fractionation process significantly reduces risk of transmitting viral disease	*Factor VIII:* To treat moderate to severe congenital factor VIII deficiency (hemophilia A) *Factor IX:* To treat factor IX deficiency (hemophilia B or Christmas disease); may be used to treat congenital factor VII or Factor X deficiency	Antibodies destroyed during processing, so compatibility not a factor

683

Table continued on following page

Appendix C — Blood Components (continued)

	Composition/Volume	Use	ABO/Rh Compatability
Coagulation Factor Concentrates *(continued)*	*Factor IX:* Lyophilized concentrate containing large quantities of factor IX; also contains factors II, VII, and X; product prepared from large pools of donor plasma, but heat treatment during fractionation process significantly reduces risk of transmitting viral disease Multiple-dose vial		

INDEX

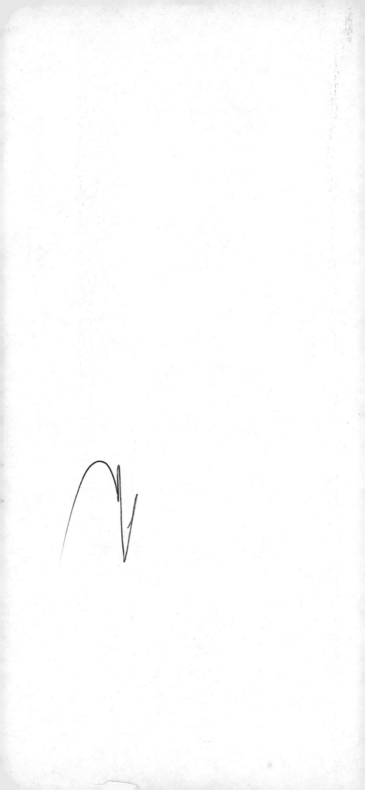